A Life *Stolen*

My Father's Journey Through Alzheimer's

Vanessa Luther

Written and published by Vanessa Luther.

"What is Alzheimer's Disease?" by David Shenk, page x, by permission of
the author.

Cover design by Vanessa Luther.

Printed in the United States of America

ISBN-13: 978-0692246979
ISBN-10: 0692246975

This book is dedicated to my daddy
who taught me to love
and live life with an
open heart.
You were always beside me
to hold my hand.
I only hope
I was there for you
when you needed me the most.

Contents

Disclaimer

This story is based on actual events that occurred as my father and I travelled the devastating road through Alzheimer's. All of the events are depicted exactly as they happened in our lives. I was completely honest in my retelling of this horrific time. The names of all doctors, hospitals, facilities, caregivers and fellow residents have been changed to protect their identity and privacy. The names of all family members have remained the same.

It is not my intent to defame anyone in this story in any way. My sole purpose is to provide awareness and insight for others placed in the role of caregiver for someone suffering from Alzheimer's or other forms of dementia as I was. In order to do this, the story had to be told in its entirety.

Preface

During the last year of my father's life, he suffered from severe dementia, namely Alzheimer's. To say that he ever had a fighting chance would be to minimize the impact that this devastating disease had on him. Alzheimer's is a horrible disease. Not only does it destroy people, but it does so in a very slow and vicious manner, stripping a person of every ounce of their dignity. It is relentless and doesn't stop until it has completely taken away a person's life. It took my father's.

When I first started down this path with my dad, I found myself thrust into a world that I knew nothing about. I didn't always do the right thing or say the correct words. Looking back, I may not have always made the right decisions. I was clearly in over my head, but I had no choice. Those were the cards we had been dealt. I knew that I couldn't change his path, so my only option was to educate myself to better care for him. I found unlimited sources of information on Alzheimer's. What I was really looking for, though, was a feeling of support within the pages of a book. Throughout this journey with my dad, I oftentimes felt so alone and overwhelmed, desperately needing the support of someone that had already travelled this road before me. I was stretched too thin to seek the help of a support group, so I had to rely on books. Unfortunately, I never found exactly what I was looking for.

At some point during the journey, I decided that I wanted to change that. I didn't want anyone else to ever go through what I was enduring. Caring for someone with this disease was hard enough, but making mistakes along the way because of a lack of knowledge was something that I found to be unacceptable and avoidable. It didn't have to be that way.

My ultimate goal is for my dad's story to provide guidance to others caring for a loved one with this terrible affliction. I hope and pray that something good can come from all of my dad's suffering. Deep inside, I have to believe there was a purpose for his tragic journey. I know if my dad thought that another caregiver or Alzheimer's patient could benefit in some way from his story, then he would want me to tell it, even if it meant divulging our personal lives and pain. It broke his heart to watch what this disease did to him and his loved ones. He wouldn't want that for anyone else.

I battled with the decision whether to reveal certain events that occurred during our journey together. They portrayed my dad, and me at times, in a light that was not very becoming. Unfortunately, that was our reality. That was Alzheimer's. After many months of deliberation, I finally realized that to omit those times would have been a disservice. It would be wrong. They were an integral part of the story and needed to be told. In order to make the difference that I wanted, I had to tell the complete story. It would take the entire journey to expose Alzheimer's for the monster that it is.

I hope that the reader will understand that this behavior was the disease. It was always the disease, causing people to act out in ways completely uncharacteristic of themselves. It makes them strangers. In his right mind, my dad would have never said or done some of the things that he did. In fact, he would have been deeply ashamed of them. My dad never mistreated anyone in his entire life. It just wasn't within him to do so. He was the kindest gentleman you could ever imagine, with the biggest heart out of anyone I've ever known. My hope is that when you strip away all of the ugliness of Alzheimer's, you will see my father for the loving, caring, generous man that he truly was.

Writing this book was undoubtedly the second hardest thing I ever lived through. With the help of medical records, calendars, daily messages with a dear friend and other documentation, I pieced together the timeline and events for this story. The details came from within me, as clear today as when they occurred. Most of what happened is etched inside of me and will never be forgotten.

If I had known the information in this book during our journey together, I am convinced that things would have turned out much differently for my father. I truly hope that our story will make a difference in the lives of everyone who reads it. My purpose is to bring about a much needed awareness to this devastating disease that seems to be taking over. Most importantly, my hope is that it will make the road for others an easier one to travel.

What is Alzheimer's Disease?

Alzheimer's is a slow, fatal disease of the brain. The disease comes on gradually as two abnormal protein fragments called plaques and tangles accumulate in the brain and kill brain cells.

It starts in the hippocampus, the part of the brain where memories are first formed. Over many years time, the plaques and tangles slowly destroy the hippocampus and it becomes harder and harder to form new memories. Simple recollections from a few hours or days ago that the rest of us might take for granted are just not there.

After that, more plaques and tangles spread into different regions of the brain, killing cells and compromising function wherever they go. This spreading around is what causes the different stages of Alzheimer's.

From the hippocampus, the disease spreads to the region of the brain where language is processed. When that happens, it gets tougher and tougher to find the right words.

Next, the disease creeps towards the front of the brain where logical thought takes place. Very gradually, a person begins to lose the ability to solve problems, grasp concepts and make plans.

Next, the plaques and tangles invade the part of the brain where emotions are regulated. When this happens, the patient gradually loses control over moods and feelings.

After that, the disease moves to where the brain makes sense of things it sees, hears and smells. In this stage, Alzheimer's wreaks havoc on a person's senses and can spark hallucinations.

Eventually, the plaques and tangles erase a person's oldest and most precious memories which are stored in the back of the brain.

Near the end, the disease compromises a person's balance and coordination and in the very last stage, it destroys the part of the brain that regulates breathing and the heart.

The progression from mild forgetting to death is slow and steady, and takes place over an average of 8 – 10 years. It is relentless and, for now, incurable.

David Shenk

(From the short film, "What is Alzheimer's Disease?", AboutAlz.org)

A Life *Stolen*

Prologue

Late November, 1996

I could almost smell the salt in the air as we neared Pensacola. Even though I left it many years ago, it would always feel like home to me, so many of my formative years spent there. Memories of family cookouts, meeting the love of my life, friendships never forgotten and endless times reveling in the white, sugary sand and clear, cool water of the beach flooded my soul. In some ways, it was where I became me.

For the first time in over a year, my entire family was together, the feeling of love in the air palpable. I couldn't have been happier. The kids were playing; the adults were reminiscing. Laughter abounded. As I looked over at my dad, I saw a peacefulness in his blue eyes that said it all. Life was good. My father was as down to earth as anyone could possibly be. He was not one for fancy cars or expensive trips. You would never find him in a ritzy restaurant. What meant the most to him could be summed up in one word...family. As he peacefully sat in his recliner with his dog on his lap, surrounded by his loved ones, all was right in his world.

Whenever our family came together, my mother always did the cooking. Ours was a traditional background. Mom was a very good cook when she was in the mood. It seemed though that the older she got, the less she enjoyed it. Some people lived to eat, but my mother ate to live.

We had ordered pizza earlier so she could have the night off. I had no sooner placed the boxes on the table than my older brother put his arms around my legs and swiftly picked me up. I immediately started giggling as he completely took me by surprise. He lifted me up so high that I could actually touch the ceiling.

It reminded me of a game that Curtis had played with me as a young girl. A friend of my father's that worked at the airport had given him the inner tube from an airplane tire. He inflated it in the corner of the backyard under a huge tree. Curtis would call all of his neighborhood friends to come over and sit on the giant tube. I would be seated in the middle of them directly under a large branch. The older kids would stand and on the count of three, they'd jump up and land on the tube sending me flying up in the air where I would try to grab onto the limb. The successful jumps were the ones that left me suspended in midair feeling exhilarated.

"Don't drop me," I said to Curtis as he held me up in the kitchen, both of us laughing. I knew he wouldn't; he was very strong. It didn't matter how infrequently we saw each other, the bond between us was immense.

An hour after dinner, as was often the norm with little boys, Preston and Shawn asked for a snack. As I stared into the kitchen cupboard, the vast assortment of items left me feeling astounded. It looked like a mini-grocery store right in front of my eyes, with every inch seemingly taken. There was so much to choose from. In the end, my healthy side took over and I chose the can of pineapple tidbits. "Are you still hungry?" my brother joked as I reached for the can. I just smiled at him.

"Uh oh, this doesn't look good," I said. Carefully setting the can on the kitchen counter, I noticed that part of it was protruding outwards. Curtis and I looked at each other. My curiosity then got the best of me and I decided to open the can. Upon the first puncture, I heard the gas quickly escape. I removed the lid and the pineapple wasn't the nice, golden color that you'd expect. The light brown shade was disgusting.

About that time, Mom walked into the kitchen. "Mom, look at this," I said. My mother was always looking for a bargain, periodically buying things from the discount cart when she grocery shopped. It was all about the price. "You need to be careful when you buy dented cans. Anytime, the can is bulging outwards, that's not good. It means that the food inside has spoiled and isn't safe to eat. You should never buy a can like that."

"Oh, I didn't notice that," said Mom. "I don't remember it being like that when I bought it." The look on her face was one of sheer embarrassment.

About that same time, Dad overheard the conversation and walked into the kitchen. As soon as he saw the can of rancid fruit, he lost it. "Are you trying to kill someone, Shirley?" he yelled, getting right in mom's face. I was shocked as I watched everything unfold, escalating in a matter of seconds. "What the hell is wrong with you? You can be so stupid sometimes!" The tirade had come on so quickly, like the flick of a light switch. Mom didn't say a word, but simply walked back into the family room. Unfortunately, Dad followed her.

As upset as I was about the dented can, I was more concerned for my mom. Her demeanor clearly said that this had happened before. She didn't seem the least bit surprised at my dad's reaction. On the contrary, she looked like someone trying to avoid a confrontation.

I then walked into the family room. The situation had not warranted getting so upset. "Dad, it's okay," I said. "Please don't yell anymore. We caught it in time. It's not worth getting so agitated over."

I had honestly never seen my father lose his temper like that. I had definitely never heard him talk that way to anyone, especially not my mother. The last thing I wanted was for my children to witness this blowup. I quickly walked back to the downstairs bedroom where the boys were playing and shut the door. I sat on the blue comforter as the tears started flowing, still hearing the shouting from the other room. It scared me. Both of my boys came to me and I hugged them tight. As I felt their little arms around me, I tried hard to block the rest of the world out.

My dad came into the bedroom soon afterwards and sat next to me on the bed. His voice was back to the gentle tone that was my father's. "I'm sorry that happened," he said, tenderly taking my hand in his. "I shouldn't have reacted like that."

"Dad, no one was going to eat it," I said. "I wasn't going to give it to the boys. But, the way you handled it, I've never seen you that way. It frightened me." He then handed me his handkerchief and I dried my eyes.

"You're right," he responded. "I lost my temper and it was wrong."

"You need to apologize to mom," I said. "She didn't deserve that." He slowly nodded his head in agreement, but didn't say a word.

"I have some pineapple that I bought," he said. "The boys can have that. Okay?"

I looked into my dad's eyes and nodded my head. I then leaned forward and gently kissed him on the cheek. My dad got up to leave the room and tousled one of the boys' hair on his way out.

My heart continued to race as I thought about what had just happened. I had never witnessed someone's emotions change so drastically before. In a matter of seconds, my dad had gone from total happiness to completely irate. I had certainly lost my temper in times past. Was this just one of those instances? As I headed out the bedroom door, I felt an incredible uncertainty inside.

The Journey

Friday, April 2, 2010

My eyes never left them as they strode through the front doors, so thankful they could still get around so easily. This was what retiring was all about. No health issues, no financial worries and endless time with grandchildren, children and each other. Not to mention they looked wonderful. To me, this was the epitome of a perfect retirement.

As they looked up, I excitedly waved to them, smiling all the while. Chris soon eyed them and made a quick dash their way. "Hey Lil' Monkey!" said Dad.

"Hi PaPa," exclaimed Chris. "It's my birthday!" Dad took Chris in his arms and hugged him tightly. "Guess how old I am, PaPa?"

"Thirty-three?" replied Dad jokingly.

"I'm seven!" laughed Chris. Dad was beaming with happiness.

Chris then turned to Mom and gave her a kiss. "Hi Grandma!" said Chris. "Mom said we can play some games before we eat pizza."

"That sounds like fun, sweetie," she said, as they made their way over to the decorated table. "I bet your Grandpa would love to play some games with you." Mom then turned to Dad and smiled. She had just volunteered him, but he didn't mind in the least.

Chris and Andrew each took one of Dad's hands and started eagerly pulling him towards the game area. He was so tickled as was written all over his face. This was happiness at its best for Dad. He loved all of his grandchildren, but definitely had a soft spot for the younger ones. These three had spent countless hours together over the years. They were best buddies. It was as simple as that.

When our three children were young, their birthdays were

traditionally spent with the family. It had always provided a relaxing and fun time for everyone. For my parents, that meant everything. In fact, it mattered so much to them that they had sold their home in Pensacola and moved to Georgia just to be near all of us. I remembered when they made the tough decision to retire and make the move. I had waited so many years for it to happen. When it finally did, I was ecstatic. We had now had them here for almost nine years and I counted my blessings every day.

I was also fortunate enough to live a couple of houses down from my younger brother Robert, who I called Bob, and his wife Monica and their two sons, Aaron and Andrew. With our hectic schedules, we didn't get to see each other every day, but it didn't matter. Just knowing they were so close made all the difference in the world. Sometimes seeing one of them drive by was all it took to fill me with that special feeling of comfort.

After placing our food order, I noticed Randy and Bob deep in conversation. "The other day, a couple of guys turned around in the intersection in front of the house and ran up in my yard about a foot," said Randy. "I happened to be looking out the window and I see the car sitting in my grass. The driver turned to his buddy, almost like he was daring him to do it. Then, he grinned and peeled out in my yard." We lived on a corner lot, so we often got people turning around and carelessly cutting into a piece of our front yard. This time though it was intentional.

"That's low," Bob remarked, shaking his head.

"Well, Vanessa took care of it," said Randy, as he smiled at me. "She had enough."

"What'd she do?" asked Bob.

"She drove down to the house that the guy was renting," Randy began. "The garage door was open, so she walked down the driveway. A young guy came out and it just happened to be the driver. She introduced herself as the one that lived in the blue house on the corner right up the road, the one where he and his buddy just wiped out in the grass. The guy actually smiled mischievously when she said this. He didn't even try to deny it. Then, he apologized like it was nothing. Vanessa calmly told him that she would appreciate it if he would keep his car off her grass. The next time, she'd let the police handle it. Then, she left the guy standing there with his mouth open and walked back to her car."

I looked at Randy and Bob and before long, we all started laughing. "He deserved it!" I said, continuing to look amused. Mom was smiling and I knew she was proud of how I had handled the situation.

Before long, the hot pizzas arrived and I sent my oldest son, Preston, to let everyone know. Mom helped me pass out the brightly colored plates and napkins. About that time, Shawn, my middle son, and Aaron made their way back. We were now only missing Dad and the two youngest boys. No sooner had I plated the pizza than they walked up, each one affectionately holding one of Dad's hands.

The evening had been very special, full of pepperoni and sausage pizza, birthday cake, singing and games. Everybody thoroughly enjoyed themselves, especially Chris. As I slowly looked around the table, I saw so many precious faces that were dear to me. I wouldn't trade this moment for anything. We had waited years to all be together. Life was very good.

Wednesday, May 26, 2010

I had butterflies in my stomach as he walked up on stage, looking so handsome in his long, green robe and gold cord. Somehow hearing his name magnified in the vastly open space made it a reality. As I sat in the arena watching the commencement exercises for Preston, I was overflowing with pride. It seemed like just yesterday Randy and I brought him home from the hospital. All of my immediate family, including my parents, had attended. I looked out over the huge graduating class, taking in the sea of green before me. The fact that my mom and dad lasted until the very end left me feeling astounded. Even Chris surprised me. I never thought I would be so happy to see 785 green caps flying up in the air.

As we walked into Longhorn Steakhouse, I felt a tremendous excitement over our celebration. Luckily, we got the best seat in the house, the circular booth in the back of the restaurant. It was private, yet gave us a full view of the other tables. We all fit perfectly. Before long, we ordered drinks and perused the menus.

I looked up and noticed that Dad's menu was still lying closed on the table. "What are you getting, Dad?" I asked.

My dad then leaned over and whispered in my ear "Will you order for me?"

I smiled at him. "Sure, do you want steak?" I asked.

He nodded his head and said "Yes." My dad had always been a meat and potato kind of guy. He was raised this way and wasn't about to change now. So, it was no surprise that he had decided on steak, a baked potato and a tossed salad.

"It's no problem, Dad," I responded. "I'll take care of it for you." He looked at me so lovingly, his appreciation evident.

The waitress took our orders and soon served us some of their famous wheat bread with butter. We were all famished. Shawn asked Chris if he could see his kids menu. I smiled knowing that regardless of how old he was, Shawn would never tire of working the puzzles. In some ways, he was so much like me.

As we all sat together, I heard "My Wish" by Rascal Flatts over the loudspeaker. How appropriate that this song was playing right now. One generation seated before me was about to embark on a college education, while another generation was enjoying their golden years. My hope for all of them was that their dreams continued to soar and their lives became everything they desired them to be.

Dinner was delicious. Before long, our waitress came by with dessert menus. I thought back about the whole ordering incident earlier and still wasn't sure what had transpired. The truth was my parents didn't go to too many different restaurants. They had their favorites...Golden Corral, Folks and Captain D's. Beyond those, they really didn't venture out much, even though my mom would probably have loved it.

Tonight, my dad seemed a little out of his comfort zone. The lighting in the restaurant was a little dim. Dad had also forgotten his reading glasses. It was quite possible he just couldn't read the menu. Whatever the reason, he clearly hadn't felt comfortable ordering for himself. I was just glad I had been there for him.

Saturday, June 12, 2010

He had just topped his coffee cup off as he gazed out the kitchen window, the neighborhood slowly coming alive. This time of the day always seemed to provide the most reflection on life. Before long, the phone rang, the caller id identifying who was on the line. Dad was having trouble with his trimmer and wondered if Randy could come by to look at it. "Sure Chester, that's no problem," said Randy. "I'll be over in a little bit."

Randy often helped Dad out. In all the years that we had been married, not once did I ever hear my husband complain about helping one of my parents. He was the perfect son-in-law to them. The bond between my dad and Randy was an especially close one. It always had been. My dad adored Randy and Randy felt the exact same way. At least once a week, he'd stop by to visit Dad where they'd have a beer together and simply talk. The relaxing times had meant the world to my father.

At a little after 1, Randy walked down the stairs to Dad's basement where he found him busily tinkering with some tools. He had the radio on listening to "Okie From Muskogee" by Merle Haggard. My dad was a country music lover and always had been. I grew up listening to the sounds of Hank Williams, Jr., Conway Twitty, Eddie Arnold and, of course, Tom T. Hall. The basement had become Dad's sanctuary.

"Hey Chester," said Randy. "How's it going?"

"Hey Ran," greeted Dad. He had given Randy this nickname over thirty years ago and continued to use it to this day. "I can't seem to figure out how to load the trimmer wire." Dad had both the trimmer and the wire lying in front of him on the cement floor. Randy soon realized that the wire Dad was using was the wrong size.

"Here's the problem," said Randy. "We just need a different size wire. That's all it is." Dad had maintained his trimmers for years. This was the first time he had ever had to ask Randy for help with one of them. "Why don't we take a ride up the road and get some more wire?"

"That sounds good, Ran," replied Dad. "You know, I used to be able to fix all these things. It's hell getting old!" he said laughing. Randy also laughed, but he could tell that inside, it really bothered Dad.

They rode to Home Depot to get the correct trimmer wire. When they got back, Randy loaded the newly purchased wire and tested it out. It worked just like new. Dad then got two beers out of the compact fridge to show his appreciation. They both sat on the patio underneath the deck to relax in the shade.

On the drive home, Randy remembered another scenario that occurred just a couple of weeks ago. The floor lamp that sat next to Dad's navy blue recliner had suddenly stopped working. Dad had taken it apart and tried to fix it, but to no avail. Randy found it lying in pieces on the basement floor in front of Dad's workbench. He assembled it back together only to find that the socket was bad. Again, he had driven Dad up to the hardware store to get the new part. It really was a minor fix, one that Dad had done many times over the years. For some reason, he had gotten confused after he took the lamp apart and ended up getting very frustrated.

When Randy got home, he told me about the visit. His concern quickly became my concern. Dad was starting to have difficulty doing certain things that he'd been doing for years. I knew to some extent it was to be expected. After all, he was 78 years old. Even so, I thought he did an incredible job maintaining things around his home.

After high school, my dad had enlisted in the Air Force. During the Korean War, he was an airplane mechanic. Many lives were entrusted to his ability to successfully maintain different aircraft. He had always been good at fixing things. It was so hard to watch what was happening to Dad. Some of the things he periodically said made it clear that it really disturbed him. It must have been so hard when you were used to doing tasks independently and then all of a sudden, you had to rely on other people.

The truth was a lot of people his age had already given up certain jobs, namely yard service. Not my dad. He mowed and edged his own yard every week. He always had. His father before him was the exact same way. Grandpa Lee had mowed his entire yard right up until he passed away.

My dad's yard was by no means considered a small yard either. Not only was it a corner lot, but it was also the first house as you entered the subdivision, over half an acre in total. Dad had the yard broken down into sections, completing one each day. By the time he had mowed the last section, it was almost time to start the cycle again. As exhausting as this was for him, it was therapeutic. It not only rejuvenated him, it made him happy.

As Dad slowly adjusted to this new phase in his life, he was relying more and more on Randy. Minor tasks that had become innate to him were now requiring assistance. Fortunately, Randy was only too happy to oblige him.

Wednesday, July 21, 2010

Mom pulled up in the driveway just as I finished the dishes. I poured the last two cups of steaming coffee and took them into the living room. As soon as I answered the front door, it was obviously not a good morning. "Hi Mom," I said, her dismal expression speaking volumes. "What is it?"

"It's your father, Vanessa," stated Mom. "Everything was fine last night. We were watching television in the family room. I was finishing up reading the newspaper. Then, your Dad just exploded."

"What made him so upset?" I asked.

"One minute we were fine," replied Mom. "The next he was telling me that I spend too much time on that computer and he was going to get rid of it. I told him that I needed the computer to manage the bills and correspond with people. He got mad, stormed out of the room and ended up going to bed early." She paused to take a sip of her hot coffee.

"This morning, he came down to breakfast and said that he couldn't find his money clip," continued Mom.

My dad never carried money in his wallet. He had a money clip that he kept his bills in and always had it in his pocket. When he would go to the store, he would pull the money clip out of his pocket when it was time to pay. I was always telling him "Dad, you are going to get robbed one of these days. You can't be flashing everyone your money." It always made me so nervous, but Dad was old school and that was just the way he did things.

"Have either of you found it yet?" I inquired.

"Not yet," she responded, sounding tired.

11

"It'll turn up eventually. It always does," I said optimistically. My dad had been misplacing things for awhile now. It was starting to happen a lot more often. About once a week, I'd get a phone call and either his money clip, his wallet or his keys would have disappeared. Usually, we found the item within a couple of days. One time, we found the keys under his bed. Another time, we discovered his wallet in a pants' pocket in his closet. About a week ago, Randy found his money hidden in a drawer in the basement.

"Are you going to be okay?" I asked.

"I feel like I'm walking on egg shells with your father," she said. "I never know when something will set him off. He works so hard in the yard and gets so hot. Then he comes in to shower and sits down with a cold drink. It always seems to happen right around suppertime. Then, the next morning, he's as nice as can be. It's as if nothing ever happened. I just don't understand what is going on."

"Mom, do you want to stay with us tonight until things settle down?" I asked.

"No honey," she replied. "In fact, I better get back. I may not have a computer when I get home," Mom joked. "Don't worry. I'll be fine." She smiled, trying to reassure me. We then hugged and I told her that I loved her.

Later that night, I got an email from my mom. Apparently, she still had her computer. In the note, she let me know that Dad had actually found his money clip in his top dresser drawer near his handkerchiefs. Once again, the missing item had been found. I felt a huge sense of relief as I turned off my laptop.

Wednesday, August 11, 2010

Silence hung in the air as we made the inevitable drive. My emotions had run the gamut today as we moved our firstborn into Lipscomb Hall at UGA. He was now officially a freshman in college. It was a lot for us to grasp, but knowing that he was less than an hour away and could come home in an emergency made it a little easier. I was so proud of Preston and knew that he would do great things. He always had.

Still, it was difficult. I knew that when I walked out of his college door, I would be leaving a part of me inside that room. Even though it was a part of life that most parents went through, nothing could have prepared me for the emotions that came with it.

Initially, Preston had planned on living at home and commuting on the days that he had classes. Unfortunately, UGA's freshmen policy wouldn't allow for that. We had even appealed it with the housing department, but they flat out turned us down. By the time all of this had transpired, his close friends already had roommates. He reluctantly ended up going into the Dawg pool and just hoped for the best.

Preston had met his new roommate weeks ago through text messages. Today, we actually met him in person. He had already moved in the previous day, as anyone planning on joining a fraternity was allowed to move in a day early. While we were there, he and a couple of his friends came by the room. He seemed friendly enough and said all the right things. Randy was impressed with the eye contact that he made when politely shaking his hand. The three friends soon left with no invitation extended to Preston to join them. He was left completely alone in his unfamiliar dorm room. An uneasy feeling that Preston and his new roommate might not be the perfect match permeated inside of me. I would have to rely on faith that he was in good hands.

Sunday, August 22, 2010

The simple act of unlocking a door was rapidly becoming a problem. He was experiencing so much confusion with the keys to get into his home. Randy had received a phone call from Dad yesterday after he had lost several of his house keys. He was having difficulty getting the remaining ones to work. The fact that each door used two different keys was fast becoming an issue.

Today, Randy and Dad had gone to Lowe's and bought five sets of deadbolt/door handle combination locks. Randy actually had the locks specially keyed so that each one used the same key. He was going to make it as easy as possible for my parents. He also bought several plastic wrist bands to put the keys on. Both Mom and Dad could wear their wrist bands and have access to their keys at all times.

It turned out to be an all day event to get all of the locks changed, but it was well worth it. Dad was thrilled. As was the norm, Randy and Dad relaxed in the family room with a cold one. Dad then slipped some money into Randy's hand. He tried to give it back, but Dad wouldn't hear of it. I didn't know anyone more generous.

Dad soon handed the remote control for the television to Randy. He was also having trouble getting to his favorite channels. Randy had already written the steps down when the same thing had happened previously. Simple things that used to be second nature were now becoming major hurdles.

When Randy arrived home, he informed me that Dad had several band-aids on his forearms. He intentionally didn't ask him about them. I think deep down inside, he knew it wasn't good.

Feeling distraught, I later called my parents' home. Mom answered the phone. "Hey, Mom," I said. "What happened to Dad's arms?"

"Last night, we were in the kitchen after dinner and he got upset with me," she replied. "I don't think he cared for the leftovers. Anyway, he grabbed the tops of my arms and squeezed them really hard. I was scared, so I dug my fingernails into his arms to get him to let go. He quickly started bleeding and then wiped the blood on my shirt. When he went upstairs to his bathroom to clean himself up, I changed clothes and tried to get the bloodstains out of my top. He stayed in his room last night and I stayed in mine. We still haven't spoken to each other."

"Mom, has Dad ever grabbed you like that before?" I asked. I heard nothing but total silence on the other end of the line. I had my answer. Apparently, this wasn't the first time. I felt sick to my stomach. My precious parents seemed to be going down a very dark road. For years, they had had a volatile relationship. One day, everything would be fine. The next day, they'd argue. I had truly thought it was just trivial disagreements. Now, I had surprisingly found out otherwise.

It was hard to know where the blame lied. Who started the arguments? According to Mom, it was always my father's fault. When I talked to Dad, he equally placed part of the blame with Mom and part with himself. I knew that there were inevitably two sides to every story. The truth was probably somewhere in the middle, with both of them playing a part. Regardless, things didn't seem to be getting any better. In fact, they were getting worse and more frequent.

I also found out that Mom had researched my dad's behavior on the Internet, convinced that he had Alzheimer's. In fact, she had secretly written a letter to his primary doctor telling him of her suspicions. I honestly knew very little about this disease, but I didn't think Dad was sick though. If he was, wouldn't he treat all of his family the same way? Wouldn't he show the same aggressive behavior towards us as he did Mom?

I had never experienced the hostility or arguments with Dad that Mom did. He never raised his voice to me or said anything other than the most loving words. He was nothing but kind to Randy and the boys as well. In no way could I believe that this wonderful man I called Daddy had Alzheimer's. There had to be something else. In my mind, he was just an aging man that argued with his wife and sometimes lost his temper.

Monday, August 23, 2010

It was 10:30 a.m. as I heard the loud rumble of my daddy's truck. You could unmistakably hear him coming long before you could see him. He had dual exhaust on his Dodge Ram and he loved it. One of his favorite pastimes was to get in his red truck and leisurely drive over for a visit. He was a perfect example of a man never being too old for some muscle in his car.

I met him at the door and kissed him hello as we both sat down in the living room. "Hey girl," he playfully said to Riley, who adored Dad. She could always sense he was on his way over long before the rest of us. She would hear his truck about a block away, lean her head to the side and start whining.

I reluctantly looked over at Dad's arms and saw the band-aids. "Dad, what happened to your arms?" I asked, already knowing my mom's version. I needed to be fair and hear his side.

The disturbing story he told me was actually very similar to Mom's. "Your momma dug her nails into my arms," he replied. "They started bleeding." As Dad had aged, his skin had become paper thin. The smallest scratch caused him to bleed excessively.

"Mom said that afterwards you wiped your blood on her shirt," I said.

"I did," Dad admitted, looking completely ashamed.

"Dad, she was really scared," I remarked. "What in the world started this?" I tried to remain calm as I delved into the cause of this latest incident.

"Your mother spends all day on that damn computer," Dad said. "Then, she comes downstairs and throws something together for dinner that I wouldn't feed a dog. I worked outside all day in the hot sun. All I wanted was a nice meal. Is that too much to ask?"

"No, it's not, Dad," I said. "When that happens, come over to my house and eat with us. Or, go grab a Wendy's burger. You just can't handle it the way you did. It makes me very nervous."

"Pootie, you know I would never ever hurt your mother," said Dad. "I may lose my temper and say things that I shouldn't say, but I would never do anything to physically harm her. I don't know why I do some of the things that I do. I don't act that way with anyone else. Your momma just knows how to push my buttons. I know I need to control my temper better."

I did believe that my dad loved my mom and that he wouldn't ever intentionally hurt her. I had no reason not to. They had been married for 53 years and he'd never once come close to hurting her before, always a perfect and devoted husband.

I had planned on going to my parents' home after dinner. I didn't know what was going on between the two of them and could never really get the complete picture when I talked to them separately. I had often thought about installing hidden cameras in their house so that I could secretly see for myself what was happening. What prevented me from ever doing that was the fear of what I might actually see.

Bob was busy watching his boys and I needed Randy to take care of Chris, so I drove to my parents' home alone. I was about to conduct my very first intervention with my mom and dad.

As we all sat down together in the family room, I began shaking. I had mentally prepared for this all day, but now that I was actually here, my voice was quivering. "The fighting has to stop," I pleaded. "You both are destroying each other, not to mention the damage you're doing to your children and grandchildren. You both have so much to be happy about." I stopped talking and took a deep breath, but not before the tears started flowing.

Dad was staring at me, looking absolutely crushed. I knew he agreed with me as his sad eyes told me so. "You are absolutely right," said Dad softly.

I looked at Mom, but she remained stoically silent. I had tried to get to the bottom of what was happening. In no time, they were pointing fingers at each other again. It seemed as though the slightest of provocations was all it took these days to start an argument. I couldn't bear to hear any more. I needed for them to listen to what I had to say. What they chose to do with it afterwards was up to them.

"You both have to be willing to overlook some things," I stated. "The things you're fighting about are so petty. In the big picture, they're nothing. You both are at a place in your lives that so many strive to reach. You're five minutes away from your children and grandchildren. It took years to get that to happen. You're already there." I looked at them for some type of reaction, but they both continued unwaveringly to stare at me. "I will do whatever I can to help. But, you both have to be willing to make some changes." An overwhelming feeling of sadness enveloped me as I wiped the tears from my eyes.

"Please don't cry," said Dad. "We'll make it better, I promise." With that, he moved next to me on the couch and lovingly hugged me. The tremendous weight on my shoulders was finally too much. I broke down and quietly sobbed into his chest. My sweet daddy had been making things right for me my whole life. I prayed that this time was no different. I undoubtedly knew at that moment how much Dad wanted the same thing. I reached my hand out towards Mom and she grasped it tightly. For the first time in awhile, a feeling of hope that my parents would overcome this obstacle in their marriage filled me inside.

As I lied in bed later that night, I tried hard to remember when everything had changed. I had a lifetime of loving memories with my parents. When had all this started? Inside, I knew that they had to hate the arguing just as much as the rest of us. Even so, I believed that they would absolutely hate living without each other even more. That thought terrified me. Would they settle for the fights just to be together?

Thursday, September 30, 2010

As he turned the page, I stared at his blue eyes, following their gaze as they traversed the words. The peacefulness of the moment reached deep inside of me, providing special comfort as I listened to his soft voice. Chris was reading me a book as he did every night before bed when the phone suddenly rang. Dad sounded so depressed. I had honestly never heard him like this. It really scared me. "Dad, did something happen?" I asked.

"Poot, I am just so unhappy," he responded. If it wasn't for the caller id, I would have thought it was someone else on the line. This despondent voice did not sound like my dad at all. "I am so tired of the arguing every day. It never stops. Is it any wonder I have high blood pressure?"

What happened next made my heart sink. This incredible man that had been the pillar of strength my entire life started crying. Not small, muffled crying either. These were deep, sorrowful sounds coming from the inner depth of my father. I just listened to him in agony as he broke down.

My dad was a virile man. I had never in my life witnessed him reach this level. In fact, I had only heard about three occasions that my dad had actually cried. Two of those times were when his parents had passed away. The sound of this precious man crying was ripping my heart in two.

We continued to talk and Dad slowly began to calm down. I was worried sick for him. All I wanted was to hold this man in my arms and soothe him as he had done for me so many times. "I think I'm going to go to bed, Vanessa," Dad said softly. I thought under the circumstances that this would be the best thing.

"I love you, Daddy," I said, as I could feel my eyes starting to water.

"I'll come over tomorrow to see you. Okay?"

"Okay, honey," replied Dad. I hung up the phone and slowly dropped to the floor. As I leaned back against the kitchen cabinet, I closed my eyes and my own tears began falling. My daddy was in horrible pain and I couldn't bear to witness it. It was killing me.

After awhile, I called my mom and told her about the disturbing conversation I had just had with Dad. "Please go check on him, Mom," I said. "I've never seen him in this state before and I'm worried about him." She agreed to look in on him.

About ten minutes later, Mom called to let me know that Dad was in bed and the lights were out. He would hopefully be okay for the night.

I knew something serious was going on with my dad. I just didn't know what. Before tonight, I had thought it was a combination of Dad getting older, him tiring of the arguments and simply that my parents were growing apart.

I thought back about the phone call from my dad and could only think of a few people in this entire world that he would have felt comfortable enough with to have divulged such personal feelings. Even then, he would have hated to have burdened them with his problems. I was one in that small group. How incredibly hard it must have been for him to come to me like he did? Was this a warning call for me? Was my dad in desperate need of help?

Thursday, October 28, 2010

I quickly searched the refrigerator in anticipation of their arrival, mentally preparing the menu. They had planned on stopping by today after his doctor appointment. He had willingly asked her to drive him as his fear of getting lost was increasing every day. It worked out well since she had a library book that she wanted me to return for her. I decided it was a perfect opportunity for me to make my parents lunch.

My mother had been instrumental in instilling a love for reading in me as she was an avid reader herself. Now that we lived near each other, we exchanged books on a weekly basis. Some of my most treasured authors were ones that she had introduced me to. Likewise, she had quickly grown to love many of my favorites.

From the kitchen window, I excitedly saw them pull up. I rushed downstairs and opened up the garage door to meet them. As Mom walked towards me, she had a flustered look on her face. "Isn't Dad coming in?" I asked.

"He won't get out of the car," she discouragingly said. I hugged my mother. "I can't stay, Vanessa. Here's the book. If you could return it for me, I'd appreciate it."

"Sure Mom," I responded. "That's no problem."

I followed her out to the car and went to the passenger side to see my dad. He didn't look happy at all. "Hey, Daddy," I said smiling.

"Hey Pootie," Dad replied.

"You don't want to come in?" I asked. "I can make you a sandwich."

"No, I need to get home," he said crossly. "Your mother didn't know where she was going. We've been gone since early this morning. I had a doctor's appointment at 10. After we left, she insisted on taking a shortcut and we got lost."

Dad was very upset as was evident by his unusual demeanor. I was treading lightly now. "Dad, it's okay," I said. "Why don't you just come inside and let me make you some lunch?"

"No, it's not okay," Dad said sharply. "I'm ready to go home and eat lunch there." He had a look of exasperation on his face that I had never seen before. I was at a complete loss for words. Never in my life had my dad snapped at me. No matter what was going on with my mom, Dad would have never taken it out on me. His words had stung.

I decided at that moment that it was probably best to let this one go. I wouldn't say another word. I then sadly watched as the car backed out of the driveway and my parents drove off, my eyes never once leaving my dad. There were no goodbyes today.

Monday, November 1, 2010

I reluctantly backed out of the driveway early this dreary morning realizing that it never got any easier. Saying goodbye was not something I was very good at. With every passing mile, the sadness within me grew. Preston and I were headed back to Athens.

I had felt elated that he delayed going back and spent Halloween with his family. There was a time when I had mixed feelings about him living on campus. After driving it today, I was convinced that he would have tired of it eventually. I think inside Preston was also glad he was forced to live on campus. He had made so many new friends and was definitely loving the unique college experience at UGA.

We usually got to see him about once a month. When he first left, I wanted to know what he was doing all the time. It was what I was accustomed to. Eventually, I realized I had to let him go regardless of how difficult it was. He also had to go through some necessary changes. God had a way of calming and reassuring the heart when you were separated from a loved one.

The only issue that Preston was currently dealing with was his roommate who had joined a fraternity and was living a very different lifestyle than Preston. Several incidents, including vomiting and urinating in the shared sink, had already transpired this year. Preston was forced to have some serious talks with his roommate and was soon to have another one. I understood about the "code" that existed amongst college students. Regardless of what they had done, you didn't rat them out. It seemed that this roommate was pushing the unwritten code to the limit. While I didn't completely agree with it, I respected Preston's decision to deal with it in his own way. It was extremely hard to bite my tongue, but I knew I had to at this point.

The unfortunate issue with his roommate had become a daily part of my prayer for him. It certainly wasn't the ideal situation, but I had to believe that there was a reason and that he'd be the better for it. Seeing one of your children not treated with the respect that they deserved was so hard. The classy manner in which Preston had handled this adversity made me so proud. Fortunately, he had already found a different roommate for the next school year.

Sunday, November 14, 2010

I kissed each of them goodbye on their way out the door. Before long, the three of them loaded up into the truck affectionately known as "Blackie", with all of them in the front seat. Randy liked his elbow room, but Chris liked sitting up front even more. As they slowly backed out of the driveway, I waved to them from the kitchen window. The boys were in desperate need of a haircut. It just so happened that Dad was their barber of choice.

My dad had cut hair for over 42 years. At the time of my parents' marriage, Dad had worked in the warehouse of McKesson and Robbins, in their liquor division. Not long afterwards, he had decided it was time he trained for a more stable career. He eagerly chose to go to barber school at night while he continued working during the day. His father before him had gone into this field and it seemed the logical choice for Dad as well.

After purchasing their first home in Hialeah, Florida, Dad began to practice barbering fulltime. He cut hair for years and eventually bought his own place, which was known as Palm Springs Barber Shop. Dad worked here throughout my childhood. I received many a haircut at my dad's shop, after which he always let me choose a soft drink out of the soda machine.

After moving to Pensacola, he purchased John's Barber Shop which was located right outside of the Navy Base and not far from their home. Being the closest one to the gate, he had several of the Blue Angels and other Navy personnel as customers. It was a landmark and he had decided to leave the longstanding name alone.

Even though Dad was retired, he still had an actual barber chair and all of his supplies. It was set up in the basement of his home like a mini barber shop complete with stereo, television and a barber pole decal on the window. He even displayed some of the exact same Navy pictures that had adorned the walls of his last barber shop. Not only did Dad routinely cut most of his grandchildren's hair, he also generously cut a neighbor and his grandson's hair. Dad loved giving to others and never asked for anything in return.

On this particular day, Shawn readily decided to get his hair cut first.

He sat in the barber chair and Dad routinely covered him with the cape. As was his custom, Dad sprayed Shawn's hair with a plastic bottle that he used for wetting. As he sprayed, he gently combed the liquid through his hair and soon noticed that something didn't smell right. "Shawn, did you put something in your hair?" asked Dad.

"No, Papa," replied Shawn.

By this time, Randy had smelled it, too. "Chester, let me see that bottle," said Randy. He unscrewed the top and carefully smelled the liquid. "Chester, this isn't water. It smells like either gasoline or some type of cleaning chemical."

Randy then quickly took the plastic bottle upstairs to the kitchen and poured it out. He rinsed it thoroughly and filled it with water before returning to the basement.

"Sometimes the grandkids play down here and I wonder if one of them might have poured something in the bottle," said Dad.

Randy then found another plastic bottle on the workbench that actually did contain water. Dad was absolutely certain that he never put any liquid other than water in the plastic bottle. He soon resumed cutting Shawn's hair. When he was finished, he gave Chris his haircut. Randy faithfully stayed in the basement and kept Dad company the entire time.

An hour later, the boys arrived home. As soon as Shawn came up the stairs, I immediately smelled what I thought was gas. "Shawn, what happened?" I asked, a little panicky.

"Papa accidentally sprayed my hair with it," said Shawn. About this time, Randy came inside and explained what happened. I immediately had Shawn get in the shower and shampoo his hair.

He came upstairs a little while later, the offensive smell still present. I then gave him some fragrant conditioner. This time, I had him shampoo twice after which, he put the conditioner in and left it for twenty minutes.

A short while later, he despairingly came back upstairs. The last washing had still not taken away the gas smell. I then started relentlessly searching the Internet. Before the day was out, we had also tried regular dish soap, mayonnaise and tomato juice. The smell was unstoppable and would not go away. Fortunately, it did lose a little of its intensity after seven washings. We would just have to give it some time and hope that with every passing day, the odor would diminish. Unfortunately, Shawn would have to carry that gaseous smell to school the next day.

Later that afternoon, I called my mother on the phone. "Mom, do you know what happened today?" I asked, extremely upset. Shawn was lucky that the spray hadn't gone into his eyes. I shuddered to think what could have happened if it had.

"Vanessa, I talked to your father," she replied. "He thinks that one of the grandchildren may have done it." Inside, I felt very skeptical. I highly doubted that the misplaced liquid had occurred at the hands of one of the boys.

As I sadly thought about the day's mishap, I realized that things had now escalated to a different level. I knew that Dad would never in a million years do anything intentionally to harm one of his grandchildren. Today, I was forced to make a tough, but necessary decision. It marked a very somber day in my life. It was the last day that any of my children would ever have their hair cut by their Grandpa Lee.

Late November, 2010

He was experiencing an extreme amount of discomfort lately, his doctor feeling his gallbladder was the probable culprit. A specialist soon confirmed the diagnosis and scheduled surgery to have it promptly removed. On the day of the procedure, Mom had driven Dad to Parkland General Hospital early that morning, planning on staying with him the entire time.

A few hours later, I happily learned that the surgery was successful. Dad's gallbladder had been extremely soft and the surgeon felt that it definitely needed to be removed. I felt hopeful that Dad's pain was finally over.

After a few more hours, Dad was routinely moved to a regular room. They intended to keep him overnight for observation. Bob had come to the hospital directly from work to spend some time with him. Dad seemed to be doing very well.

Mom realized that evening that she had forgotten some things at home. She had planned on following Bob to Buford Drive once he decided to leave. From there, she'd be able to successfully make it home to pack a few items and then return to the hospital. Dad was sleeping peacefully, still having drugs from the surgery in his system. Hopefully, Mom would be back before he ever awoke.

When Mom had called me earlier, I asked her to let me know when she was leaving to go back to the hospital. As 11:00 p.m. steadily approached, I still had not heard from her. I began to worry, so I called her at home.

"Hello," she said, sounding very tired.

"Mom, were you asleep?" I asked.

"Yes, I got home and was absolutely exhausted," she replied. "I decided to just get a good night's sleep and then go back to the hospital first thing in the morning."

"Are you sure Dad is going to be okay?" I inquired.

"I think he'll be just fine, honey," said Mom. "The nurses will take good care of him." Somehow, I didn't feel quite as certain as Mom. In fact, I actually felt a little worried.

At midnight, Mom's sleep was interrupted once again. The hospital called to inform her that Dad was very upset. He had awoken unexpectedly and become very confused, as he didn't know where he was and didn't recognize anyone. They were trying to calm him down, but he was demanding that they contact his wife. They desperately needed her to come back.

Mom quickly got up and dressed. She then returned once more to the hospital. By the time she got there, Dad was sitting up in his bed, one of the nurses currently by his side. He was fairly quiet and had calmed down somewhat since the call. He was still out of sorts, but seeing Mom had definitely helped to ease his anxiety.

The next day, Dad was released from the hospital and my parents returned home. The surgery was behind him and hopefully, so was his trouble. One thing was for certain. Something about Dad staying in a hospital did not bode well with him. He'd be fine for awhile, but inevitably, his apprehension would take over. The visits involving surgery and anesthesia were even worse.

Dad did not ordinarily do well with drugs, at least not when he was coming down from them. They consistently did odd things to him. I remembered how he acted after his knee operation years before. The doctor had prescribed some pain medicine, which Dad had unwittingly taken the very first night after the procedure. In the middle of the night, Mom had found him at the bottom of the stairs in the foyer trying to traverse them. He was hallucinating and talking about incidents that had occurred years prior.

It seemed that the heavier narcotics used during surgery caused Dad to lose touch with reality. It was almost as if the nerve endings in his brain that were severed during anesthesia did not reconnect normally afterwards. I'm not sure what it was about Dad that caused this, but I truly prayed that this would be the last time he had to be hospitalized and put under for awhile.

Thursday, November 25, 2010

I loved wearing shorts in November. Today was one of those absolutely beautiful days in the low 70's. We were celebrating Thanksgiving at Bob and Monica's. Mom and Dad had already arrived more than an hour ago. I silently watched them drive by earlier and assumed they were helping with the preparations. Then, I thought better. Punctuality had always been important to my dad. Lately though, he had taken it to a new level. It was not uncommon for him to get ready for an outing a couple of hours in advance. We had all gotten used to this and simply accepted it.

I soon made my way over to my parents as they stood in the dining room, lovingly kissing them both. I then looked over at my dad. "How are you feeling, Daddy?" I asked.

"I feel good," he replied. "I just may have to do some yard work tomorrow," he said jokingly. Dad laughed, but inside I knew there was some seriousness to that comment. I lovingly gave him a stern look.

"Now, Pootie," he said. Dad had consistently called me by that nickname my entire life. I asked him several times how it had come to be and was always given the same story. I was a toddler at the time. One day, I was comfortably sitting on Dad's lap and he called me "Pootie". There was no rhyme or reason as to why. It had just come out of his mouth.

Dad had called me this pet name in front of other people so many different times over the years. The person would immediately look at me with eyebrows raised. I would usually get onto him about it and he'd promise not to say it in public anymore, but he inevitably still did. He just couldn't help himself. He had routinely used the special nickname for so many years that it had become second nature to him. It was a rare occasion when he actually called me "Vanessa".

After a wonderful dinner, Dad gradually made his way over to the comfortable recliner by the living room window. The grandchildren were playing and laughing. Dad looked as content and happy as any one person could possibly be. Things seemed to be looking up and for this, I was very thankful.

Saturday, December 4, 2010

As I leisurely drove that familiar road to my parents' home, the look of excitement on my face said it all. I could hardly contain myself. Tonight, we were celebrating Dad's 79th birthday. Mom had been planning the special evening with pizza and cake for over a week. The big surprise was that Bob would be bringing one of his dogs over as a special present to Dad. The thought of it made me smile uncontrollably as I'd looked forward to this for such a long time.

It was no secret that Dad adored dogs. His last pet was a black, cock-a-poo named Porky. They had been together for over thirteen years and were inseparable. Porky customarily went everywhere with Dad. I would never forget the time my parents came to Atlanta for Christmas. Randy and I lived in a 3rd floor apartment near Gwinnett Place Mall. That year, we had bought a real tree which smelled incredible. We had decorated it so pretty in our living room. I had already wrapped all of the presents and had them arranged under the tree just so.

As my parents arrived late that afternoon, Dad knocked on our front door. Randy let them in just as I came out of our bedroom. Porky swiftly ran inside and surprisingly made a beeline for the Christmas tree. Before

I could do anything, he hiked his rear leg up and uniformly sprayed all of the presents. Dad quickly reprimanded him, but it was too late. I was in disbelief. My dog Scooter had never done anything like this. It never dawned on me that this could be an issue with Porky. Years later, I would think back on this memorable incident and laugh. I could only imagine what was going through Porky's little head. "I love this place. It has indoor trees!"

When Porky had suddenly died, my dad was crushed, definitely taking its toll on him. It would be years before he was over Porky enough to even look at another dog. For so long, we had routinely dropped hints and kept our eyes open. We all agreed that he had undoubtedly reached the point in his life where he was ready for another pet. It would be good for Dad and for the first time in years, Mom was also on board.

Barron was a black, shitzu-poo that looked surprisingly very similar to Porky. His best feature by far was his front teeth. He had an under bite that was evident every time he opened his little mouth.

As we were all seated near the fireplace, Bob and his family arrived. Dad was sitting comfortably in his favorite recliner. Barron immediately made his way over to him and eagerly jumped up on his lap. Dad was so elated to see him, but still had absolutely no idea that Barron was now his. "Happy Birthday, Dad!" said Bob, eyeing the little, black dog.

"Is this for me?" he asked.

"This is your birthday present," Bob replied. Everyone's eyes were glued to the scene unfolding as we smiled, watching Dad and his new friend. He was speechless and evidently very moved. We all had felt that Dad needed another dog to keep him company. It had definitely been a long time coming.

As the excitement wound down, I noticed that Mom was no longer in the room. She wasn't in the kitchen either. I started up the stairs to her bedroom when something startling caught my eye. She was quietly lying on the couch in the living room, the area completely dark. "Mom, are you okay?" I asked.

"I started feeling dizzy," she responded. "I just need to lie here for awhile."

"Okay," I said, "I'll try to keep the boys quiet for you. Were you planning on having pizza for everyone?"

"No, I hadn't even planned anything for dinner," she answered.

I was dumbfounded. I had just spoken to Mom earlier in the week and she specifically said that she was going to provide pizza for everyone. Something was clearly going on with her and it wasn't good. "Mom, would you like for me to take care of dinner?" I asked.

"Sure, honey," she said. "I'd really appreciate it."

With that, I proceeded to look in the freezer in the kitchen. I luckily found one frozen pizza. I then went downstairs to the basement and checked the upright freezer, finding a total of two large pizzas. I knew there was birthday cake and ice cream for later. Hopefully that would be enough.

I soon got the pizzas cooking in the oven. About that time, Dad came in and curiously inquired where Mom was. "She isn't feeling well, Daddy," I said. "She's lying in the living room. I'm going to take care of dinner for her."

Dad looked worried as I followed him into the next room. "She got dizzy all of a sudden and needed to lie down," I added. "Maybe a slice of pizza will help." I left them together and went back into the kitchen. The concerned look on Dad's face clearly showed how much he loved Mom. He just wanted to take care of her.

As I cut the pizza, Mom slowly made her way into the family room. I then brought a hot slice to her. Not long after she ate it, the color began to return to her face, apparently starting to feel better. As she made her way into the kitchen, Dad dotingly followed behind, still so concerned about her. "Mom, how long have you been feeling dizzy?" I asked.

"It actually started on Tuesday," she replied. "I was coming out of Walmart and got lightheaded. I had to sit on one of the benches in front of the store for a few minutes. Today was the first time since then."

Mom had always exhibited such strength. For the first time, I saw a surprisingly frail woman before me. I had her sit in the recliner in the family room while everyone finished their pizza. Meanwhile, I got the cake and ice cream ready.

Mom had ordered a huge sheet cake for the party. It was chocolate with white frosting. On the top was written "Happy Birthday, Gump!", which had been my dad's nickname ever since he was a young boy.

My dad had played baseball on a team that his father had coached.

Another baseball player in the same league was named Gump. My grandfather always thought Dad looked like him, so one day he jokingly began calling my dad Gump. The name had somehow stuck throughout all of these years.

I served my parents their dessert first. Dad took his dish to the dining room table where Randy, Chris and Andrew were sitting. Before he could get the first bite down, he abruptly excused himself.

When Dad hadn't returned in fifteen minutes, I nervously went upstairs to his bathroom. The door was closed. "Dad, is everything alright?" I questioned.

"My stomach's not feeling too good, Pootie," he said.

"Do you need me to do anything?" I asked.

"No, honey," he replied. "Give me a couple more minutes and then I'll be down."

With that, I reluctantly went back downstairs. I put Dad's ice cream and cake in the freezer to keep it cold. About five minutes later, Dad came back down, not looking good at all. Then, Dad offered Randy his cake and ice cream. There was no way he could eat anything right then. That behavior was so uncharacteristic of my dad, always loving his cake and ice cream. He'd routinely eaten it every night for years.

We ended up leaving his dessert in the freezer. Mom and Dad sat silently in the family room while everyone finished eating. I hurriedly cleaned the kitchen and put the food up. It was getting late and I could sense that my parents were tired. I lovingly kissed and hugged them goodbye, feeling very uneasy leaving them.

On the way home, I thought about how drastically the evening had changed. I originally came over envisioning two, healthy parents having a wonderful night at a birthday party. I sorrowfully left with an image of two, fragile people declining before my very eyes. The sudden realization that my parents were not doing well was disheartening. What had happened to them? It appeared that they had aged dramatically overnight.

Sunday, December 5, 2010

As I drank my morning coffee, a troubled feeling grew inside of me, remembering the disturbing events of last night. I felt deeply concerned over my parents' health and decided to check on them first thing. Mom answered the phone and let me know that she was actually doing better. Dad, on the other hand, was still feeling terrible. In fact, he had now asked to go to the emergency room. "Vanessa, I still don't feel well enough to drive him to the hospital," said Mom.

"Let me talk to Randy and I'll call you back," I said. A few minutes later, I let Mom know that Randy was en route.

On the way to the hospital, Dad was very anxious and looked awful. When Randy asked him what was bothering him, he told him he was having chest pains. He remarked "Don't ever get old, Ran. It's hell." He often said this.

As the hospital clerk was admitting Dad, he became very quiet. Randy ended up answering all of the questions for him. When the nurse checked him, he again said that he was having chest pains. He also told her that one of his grandchildren had accidentally kicked him in the groin area and that it was sore.

While they were waiting on the doctor, Dad suddenly began to feel nauseous. Randy held the trash can for him and Dad actually got sick. When the doctor eventually entered the room, he asked Dad what seemed to be the problem. Dad told him about the groin area, but surprisingly said nothing about the chest pains. "Chester, you've been complaining about chest pains ever since I picked you up," Randy said. "Have they stopped?" he asked, very concerned and stunned. Dad slowly nodded his head yes. He had completely forgotten about them.

The doctor listened to Dad's heart. He then obligingly checked his groin area, but saw no swelling or bruising. Based on his limited exam, the doctor didn't find anything wrong with Dad.

"I'm actually feeling better now," Dad said.

"Are you sure, Chester?" Randy asked, feeling very troubled. Dad assured Randy that he was fine and then proceeded to get dressed.

On the drive home, Dad had relaxed considerably and looked more like himself. It was strange. He was adamant about going to the hospital, but once he got there, he couldn't wait to leave. As Randy cautiously peered at Dad, he actually seemed to be doing much better since getting the good report from the doctor. Maybe that was all that he needed today. Once again, Dad looked over at Randy and said his standard line "Don't ever get old, Ran. It's hell."

Wednesday, December 8, 2010

I quietly sat across from her in the waiting room at Parkland General Hospital. A cardiac catheterization was scheduled for early this morning. Mom had taken Dad to the emergency room yesterday after the chest pains had once again returned. She had told me that the plan was to put a pacemaker in this morning, but overnight the course of action had drastically changed.

We soon heard voices and I excitedly realized that it was my daddy. He was steadily getting closer. I quickly got up and made it to the aisle just as she was wheeling him by. The nurse then stopped the stretcher. He had a big grin on his face. "There's my girl," said Dad.

"Hey Daddy," I said. "Everything's gonna be fine." I held his hand tightly.

"Your father is a character," said the nurse, who then repeated an amusing joke that my dad had told her earlier in the room. Dad and I both laughed. The drugs had apparently already started to take effect.

I gently kissed him on the cheek and stepped back as Mom made her way forward. They talked in private for a minute before the nurse began pushing the stretcher again.

Soon after, Bob and Monica joined us in the waiting room. Mom was busy looking through the newspaper. I tried to concentrate on a book, but to no avail. I felt more than a little nervous.

It seemed like forever, but in actuality, it was just a couple of hours later. The door opened and the doctor came out asking for the family of William Lee. We all hesitated for a couple of seconds. My dad's full name was William Chester Lee, Jr. To all who knew and loved him, he was Chester. It always caught me off guard when someone referred to him as

William.

We all crowded around the doctor as he solemnly delivered the long-awaited news. It was not good. "One of your father's arteries is 100% blocked and two others are 80% blocked," the doctor said. "In addition, the arteries are highly calcified. This severely limits what can be done. There really is only one option available. He needs to have triple bypass surgery immediately." We all just stared at the doctor in shock. "Without surgery, it will just be a matter of time. He won't survive."

"What do you think my dad's chances are of making it through the operation?" I asked in anticipation.

"Because of your father's age and his diabetes, the surgery is definitely more risky," he replied. Neither option was sounding good at the moment. "In my opinion, not having the surgery at all is the riskier of the two options."

The doctor eventually left and we all took our seats again. About that time, my cell phone unexpectedly rang. As I relayed the devastating news to Randy, I tried to keep my composure. And I did until the part about the operation being so risky. As the tears began to flow, I stopped talking. Half of me was hearing the words of compassion emanating from my husband and the other half was thinking about the possibility of losing my daddy. He was really sick and probably had been for a long time. And yet, he had somehow still managed to be there for me.

There really was but one option. Dad was in far too much pain to simply ignore it. And as much yard work as he did, he would probably end up having a heart attack. I couldn't stomach that thought. We all knew what needed to happen.

A little while later, we visited Dad in his recovery room. He was wide awake and looked good. It was obvious that a lot of drugs were still in his system. Prior to the procedure, he thought he was getting a pacemaker. Now, he was hearing completely different. We had explained the results of the catheterization. We also told him unequivocally that he needed to have surgery to fix his arteries.

Dad was extremely confused and began to get paranoid, feeling that everyone was keeping secrets from him. He looked directly at me. "Pootie, what is going on?" he asked seriously. "Someone is not being truthful with me."

"Honest, Dad, I just found out all of this as well," I replied. "I had been told that they were planning on putting a pacemaker in you. They had no idea how serious your blockage was until today's procedure. The only option is to operate." I tried my hardest to reassure him, but the look on his face told me otherwise.

The ultimate plan was to transfer Dad to North Georgia Heart Institute later this afternoon. This particular facility was indisputably one of the best hospitals for cardiac care in the country. He would be in good hands.

Initially, Mom had not planned on staying at the hospital with him. I didn't think she truly grasped the severity of the situation. "Mom, you can't leave Dad alone at the hospital," I said. "Do you remember what happened the last time?" She remained silent. "I will come every day to help, but you need to stay with him."

I soon left to pick up Chris and Shawn from school, while Bob went back to work. Monica took Mom to her home so that she could pack some things before she drove her to North Georgia Heart Institute. Dad would eventually be transported by ambulance. A plan was in place.

That evening, I got a phone call from Randy. The hospital had just called him at work. For some reason, they had Randy's cell phone number in Dad's record. They had put Dad on the phone, sounding very confused and upset. "Ran, I need you to come get me," said Dad. "Shirley and Vanessa dropped me off at this motel and left me. Now, I have no clothes. They're in the trunk of the car. These people won't let me leave."

"Chester, you're at the hospital," said Randy. "Those people are trying to help you."

"No, I need to get out of here," insisted Dad. "I don't trust them." Randy could hear a lot of noise in the background, sounding unbelievably chaotic.

"Shirley should be there soon," said Randy, trying to reassure him. As he later hung up the phone, he felt a tremendous sense of uneasiness. A minute later, Randy called me and gave me the phone number for my dad.

When I hastily called the number, one of the nurses answered. "Hi, I'm calling to get some information on Mr. William Lee," I said.

"Hi, is this Mr. Lee's daughter?" asked the nurse. They seemed to be expecting my call as Dad had apparently been trying to reach me.

"Yes, this is Vanessa," I replied.

"Vanessa, your dad got very confused after they brought him in," she said. "We were trying to keep an eye on his heart rate and he kept taking the monitor off. He became very irate. We couldn't get him to take any of his medications. At one point, he grabbed my wrist." I held my breath for what would come next. "We had no choice then but to call security to restrain him. They had to tie his arms to the bed." I could clearly hear a male voice in the background talking to my dad. It was obviously one of the security guards.

"Is he going to be okay?" I asked terrified, my voice now quivering.

"He should be fine," she responded. "We've seen this type of behavior before." Somehow, I didn't think they had anticipated this conduct from my dad. "Is anyone in the family going to be coming to the hospital?"

"Yes, my mom and sister-in-law are on their way," I said. "I'm surprised they're not there already. Could I talk to my dad?"

"Sure," she answered. "Mr. Lee, your daughter is on the phone." I could then hear her passing the phone to my dad.

He was extremely upset and sounded completely disoriented. "Pootie, why did you all leave me here?" he asked. "I don't know any of these people." His bewildered voice was getting louder.

"Dad, please calm down," I pleaded. "You're at the hospital. Mom is on her way right now. Remember earlier today when we talked about the surgery you needed?" I could hear several different voices in the background accompanied by numerous beeping sounds, so much currently going on in the room. It sounded absolutely crazy. It was all clearly too much for my dad.

"I told you I don't want this on," Dad angrily yelled at one of the nurses. "You are so stupid!" I could hear several voices trying to talk to Dad. "This is my daughter. Don't you say one damn thing about her!"

"Dad, please you have to calm down," I begged, not sure if he could even hear me. "I don't want anything to happen to you. You're scaring me." My dad was a very strong man and in his current state, there was no telling what he might do.

"Pootie, I need for you to get me out of here," he stated. "I don't belong here." The chaos continued as someone had apparently entered his room with some new medication. "I am not taking anything from you. Get the hell away from me!" Dad yelled.

I held my hand over the mouthpiece and whispered frantically to Shawn to call Randy from his cell phone, desperately hoping that he could go to the hospital. Dad was out of control and I was terrified that they were going to hurt him. I watched Shawn run down the hall towards his bedroom. A minute later, I could hear him talking to his father in the distance. Not long after that, he returned to my side and nodded his head slightly. I knew that Randy was on his way to the hospital. He was the other man in my life that had always been there for me.

"Daddy, I'm begging you," I said trembling. "Please do what they say. They're only trying to help you." I couldn't hold the tears back any longer.

"Pootie," remarked my dad, "you disappoint me. You really disappoint me." And with that, the phone went dead. I put my head down and covered my face with my hands, crying deep heavy sobs. I was having a difficult time breathing. My daddy was becoming a stranger to me.

Suddenly, I felt arms around me. I looked up and Shawn was sitting on the edge of the chair next to me. Just as it devastated me to witness my dad going through so much anguish, it was killing Shawn to watch his mother's heart breaking. We hugged each other tightly. I don't even remember for how long. I then looked up to see Chris staring at me, his eyes wide with fear. He had absolutely no idea what had just happened. He quickly came over to me and I held him, too.

Thirty minutes later, Randy nervously approached Dad's room. He could see that Mom and Monica had finally made it. What he saw next left him speechless. Dad's eyes looked wild and his hair was in complete disarray. Randy had never seen him like this, looking like a mad man. Dad was arguing with Mom, as he continued to pull on the restraints.

The nurse that had recently come on duty entered the room with some new medication. "Hello, Mr. Lee," she said smiling. "I'm Nadia. I've got something for you." She had a very compassionate demeanor and a soft voice. Dad seemed to be responding well to her. He actually took the pills with no argument.

The medicine soon started working and Dad slowly became quieter. He still looked wild, but he had begun to calm down considerably. The arm restraints were eventually removed as Dad was gradually returning to normal.

As things continued to settle down, Randy decided to leave the hospital. Mom was there and hopefully, that would be enough to keep Dad's confusion and irrational behavior at bay.

That night as I lay my head on Randy's chest, I began to softly cry. Everything was happening so fast. I was seeing a side of my dad that I had never seen before. I couldn't begin to fathom the things that were currently going on inside of him. I desperately wanted our lives to return to the way they had been. But mostly, I wanted my daddy to be okay. Would he survive this ordeal? Would he ever be the same again? I began to feel extremely dismayed.

Thursday, December 9, 2010

My nerves were on edge as I cautiously drove to the hospital, the traffic as I passed through Spaghetti Junction not helping the situation any. I always hated getting on I285 as it seemed to operate on its own set of non-existent rules. The previous night had been an absolute nightmare. I had no idea how much of it my dad would remember or what precarious state I would find him in today. I was a complete wreck.

When I arrived at his room, I could hear the television playing from inside, the white door partially closed. As I slowly poked my head in, I noticed Dad sitting upright in his bed. He looked up at me, but no words were said. I then kissed him gently on the cheek. "Hey, Dad," I said.

"Hey, Pootie," Dad replied. Mom was on the other side of the bed busily getting his breakfast tray in order. She stopped for a moment as we lovingly embraced each other. The room was small, but cozy. I made my way over to one of the chairs by the window and set my personal belongings down.

As Mom walked into the bathroom to rinse her hands, Dad looked over at me. "I'm so sorry, Pootie," he said. He apparently did remember what had happened after all. "You know I didn't mean it." My old dad was back. I bent down and hugged him tightly. A tremendous weight had just been lifted off of my shoulders.

I then helped Dad with his breakfast. There was far too much food for just one person. It worked out well as I knew that Mom also needed to eat. Whatever Dad didn't want, Mom gladly ate.

As I watched Dad, I noticed he still looked unkempt. I found a wide-toothed comb in the basket of supplies and gently ran it through his hair. He sat so unbelievably still for me, almost as if he was afraid I'd stop if he moved. I could clearly hear one of the judge programs on the television behind me. Watching their favorite court shows was a part of my parents' daily routine. The tiny room was starting to feel a little more like home.

When I was done, I placed the comb back into the basket. "Thanks, Pootie," my dad said, smiling and scrunching his nose. That was his trademark look which he'd been doing forever. It was his way of saying he loved someone without actually uttering any words. I smiled at my dad and happily noticed that the sparkle in his blue eyes had returned.

About that time, the day nurse assigned to Dad came in, smiling as she said hello to me. I noticed that the name on her badge read Maria. She was a pretty, Hispanic girl with mesmerizing brown eyes. She joked with Dad and he called her "Honey". They were seemingly getting along just fine.

Mom, however, didn't look that well. She almost seemed like she was in another world. I cautiously watched her as she moved slowly about the room. She had lost so much weight in the past few months, really causing me to worry. I soon decided to take her to the hospital cafeteria and make her get something to eat. She chose the buffet and made herself a healthy salad. I knew that I had to keep an eye on her as well as my dad.

I helped Dad fill out his order form for his upcoming meals. So far, I had seen him eat breakfast and lunch, thoroughly enjoying both of them. Dad had always loved eating. I was thankful he still had his appetite.

Today, they were running some tests on Dad to make sure that he could, in fact, handle the operation. If all went as planned, he would have triple bypass surgery on Monday. I completely understood how serious this type of surgery was, especially for a 79-year old. When you factored in the diabetes and high blood pressure, it became even riskier.

I spent as much time as I possibly could at the hospital, feeling so incredibly torn. I wanted to stay with my dad every minute of the day, but

I knew I couldn't. I had children at home that also needed me. Still, I knew that Dad could not be left alone while he was here. We needed to do whatever was necessary in order to prevent another outburst. As I carefully watched him, it appeared that he had taken something to keep him relaxed. I'm sure the hospital staff did not want a repeat of last night. I tried to keep him occupied and calm. I could only hope that when I eventually left, his disposition would remain the same.

January, 1962

She had been vomiting for several days now. No matter what we gave her, she couldn't seem to hold anything down. We had taken her to the doctor earlier in the week. He didn't know what was wrong with our baby girl.

She also had not had any bowel movements in days. Her grandmother had brought a suppository over and carefully given it to her. Her tiny body had still not responded.

On Friday, she was taken back to the doctor. By this time, her little tummy was as hard as a rock, her blue eyes rolling back in her head. She was completely listless. It was heartbreaking to see our helpless little baby spiraling downward.

The doctor said it was imperative that I contact a surgeon immediately. I didn't know any, so the pediatrician recommended one. When I got home, I quickly called the number and left a message. Then, I waited patiently for the return call.

On Saturday, I gently put her down for a nap. I lovingly watched her precious face, the smooth rhythm of her breathing. She was still my perfect angel, even though I had absolutely no idea what was happening to her. As I left her room, I wondered where Chester had gone. I approached our bedroom and heard the faintest of sounds. I immediately stopped in the doorway. My sweet husband was sitting on the bed, his back to me. I could see his strong body trembling. I soon realized that the weary sound I heard was him praying. As I slowly walked around the bed, he looked up at me. I had never seen his beautiful eyes look so sad, tears streaming down his cheeks. I knelt beside him and tenderly took him in my arms. I had also never witnessed my husband cry before. We were losing our baby girl and it was ripping our hearts out.

Her grandparents came over the next day. "She doesn't look good," said Grandpa Lee.

"We're still waiting to hear back from the surgeon," I replied.

About an hour later, he finally called. I grimly described to him the latest condition of our daughter. He said to meet him at Variety Children's Hospital immediately.

We waited in agony while the doctor thoroughly evaluated her. After what seemed an eternity, he came and sat near us, his face looking dismal. "She is suffering from a condition called Intussusception," he said. "Basically, a part of her intestine has telescoped over another part. It's created an obstruction and nothing can get past it."

He looked back and forth between the two of us. We didn't know what to think. "We've given her a barium enema," he continued bleakly, "but it was unsuccessful. We have no choice but to operate. It's that serious."

I wiped the tears from my tired eyes. This absolutely couldn't be happening. She was only four months old. I peered down at my watch. It was almost midnight. I then looked back to the doctor. "Please save our baby." It was all I could say before I inevitably lost control. Then, I wept.

Grandpa continuously paced the floor. "That baby's not gonna make it," he said. "That baby's not gonna make it." We were all so scared. Inside, I prayed deeply for our precious newborn.

Several hours later, the dedicated surgeon emerged. We waited in anticipation. "She made it," he finally said as he smiled. "You have a strong daughter." Chester and I held each other closely. Then, he lovingly hugged his father. Tears of joy flowed from my eyes. I had never in my life felt such relief. We looked gratefully back at the doctor. "The blockage was so severe that gangrene had set in. We had to remove seven inches of her intestinal cord. You got her here just in time. She wouldn't have made it until morning." With the devastating news delivered, he turned and left the room.

I looked at Chester. We had come so close to losing our little girl. "God answered our prayers," I cried. Then we held each other again. Inside, I thanked my Heavenly father for miraculously saving our precious Vanessa.

Friday, December 10, 2010

Happiness was in the air as I strode into his room. "There she is," said Dad, as I lovingly kissed him. It was such a welcoming sight. The television was on, but he was clearly not interested in the news. I flipped through the channels with the remote and eventually found an old rerun of *Gunsmoke*, which quickly got his attention. His two favorite shows were *Gunsmoke* and *Law & Order*. I had watched them with Dad for as long as I could remember. As I looked at his handsome face, he was the picture of contentment. What a difference a day had made!

Dad hadn't had a shower since Tuesday night and was starting to look a little disheveled. Even worse, he was beginning to feel that way. Looking around, I noticed a plastic cup sitting on the counter. I generously filled it with water and brought it and the comb over to his bed. I carefully wet his hair and ran the comb softly through it. It did wonders for him.

In the complimentary supply basket, I found a blue, plastic razor. "Dad, do you want me to try and shave you?" I asked.

"Sure honey," replied Dad. I also spotted a miniature bar of soap in the basket. I then covered Dad's neck and chest with a large towel. Using the water in the cup, I did my best to get a soapy lather on his face. I gently ran the razor along his stubbled cheek. It certainly wasn't the best trim, but it was better than nothing. I took a compact mirror from my purse and handed it to Dad. As he carefully looked himself over, he said "Ah, yes. You did good, Poot." Then, he scrunched his nose and gave me that wonderful look that said everything was good with us.

Later that day, as Mom was trying to help Dad with his lunch, he snapped at her. It was really over nothing. Mom was dotingly trying to butter his roll and Dad felt he could do it himself. Fortunately, I managed to calm him down before it escalated any further. It seemed that his anxiety level rose as the day went on. He was completely fine when I arrived this morning, but sometime in the late afternoon, he started to get a little restless. It invariably seemed to get worse after that. I knew that the noisy atmosphere and the constant hustle and bustle of the hospital did not help the matter any. I just wasn't sure what was going on with Dad. I surreptitiously overheard one of the nurses talking in the hall and she specifically used the term sundowning which I had never heard before. Could she have been talking about my dad?

Saturday, December 11, 2010

While making the long trip to Buford, I was deep in thought over the intense events of the past several days. It felt odd travelling to their home when I knew they were currently in the opposite direction. Mom had needed me to go by and get some things that she'd forgotten. As I walked through the quiet house, it felt so empty without my parents here. So much of how they had spent their last few days was visually evident in each room. I gathered the necessary items and quickly went back downstairs.

After I locked the front door, I saw Larry, their neighbor from across the street whom I had heard so much about. He was my dad's buddy. Now, I would finally meet him. He was currently standing at his mailbox and smiled as I approached. "Hi," I said. "I'm Chester and Shirley's daughter, Vanessa."

"Hi Vanessa, I'm Larry," he said. "How's Chester doing?"

Before I could stop myself, my emotions got the best of me. With tears in my eyes, I said "Not too good." I took a moment to compose myself. "He had been having a lot of chest pains. He's going to be having triple bypass surgery on Monday."

"I'm sorry to hear that," Larry said compassionately.

"Thank you. Could you keep an eye on their house?" I asked. I then gave him my cell phone number in case he needed to get in touch with me, after which he gave me his. Dad had been right. He seemed like a very nice man.

Later that day, Randy and I went to the hospital. Dad was thrilled to see us. He actually looked better than he had in days, slowly gaining his strength back. Randy gently helped him out of the bed to use the restroom. Dad was able to manage the rest on his own.

While leisurely sitting in the room, one of the nurses called me outside in the hall. She wanted to tell me that Dad was getting increasingly agitated in the evenings. Some nights, it was bordering on aggressive behavior. Although not completely surprised, this was not the news that I had wanted to hear. Then, she specifically told me that his type of behavior was common in patients with Sundowner's Syndrome. She also mentioned him having dementia.

I felt a little taken aback by her presumptuous words. I was distinctly aware of the high blood pressure, high cholesterol and diabetes. But as far as I had known, my dad had not been determined to have dementia or Sundowner's Syndrome. I knew that Mom had suspected Alzheimer's, but he had never officially been diagnosed with it. What were they basing their assumptions on? Did my dad's problems reach far beyond his heart?

Sunday, December 12, 2010

I pulled my black coat tightly around me as Bob and I made our way into the hospital, the cold weather making me shiver. Venturing up to the third floor was now becoming second nature to us. As we walked into the room, Dad was just finishing his lunch. Once again, the plates were completely clean. It warmed my heart to see him doing so well, truly a wonderful sight.

For the first time since Dad had been at North Georgia Heart Institute, he was going to get a much needed shower. He was absolutely beside himself. Bob gently helped Dad into the stall where he sat on a plastic stool, actually able to do most of the bathing on his own. For a long time, he just sat in the large shower and let the warm water run freely over him. It was exhilarating.

For the pièce de résistance, Bob gave him a shave. It wasn't a second-rate job with a cheap razor like I had previously done. Bob brought some of his personal supplies from home. Dad was in Heaven. Afterwards, he looked like a new man.

We had talked to Dad extensively about the upcoming surgery. He hadn't asked a lot of questions, but seemed to fully understand what was going to happen tomorrow. He had definitely put a lot of trust in us to make the right decisions for him.

At 6:30 in the morning, Dad would be promptly taken to surgery, with the entire procedure lasting approximately four hours. Afterwards, he'd be moved into an ICU recovery room with four other heart surgery patients where he would remain for 24 hours. We would be right outside in an ICU waiting room. We'd be allowed to visit him for thirty minute segments, five times a day. If all went well, he'd be moved to a private room on Tuesday where we could conveniently stay with him 24/7.

That night as I carefully packed for my hospital stay, I knelt at my bedside. Never before had I prayed with such intensity. Never before had the words been more heartfelt. I absolutely couldn't imagine my life without my dad, nor could I imagine my children living without their grandfather or my mother living without her husband. There came a point in time where all you really had was your undying faith.

There would be a skilled surgeon in the room, as well as an anesthesiologist and a complete team of experts. When they walked into that operating room tomorrow, they would all have one common goal, to perform a procedure that was nothing short of miraculous. Beyond that, its success ultimately lied with God. We never completely knew what God's will for us was until after it happened. Maybe my prayer was selfish, but I prayed that God's will was not to take my daddy just yet. He was still so needed here on Earth, making such a remarkable difference in the lives of everyone he touched. I knew unequivocally that God was listening. I could feel Him. I also believed in the power of prayer and knew that with God, all things were possible.

Monday, December 13, 2010

As I nervously backed out of the garage, everyone inside was fast asleep, the neighborhood streets desolate. It was still completely dark outside when I arrived at the hospital. Inside, however, was a different story. Dad was wide awake and seemingly doing fine, appearing a little quiet which was to be expected. Mom busily packed all of their belongings. My parents had accumulated so much in just five days, the number of additional bags surprising. At the point in time when Dad was actually taken away for surgery, they would have to be completely moved out. Holding a hospital room for 24 hours was just not plausible.

At 6:20, a male orderly promptly arrived at the door to take my father. Several nurses smiled and said goodbye to him on our way out. We rode the cramped elevator down with Dad. After arriving at our floor, the orderly firmly pushed the stretcher out of the elevator car. Dad seemed very calm, but my heart was racing as I tenderly looked at him. "You are going to do wonderful, Daddy," I said. "I just know it. I love you." Then, I gently kissed him and prayed it wasn't for the last time.

I turned to face the elevator door to give my parents their privacy. A few minutes later, we nervously watched as the orderly wheeled him away. A lone tear ran down my cheek. I closed my eyes and again begged God to take care of my precious daddy.

Mom and I then made our way to the ICU waiting room on the second floor. There, we would try to remain as calm as possible for the next four hours. Not many people were waiting, so we actually got our pick of seats, optimally choosing a corner couch next to two recliners. A few minutes after we sat down, Bob arrived and joined us. We all got comfortable as it was undoubtedly going to be a long day.

I tried unsuccessfully to stay busy with the reading material I had brought. It seemed as though with every other sentence, my mind was wandering and thinking about what was currently happening in the operating room. I had talked extensively to the nurses and done enough research that I had a good idea. The heart surgeon would make an incision in the center of my dad's chest. Then, he would cut the breastbone and open up the rib cage in order to reach his heart. It was absolutely mind boggling. My understanding was that his heart wouldn't actually be stopped. Instead, the surgeon would use a mechanical device to help him steady the heart while he operated on it. For each of the three arteries involved in the intricate operation, a vital section of a long vein from my dad's legs would be removed and used to bypass the portion of each artery that was blocked. It was a greatly simplified explanation, but one that I could easily understand. It was both incredible and scary at the same time.

After several hours, a nurse came out and gave us the long awaited news that Dad had successfully made it. I felt so unbelievably elated and found it hard to concentrate on anything else after that. Returning to my seat, I immediately called Randy to tell him the wonderful news. I was in a daze of happiness and amazement.

An hour later, the same nurse came back to get us. We were taken to a small, but comfortable office and told that the heart surgeon would be meeting with us shortly. He entered the room not long afterwards. I would be forever grateful to this incredible man for saving my father's life. We politely shook hands with him and sat down. He briefly explained the operation and said that Dad was doing fine. No unforeseen complications had developed during the surgery. As I sat and intently listened to the doctor, I couldn't help but be mesmerized. Just a few hours earlier, this man had literally touched my dad's heart. And then he had put him back together again. Now, he had forever touched my heart.

Not long after we met with the surgeon, another woman came to take us to Dad. There would be a total of five visits per day for thirty minutes each. They unfortunately only allowed two visitors at a time, so Bob had me go with Mom for the first fifteen minutes.

As we slowly walked into the secured room, I looked around in awe at all of the intense activity. The room was large enough to accommodate many heart patients, but at the moment, only two were here. Medical equipment was everywhere, the sounds overwhelming. Dad currently slept, looking pale and very swollen. The breathing tube was still in his mouth, in addition to being hooked up to several other medical devices. I knew it was my dad, but in his current state, it really didn't look like him. I took his hand and gently caressed it. Mom and I both talked softly to him, but he didn't move. I wasn't at all surprised as drugs often had this lasting effect on him after anesthesia. I stayed for fifteen minutes and then went back to our area so that Bob could visit with Dad.

While in the waiting room, we met a very sweet lady who was constantly there for her husband. She would not leave the hospital even though her children begged her to. When she had left the room earlier, her daughter confided in us that her father, the woman's husband, was sadly not doing well at all. They actually didn't think he was going to make it, but the woman just couldn't accept it. It broke my heart. This shouldn't be the place where someone's sweet life ends. We were getting to know this family very well.

A few hours later, it was time for another visit with my dad. I let Bob go first this time. As soon as it was my turn, I optimistically went through the door and looked across the room, hoping to see a change. Dad looked exactly the same as he had earlier. I brushed his soft hair off of his forehead and then ran my finger along his cheek. "I love you, Daddy," I said. It might have been my imagination, but I distinctly thought I heard a moan come from my dad. I hoped that it meant he had heard me and felt our presence.

Bob had decided to go home after the last visit. Since Mom and I had only eaten snacks that day, we decided to get something for dinner. We left our bedding to clearly indicate to others that these seats were taken. The waiting room was now crowded and we weren't ready to give our location up just yet. We eagerly walked to the cafeteria and both of us got a hot meal which we brought back to the waiting room.

That evening during our last visit of the day, I had hoped beyond hope that Dad would be awake. As we cautiously entered the room, I saw that he was still asleep. Dad moved a couple of times and actually fluttered his eyes, but he was still too tired to wake up. The man next to him was sitting in a recliner with a red, heart-shaped pillow pressed against his chest. I felt a little concerned that Dad had yet to wake up. The drugs had apparently really knocked him out.

I retrieved several blankets and pillows for our nights stay. I made a soft pallet on the couch for my mom so she'd be as comfortable as possible. I then called home and said good night to my children and my husband. Tonight, I would stay with my mother and father and Randy would take care of our boys.

Tuesday, December 14, 2010

It hadn't dawned on me that the incessant ringing I was hearing was from my own cell phone. I had set the alarm for 5:30 a.m. the night before. As I tried to open my tired eyes, it felt more like 2:30. Sleeping in a hospital waiting room did not lend itself well to a good night's rest. We had turned off all of the overhead lights in our section, but the hallways and common areas remained alive with activity. We could do nothing about them. Between the night staff, cell phones ringing and the normal beeping within a hospital that seemed to come from every corner, I was exhausted.

I gently nudged my mother before I made my way to the restroom to wash my face. Our first visit this morning would be at 6:30. I truly hoped that Dad would be awake after sleeping all night.

As Mom and I entered the special recovery room, I noticed that Dad was beginning to stir. His eyes fluttered and before long, he actually opened them. I tenderly kissed his cheek and smiled at him. He looked at me, but I couldn't be absolutely sure it had registered yet who I was. And then in an instant, he shut his eyes for one more nap.

Our next visit was scheduled for 10:30 a.m. The nurse informed us that Dad had been moved to a special ICU recovery room down the hall which was designed for a single patient. Not only would it be more private, it would hopefully be quieter as well. As we timidly walked into the room, it seemed so much smaller than the regular rooms. Maybe it was all of the sophisticated equipment that lined the walls.

Dad lied in bed, fully alert and looking our way as we walked into the room. "Hey, Daddy," I said, gently kissing him on the forehead. He actually smiled at me and called me by name. It was a blessed moment.

"Are you feeling okay?" I asked.

"Yes," he replied softly. I continued to ask Dad questions, his responses short and to the point. He was apparently still very tired, so I decided to let him rest.

Dad lovingly looked back and forth between the two of us. He was very quiet, but undoubtedly recognized us. He began to stare at me and I sensed that he wanted to say something. "You are so beautiful," he finally said.

My heart absolutely melted. Two days ago, I wasn't sure whether I would lose my dad or not. I had seen an unfortunate side of him that I never wanted to see again. Now today, he said these incredibly loving words to me. This was truly him speaking, as heartfelt as it got. I loved this precious man so much.

Then, he looked at my mother so affectionately and smiled, extending his hand to hers. She took it and held it tightly. The moment could not have been more perfect.

A short time later, Dad began to squirm in his bed. He was lying at an angle and looked very uncomfortable. I took the bed controls and tried to change the position, but unfortunately it didn't seem to be making a difference. He was starting to get more restless, his eyes taking on a distant look.

After about ten minutes, his anxiety had reached an alarming level. He was now in an agitated state. "You two really disappoint me," he remarked. "You can't do anything for me."

I was absolutely speechless. It had seemingly come out of nowhere. The man that I was looking at was clearly my father, but the person that just spoke those harsh words was a stranger. In just fifteen minutes, the conversation had gone to two extremes, almost as if I had talked with two different people. I looked at Mom and she seemed to be handling the situation a lot better than me.

I stepped back near the sliding glass door, one of the nurses soon appearing at my side. As I sadly looked at her, my eyes filled with tears. She tenderly put her arm around me at which point, they began flowing. There was something about a loving hug that signaled the body to simply let go. "What is happening with him?" I asked her.

"It's the drugs that are making him act this way," she replied. "He still has a lot of them in his system." She seemed to uncannily sense exactly what I needed to hear. "Try not to take it personally. It's not him."

Dad was getting more upset with each passing moment. I felt like I was doing more harm than good. I dismally looked at Mom and said "I have to leave." With that, I quickly walked through the door in tears. I had waited for hours to see my dad and now I hadn't even made it for the full thirty minutes of our visit.

I patiently waited for Mom outside the door. We soon walked back to the waiting room together. I had a terrible feeling in my stomach that things were currently not going well in my dad's room.

I despondently left the hospital a couple of hours later to go to Chris' school. His class was having their Christmas party and I really wanted to be there for him. It felt like I had missed so much with him lately and I couldn't allow today to end up the same way.

By the time I arrived, I had completely composed myself. No one at this party needed to know what was going on inside of me. I knew so many of these children through my involvement with the school. Their loving hugs could not have come at a better time.

Randy had gone into the office for awhile. He'd be coming home soon to work from home so that I could go be with Mom and Dad once again. Bob had returned to the hospital earlier and while in the waiting room, he had surprisingly received a phone call from the staff. Dad was not cooperating. They allowed Bob to go back to Dad's room.

When he got there, Dad was sitting upright in the aqua recliner, seeming to like this position much better as it allowed him to breathe easier. They had brought some soft food and were trying to get Dad to eat, but instead he got very agitated. They were close to calling security and restraining him again.

Bob calmly talked to Dad and eventually got him to settle down. He also talked with the staff and they agreed that they would make an exception to the visitation rules for Dad and not only allow us to come back anytime, they'd let Mom stay in his room 24/7.

When I returned later, I talked briefly with one of the nurses before entering Dad's room. He had run into some complications earlier. His right lung was not expanding enough and they had found some fluid in it. They had to insert a tube to remove the fluid and to help with the breathing. It was very uncomfortable for him, which caused him to be combative. They didn't want to give him any more morphine because it made him so sleepy. He needed to be awake and sitting upright so that he could breathe easier. They were now giving him Tylenol to help with the pain. It was definitely not a good situation and for awhile, it seemed like he was giving up. As the day progressed, he slowly began to adjust to the new regimen and seemed to be improving.

As I nervously walked through the door, I noticed that Dad was once again in his bed, almost asleep. It had been a long day. Mom was lying in the recliner with curlers in her hair, trying to make the best of a bad situation. The small room was really not set up to accommodate two people comfortably. If Dad was sitting in the recliner, then Mom had to sit on his bed. This setup was clearly wearing Mom down. I prayed that God would help my dad's body and mind to heal. I also hoped he'd be moved into a regular room soon, for the sake of everyone involved.

Wednesday, December 15, 2010

I smiled as I pressed the elevator button for the third floor. I felt a certain comfort inside knowing I was returning once again to a familiar setting. My prayers were answered as Dad had been moved from ICU to a private room this morning. He was steadily progressing. The new room would allow him to have unlimited visitors 24/7. It also had more chairs and a recliner that lied back for sleeping which would be much more comfortable for everyone, especially Mom.

Most of the medical tubes were already removed. Dad had been eating solids for a little over 24 hours. His extreme pain had diminished greatly. They were no longer giving him morphine, but he still had some residual drugs in his body. My dad had always had a high sensitivity to narcotics. Not only did they impact him intensely, they also stayed in his system longer than normal.

When they had moved him earlier, the room and nurses both looked unfamiliar to him causing him to ultimately get very confused. He thought he was at home and rightfully wondered why nurses were there. As my mom tried to explain things to him, he started getting combative with her.

When Bob and I arrived at the hospital, we also tried to explain things to Dad. After about thirty minutes, he seemed to have calmed down. It was always a slow process with two steps forward and one step backward, some days harder than others. My mom was normally a strong woman. She seemed like she was holding up okay, but I knew she was exhausted. It would be so much easier for all of us once Dad was home. They only lived ten minutes from us, whereas the hospital was an hour away. I felt very optimistic that things would improve once that happened.

Bob and I left the hospital tonight a little earlier than normal. I knew beforehand that the roads were going to be treacherous and I had ridden to the hospital with Bob. Both Mom and Dad were understandably worried about us driving on them. They wanted us to leave early and get back home safely. Around 9:30 p.m., we decided to do just that. The parking deck had already begun to ice over in spots. Unfortunately, we got caught on the icy roads, the perilous storm hitting hours before the DOT had anticipated it would. It inevitably took us two hours and 45 minutes to get back to Lawrenceville.

I felt wonderful as I stepped foot into the warmth of my home. It could only be matched by the comforting thought that my parents were safe and sound inside their hospital room. Regardless of some bad times, Dad was continually getting stronger every day. I didn't believe that God would put him through all of this if he wasn't meant to survive it. I desperately held on to that thought every day.

Thursday, December 16, 2010

As I joyously watched him eat, I saw the familiar man that I knew as my father. He periodically looked around the room as he ate his meal, slowly returning to his normal self. Every now and then, he'd generously offer me part of his food as was his typical personality. Earlier today, Dad had begun his rehabilitation therapy, the cheerful therapist coming by to introduce herself. Dad was in such a good mood as I carefully helped him out of the bed. With the aid of the walker, he successfully managed to walk out the door and around the nurses' station, the therapist walking beside him the entire way. Several of the nurses said "Hello, Mr. Lee" as he slowly walked by, smiling at each one of them. I was so unbelievably proud of his progress.

A little while later, Dad's nurse came in and gave him an incentive spirometer. I had actually never seen one before. Basically, it was a device that would help Dad to exercise his lungs. It was extremely important to keep them healthy while he healed from the surgery, pneumonia being a strong possibility in his current state.

The spirometer would need to be consistently used every couple of hours. The first time he tried it, he got very confused and blew air into it instead of inhaling air from it. After several attempts, he successfully managed to breathe in and get the ball in the middle of the spirometer to rise to the designated marker put there by the nurse. "You did it, Dad," I squealed, seemingly more excited than he was. He took his mouth off of the tube and laughed.

An hour after lunch, Dad leisurely began watching an episode of *Gunsmoke*. Halfway through the show, he fell asleep. Mom came and sat next to me in the recliner. "Your father had a difficult time last night," she whispered. "A young man came in to check on him. Your father had to use the restroom. The man tried to assist him, but your father didn't want any help. I don't know if the man was being rough or if your dad was just tired. He got very upset with the man and said some things that were a little out of line. The man ended up leaving the room."

Apparently, Dad had become very agitated and given a member of the staff a hard time. Fortunately, his nurse had heard the commotion and quickly come into the room, managing to rectify the situation before it got out of control.

Several nurses had said that in the evenings, my dad suffered from sundowning. I had thoroughly researched this when it was first mentioned. Sundowner's Syndrome was a serious disorder that caused symptoms of confusion to unfold after "sundown". It was very much a mystery why the symptoms began at night or late in the day. Some doctors felt that hormonal imbalances occurring at night caused it. Others felt that the reaction that a person had to their senses during the day accelerated and finally reached a point that was overwhelming to them. Still some believed it was simply due to the accumulation of fatigue throughout the day. Regardless of what caused the heightened confusion, the person usually dealt with the stress by getting very agitated. The behavior from my dad that mimicked this condition seemed to be occurring more often. I had also learned that Sundowner's Syndrome was most common in patients with Alzheimer's.

The other term that I had heard repeatedly regarding my dad was dementia. Dementia itself was not actually a disease, but was instead a group of symptoms that caused individuals to have difficulty functioning in their daily lives, with the most common of these being memory loss. A good analogy would be to compare it to the word "fever" which was nothing more than a temperature that had risen beyond a reasonable level. The fever itself was not the problem. It just signaled that there was a problem, with something underlying causing the fever.

Similarly, the word "dementia" was not the actual disease or the cause. It simply indicated that something was seriously wrong with an individual's brain. The cause could be from many different conditions. I had learned that the most common cause of dementia was Alzheimer's Disease.

As I vigilantly studied these medical terms, I had a lot of concerns. A common thread clearly existed between the two of them. It was undeniably Alzheimer's. This knowledge was breaking my heart. The sad truth was that I did recognize some of the symptoms in my dad. I was slowly coming to the realization that there might be a lot more going on with Dad than I ever imagined.

Friday, December 17, 2010

Some of the nursing staff stopped and smiled as he humbly walked by them so effortlessly. It might not have been apparent on the outside, but I knew this recapturing of independence made Dad very happy. The three of us gradually headed to a conference room for a discharge class. Dad actually made it there completely on his own with only the aid of his walker. He did surprisingly great! I brought his red, heart-shaped pillow that was standard issue for all heart surgery patients. Two other men were in attendance and they also had their pillows close by.

We learned about the types of food Dad needed to be eating, as well as the ones that he needed to steer clear of. Unfortunately, some of those were undoubtedly already sitting in their pantry at home. When the nutritionist asked for questions, Dad motioned that he had one. It ended up being a good question about low fat cheese versus regular cheese to which she gave him a thorough answer. I had felt a little trepidation the moment that Dad had raised his hand, having no idea what was about to come out of his mouth. Some of his aggressive behavior this past week had made me paranoid. I also felt a little nervous that he wouldn't be able to sit in the same chair for over an hour. He proved me wrong as he actually did fine. Maybe things were finally getting better.

Before lunch, Dad again did some rehab, only this time without the walker. The therapist put a large, leather belt on Dad that she was able to grip from behind. He walked on his own with the therapist trailing after him, having improved so much. He also loved the added attention that he got from the female nurses on the floor as he passed them.

Today, I learned how to check my dad's blood sugar. I felt a little nervous at first, but it actually seemed fairly easy. The small monitor they gave us was a One Touch Ultra Mini. The nurse patiently showed me how to load and unload the lancet, as well as the test strip. During Dad's stay in the hospital, he had received insulin. When he went home, he would once again return to taking his diabetes medication.

Later that afternoon, my Uncle Ronnie who was my mother's younger brother and his wife Terry came by the hospital. I sat on the end of Dad's bed while they took the chairs, everyone joining in on the conversation. Dad successfully answered questions when they were posed directly to him. Otherwise, he remained quiet. After awhile, I noticed that he was getting a little restless. I immediately turned my attention to him to thwart off any future problems.

While everyone was happily visiting, one of the head nurses came in to talk about Dad's medications. "Who is going to be administering Mr. Lee's medicine?" she asked, clearly concerned that Dad couldn't manage them by himself.

"I'll be doing that," replied Mom confidently. I looked at my mother skeptically, knowing that she had actually tried to take on this role months earlier. Dad took so many pills each day and he didn't seem capable of managing them by himself anymore. I attentively listened to the nurse as she went over all of Dad's medications, both existing and new. I wasn't sure whether my mom would be able to successfully oversee this or not, but I knew I needed to be ready to take over, just in case.

After the nurse left, I dismally thought about all of the patients discharged from hospitals everyday that didn't have someone to take care of their meds for them. How did they possibly manage? Sadly I knew the answer to that question, some of them didn't. In those cases, crucial meds could potentially go untaken. I promised myself that wasn't going to happen to my dad.

Saturday, December 18, 2010

As I began to get ready for my day, I thought about all of the recent events that had occurred, some good, some not so good. He had endured so much to get to where he currently was. It had been a long week and a half, but the day we had all looked forward to had finally arrived. Dad would hopefully be released sometime between 2 and 4. Bob had gone to the hospital today to be with Mom and Dad and eventually drive them home. I knew based on Dad's demeanor how absolutely ready he was to leave the hospital.

One of the things that he continuously mentioned missing was having a clean shave, something that Dad would ordinarily have done every morning at home. Now, he'd be able to do that once again. I had made a chart for his daily care that had become quite extensive. My mom was a little nervous about taking care of Dad, but I assured her we would all help.

I had previously gone to the grocery store to get them milk, orange juice and some other miscellaneous items. I wanted their long awaited homecoming to be perfect. I had also bought them a small Christmas tree complete with decorations. My mother had always decorated their home to the hilt during this time of the year. By the time she was finished, every single room in their home would be adorned with something. I knew they couldn't do that this year, but I really wanted them to feel the Christmas spirit in their home. They had been through a lot recently.

Late that afternoon, I received the anticipated phone call from Bob saying they were on their way. Shawn and I quickly headed over to my parents' home in Buford with the newly purchased items. The fact that my son genuinely wanted to spend part of his weekend helping to make my parents' arrival that much more special warmed my heart. He was very special to me, as were all of my children.

As I put the groceries up, Shawn started assembling the miniature Christmas tree. Before long, I heard the front door opening. Dad blissfully walked through the entranceway first. "Hey, Pootie," he said. "Hey, Shawnee." This had been Dad's nickname for him ever since he was a little boy.

Dad was beaming as he sat down at the breakfast area table, obviously looking forward to this moment for awhile now. "Welcome home," I said happily.

Within a couple of minutes, Dad picked up the stack of mail that had accumulated while they were gone. He sat back down at the table and eagerly started to open the envelopes. Mom decided to run up to Walmart and get Dad's new prescriptions filled. While she was gone, Bob and I rapidly cleaned out the refrigerator. A lot of things definitely needed to be thrown out.

No sooner had we finished than Mom walked into the kitchen with the new medications. It was getting late and Bob soon decided to leave. I then had Mom bring me all of Dad's medicine which was contained in a small, plastic crate. I meticulously looked through all of the pill bottles, trying to cross reference them back to the list that I had received from the hospital. It was a complete mess. Pills were in the bin that were not on the list. Likewise, a couple of medications on the list weren't in the crate. I decided that the first thing I needed to do was collect all of Dad's current medicine.

I went through the entire house and gathered everything that had my dad's name on it. I then brought them all down to the large coffee table in the family room. Mom and Shawn sat next to me on the couch, the three of us attempting to get a handle on Dad's medications. Not only had I found lots of pill bottles, I also found several blood sugar monitors, lancets and test strips that had surprisingly never even been used. I didn't think Dad had ever checked his blood sugar and I highly doubted that Mom had either. I had absolutely no idea that they hadn't been on top of this.

Meanwhile, Dad had gone upstairs. He soon came back down

anxiously looking for a light bulb for his small, bedside lamp. He was starting to get a little antsy, so I decided it was best that I took a break and tended to him. We looked in one of the drawers in the dining room and finally found a bulb that would fit. I then went up to Dad's bedroom to put it in. What I found was a little disheartening. The previous bulb was broken and all that was left in the lamp was its base. I didn't know how or when this had happened, but I couldn't deal with it right now. It was not as critical as getting the medications straightened out.

"Dad, I'll have to fix this in a little bit," I said. "It isn't as simple as replacing the bulb. I'll have to get some pliers to get this out of here. How about we just leave the lamp over here in the meantime?" I placed the small lamp on the floor next to his nightstand so he would hopefully remember not to use it. Dad seemed fine with that.

I then returned to the family room to continue diligently working on the medicine. Before long, Dad came back downstairs and stood watching us. He wouldn't sit still and I couldn't get my hands around all of the meds because of having to take care of him. I noticed that he was getting very agitated over the pills.

"Do you all know what you are doing?" he questioned, clearly getting worried.

"I'm trying, Dad," I replied. By now, I was getting frustrated and trying very hard to hide this from Dad. "I just need some time to go through all of this."

"I just want to make sure that I'm taking the right things," Dad said. "Maybe we need someone here to help us out." I knew he would have definitely felt more comfortable if he still had a nurse assigned to him, but unfortunately that was not an option.

"Dad, I promise you," I said. "We'll get it right."

"Okay," he responded, sounding defeated. I wasn't convinced that he actually believed this. He then reluctantly walked off and headed back upstairs. I could clearly sense that he felt not in control. All he had wanted to do since he came home was be solely responsible for something. First, it was the mail. Then, it was the lamp. Now, it was the medicine.

Our continued progress was soon hindered once again. Within five minutes, Dad had returned downstairs. I tried to focus on the medicine, but it was hard when Dad kept continuously interrupting us. "Dad, why don't you go ahead and get ready for bed," I said. "I know you must be tired."

"I'm worried about what is going on down here," he remarked.

"Dad, you have got to settle down," I urged. "You are not helping the situation. I can't concentrate when you keep coming down here every five minutes."

"Pootie, I'm worried you all are going to do something wrong and I'm going to end up dead," said Dad.

At this point, I stopped what I was doing and just stared at my dad, my heart racing. "Are you kidding me?" I asked, as my voice started to rise. "I have spent every minute that I could for the past week and a half at the hospital with you. I have neglected my family and my health and put you first. I am doing everything I can to get this right and take care of you. Do you honestly think I would do something to cause you to die? Really?"

I didn't know what else to say. I was utterly shocked. My frustration level had crossed that safe line, our eyes remaining locked on each other. Nobody said a word. I tried to breathe deeply and calm myself down.

"Alright, I'll trust you," said Dad. I eventually convinced him to go upstairs and get ready for bed. As he slowly walked off, I could only hope that this really was the end of this issue tonight.

After five minutes had passed, Dad had yet to return downstairs. My heart felt so unbelievably heavy. I went upstairs to his bedroom and found him peacefully lying in his bed. His eyes were open and he had such a look of innocence about him. I felt absolutely terrible about my earlier comments. "I promise that I'm going to take care of you, Daddy," I said. "You have to trust me. I would never do anything to hurt you." He then smiled and nodded his head as I gently kissed him goodnight.

I went back downstairs and continued the arduous process of going through Dad's pills. The house was now very quiet. I found lots of old prescriptions that were somehow not on the list. I didn't even know what they were for. I ended up having to go back upstairs and get on the computer to look them up.

After awhile, I returned to my spot on the couch downstairs. Mom was physically drained and mentally, she was starting to slip. I asked her some questions about Dad's medicine, but unfortunately she was unable to give me the answers that I needed. I soon realized that this was the crucial point where I took over. My Dad took a lot of medication and I could no longer in good conscience let her take care of it.

An hour later, I had managed to make some major headway. I placed all of the expired pills and the ones not on the list in a plastic bag to be taken home with me for safekeeping. I placed all of the current and new medications in the blue crate and secretly hid it under the dining room table in one of the chairs. I then hugged my mother goodbye as she looked absolutely exhausted. Shawn and I were also very tired. It was inevitably time for us to leave.

Once I got home, I carefully added all of Dad's medications to the daily chart. His current medicine included aspirin – 81 mg. (for a blood thinner), Carvedilol 25 mg. (for high blood pressure), Caduet - Amlodipine 10 mg./Atorvastatin 40 mg. (for high blood pressure and high cholesterol, respectively); Lisinopril 40 mg. (for high blood pressure), Sertraline 50 mg. (for depression), Glipizide 10 mg. twice a day (for type 2 diabetes), Finasteride 5 mg. (for enlarged prostate), Potassium 20 mEq and Risperdal 1 mg. (for aggression). He also had several medications that were specifically as a result of the heart surgery and would only be temporary. They were Ferro-sequel (iron supplement), Plavix (prevented blood clots), Colace (stool softener) and Prilosec (heartburn). The list was daunting.

Earlier today, I felt like I was undoubtedly in over my head. I had no idea at the time about the massive learning curve that lied ahead of me. For the first time all day, I finally began to feel like I had a handle on things, but it had definitely taken a toll on me.

Tomorrow would begin a new chapter in our lives. My dad would have a strict daily regimen that would have to be followed to the tee. I felt hopeful that once we got him into the routine, things would settle down and his body would become stronger every day. Now that the heart surgery was behind him, I prayed that this would truly be a new beginning for him. As I closed my eyes, the last image that I remembered was that of my daddy sleeping peacefully.

Sunday, December 19, 2010

6:45 a.m. came early as I grabbed my coffee mug and quickly headed to Buford, my children and husband still sound asleep. Riley silently stood at the top of the stairs seeing me off as she customarily did every time I left the house. I felt a little sad that I was leaving them so early, but I needed to get to my parents' home before Dad had a chance to eat or drink anything. It would ultimately be my first day testing his blood sugar.

As I unlocked the front door, the house was completely quiet. I retrieved the crate full of medicine and began preparing Dad's morning doses. Before long, I looked up to find him cheerfully walking towards me, fully dressed and looking refreshed.

"Hey Daddy," I said, lovingly kissing him on the cheek. "I need to check your blood sugar." I then had him sit in his blue recliner in the family room, feeling more than a little nervous. In the hospital, I had only watched the nurse. Now I was actually doing it myself.

I pulled the monitor and the lancing device out of the small, black bag and got a new test strip. I then wiped Dad's second finger with the alcohol swab. As I carefully placed the lancing device snugly against his finger, I pressed the button to release the lancet. Dad amazingly didn't flinch at all. I pulled the device back and, to my surprise, a drop of blood appeared. I gently squeezed his finger until enough came out for the test. Then, I securely placed the test strip into the glucose monitor and positioned the end of the strip against the blood. I watched the red fluid rapidly slide up the marking. When it was completely covered, I held the monitor up and waited in anticipation for the number. Within a matter of seconds, 117 suddenly appeared on the display. I recorded the number in Dad's chart and then put everything up. I knew this accomplishment was miniscule in the big picture, but I felt incredible. I couldn't hide my joy. I smiled at Dad and he smiled back at me. We had just made major headway.

I then poured Dad a glass of orange juice and handed him his morning pills, never before realizing just how many he took. I watched him as he attentively moved them around in the little cup. He preferred grouping the smaller ones together and taking them at one time. The potassium pills were huge and he had a difficult time with them. I decided from now on, I would cut them in half. Before long, he had washed them all down. "Do you want some coffee?" I asked.

"Ah yes, Pootie," replied Dad. "That sounds wonderful." I hadn't seen Dad this happy or content in a long time. It was so good to have him back home, seemingly much better than he'd been the previous night. He was completely calm.

I then showed him his new chart and explained in detail the different items on it. The confident look on his face told me he was feeling a lot more at ease this morning. "This looks good, Poot," he said. "You're doing a great job."

Mom soon made her way downstairs, looking exceptionally tired. "Mom, do you want some coffee?" I asked.

"That sounds good, honey," she responded. As I soon handed her the cup, I sat down with my coffee. I used the remote control and turned on one of their favorite judge shows. I opened up the blinds to let the radiant, morning sunshine in. This time together felt especially nice.

As the final credits rolled for the current program, I decided to make them breakfast. Dad wanted a bowl of corn flakes cereal with some peaches on top, which was his typical breakfast. Along with his cereal, he liked eating a small sweet roll. Knowing that the diabetes was a growing concern, I decided to cut the sweet roll in half and put the rest up for tomorrow.

I then asked Mom what she wanted for breakfast and her reply was that she wasn't hungry. I actually had to force her as I knew she hadn't eaten anything since she was at the hospital yesterday. She had lost so much weight that she now in fact weighed less than me. I made her a bowl of cereal with blueberries on top and attentively watched to make sure she ate it. Dad, on the other hand, had eaten every spoonful without any prodding.

After breakfast, I had Dad practice using his incentive spirometer again. Just like in the hospital, he got easily confused. I reiterated the steps and he finally got it. For some reason, the natural thing for him to do was to blow air out after he put the mouthpiece in. He eventually managed to get the ball to the correct level.

Before Dad ate lunch, I carefully checked his blood sugar again. This time, it was 238. His doctor had told me that Dad's blood sugar generally tended to run a little high. If it hovered around 100 first thing in the morning and between 200 to 300 before lunch and dinner, then I didn't need to worry. Again, I recorded the reading in his chart.

After lunch, Dad was a little tired, so he decided to go upstairs for a nap. I ardently called home to check on my family. They completely understood that I needed to be here today to take care of my Dad. I really missed them though.

That afternoon, I tried to get Dad to do some light exercises. I had him successfully do some ankle circles and knee lifts while he was sitting in his recliner. Next, he stood with me and we did arm rotations. Then, I got him to slowly walk with me around the downstairs level. He did exceptionally well, but was soon ready to rest.

I busily spent all day with my parents getting our new routine down. I couldn't help but feel like Dad's personal nurse. I checked his blood sugar one more time before making them a quick dinner of chicken noodle soup and a sandwich.

I left Mom with clear instructions for the evening. She'd have to check Dad's blood sugar one time before he went to bed. I had gone over the instructions with her several times and even had her watch me when I checked it last. I hoped she'd be successful with it.

Dad's evening pills were already packaged in a small container and labeled. Mom would need to give them to him before he went to bed. Feeling confident that she could handle things independently for the rest of the night, I decided to leave. It had definitely been a long day.

On the drive home, I happily thought back over the day that I had just spent with my parents and felt good about it. My dad hadn't had any bouts of anxiety. Everything had gone exceptionally well. It was actually the most enjoyable day I had experienced since this whole ordeal began.

Later that night, I nervously called my parents. Dad was already asleep in his bed. Mom had successfully gotten him to take his evening pills. Unfortunately, when she tried to check his blood sugar, she got a little confused. I'd have to show her again tomorrow how to use the devices.

Randy walked into the kitchen as I hung up the phone and gently kissed me on the forehead. "So, is your Dad doing okay?" he asked.

"Yeah, actually he is," I replied. "Everything went really well today. He seems to be doing much better now that he's home." With that, he pulled me close to him.

"I'm really glad," he said. "The past few weeks have been rough for your dad. It'll be nice to have him get back to his old self." I couldn't have agreed more. I missed my daddy so much.

Monday, December 20, 2010

I lovingly blew my husband a kiss as we both backed out of the driveway at the same time this morning, him for work and me for my parents' home. The boys were still sleeping soundly and probably would be for awhile. I was so thankful for Preston and Shawn stepping up to the plate when I needed them to the most. They would see to it that Chris ate breakfast, in addition to everything else that he normally did each morning. I was really proud of my boys.

On the way, I dutifully stopped at the grocery store to pick up some items for my parents. While in the store, my cell phone rang. I immediately recognized the somewhat eerie ringtone that was designated for my mom and dad. I had actually received the ringtone last Halloween. For some reason, I had chosen it for my parents' home phone.

"Hi Mom," I said, feeling a tinge of panic. "Is everything okay?"

"We're fine," she answered. "Is it too late to get you to add something to my list? We need some cokes."

"That's no problem, Mom," I said. "I'll see you in a little bit." With that, I quickly turned the cart around and headed to the soft drink aisle.

I arrived at my parents' home fifteen minutes later, managing to get all of the bags inside in one trip. Dad was still in bed, which allowed me to get his morning medicine ready before he came downstairs.

While shopping at the grocery store earlier, I had bought Dad a crossword puzzle book. He had religiously worked the daily crossword in the newspaper everyday for as long as I could remember. He was exceptionally good at it, too. I had noticed that he didn't seem to read the paper as in depth as he used to. I hoped the puzzles would be good exercise for him. I eagerly placed the book and a pencil on the table next to his blue recliner.

Later that morning, Mom got a phone call. As I intently listened to her side of the conversation, she made an appointment for Wednesday. After she hung up the phone, I asked her who it was.

"That was someone with Dr. Martinez's office," Mom said. "I need to have a thyroid test. It's set up at Parkland General Hospital for later this week."

"Mom, what kind of problems are you having with your thyroid?" I asked.

"I'm not sure, Vanessa," she replied. "My mind is just so foggy right now. I can't think." I was beginning to get very alarmed at my mom's behavior. This was not like her at all.

As I tensely sat on the couch, I tried to remember any conversation that I had had with my mom about her thyroid. I vaguely recalled some phone calls with her awhile back. I decided to go up to her computer and look through her old emails hoping to find some information that way.

Fortunately, Mom already had her email account open. I entered "thyroid" as the search criteria and a list with several emails opened up. I then began perusing each one. The emails eventually jogged my memory. Mom had successfully found a doctor in the Atlanta area that specialized in thyroid procedures, actually considered to be one of the best in the country. She had asked me if I could drive her down to the appointment if she scheduled it. The emails went back and forth with this doctor. The condition referenced in the emails was hypothyroidism. A lot of discussion about the different options for handling this condition had ensued. The emails suddenly stopped and it didn't appear that any further decision was ever made.

I went back downstairs to talk to Mom, but she couldn't remember too many of the details. She was getting a cold and didn't feel well. I reluctantly decided to call her endocrinologist. His assistant informed me that they couldn't give me any information until Mom came in and signed a privacy form. Unfortunately, I couldn't do anything about that today. It definitely didn't leave me with a comfortable feeling. I clearly knew I had to keep an eye on Mom, as well as Dad. Hopefully, I would get some answers after Wednesday's test.

Later this afternoon, an older gentlemen that lived a block away in their subdivision phoned their home. Dad had generously cut his hair for years. The neighbor wanted to check if Dad could perhaps give him a trim today. When I informed him of Dad's recent surgery, he was surprised. Dad hadn't been in the yard lately, but the man had absolutely no idea why. He had me relay good wishes to Dad. I didn't say so on the phone, but I had a feeling that Dad's barbering days were over.

Today we continued to solidify our new routine, with Dad doing better every day. We watched one of his favorite movies, A Fistful of Dollars with Clint Eastwood, earlier. Dad had probably seen every one of his movies. He unfortunately only lasted about thirty minutes before he fell asleep on the couch. As I lovingly watched him rest, I noticed how content he looked. Things were definitely settling down and I was resting a lot easier where my dad was concerned.

It was my mom that I was now becoming exceedingly worried about. It seemed as though the entire time she was taking care of Dad, she had completely neglected herself. She was usually a pillar of strength. Lately, however, she had begun to look very fragile. I had been so consumed with my dad that I never saw it coming. When did this happen?

Wednesday, December 22, 2010

We both watched her with concern as she slowly put her coat on, having a distinct air of confidence about her. I had verbally gone over the directions to get to the hospital a couple of different times. She had assured me repeatedly that she'd be able to manage on her own. Today was the appointment to have her thyroid tested. "Mom, are you sure you can make it by yourself?" I asked.

"I'll be fine," she responded. I made her tell me one more time the route that she was planning on taking to get there. As she successfully repeated the directions back to me, I finally began to feel at ease.

"Take your cell phone in case something happens," I said. She lovingly kissed us goodbye and then left with plenty of time to get there.

Meanwhile, Dad had his customary breakfast and his morning coffee.

He was unusually quiet and I knew he was thinking about Mom. "Try not to worry, Dad," I said. "She'll be home soon." We then watched one of his judge shows to occupy our time.

Before long, I happily heard the garage door open. I looked over at Dad and knew he felt the same relief that I did. Mom had made it back home safely.

She soon made her way into the family room and sat on the couch. "Did everything go okay, Mom?" I inquired.

"Well," she replied, "I got there and they called me right back. We filled out some paperwork and then they put this plastic bracelet on me." She lifted her hand up to show us. "Then, they led me into a room and started explaining what was going to happen. They were going to give me an iodine pill and I wouldn't be able to be around any children or pregnant women for a week. I told them that Christmas was in three days and I couldn't possibly go without seeing my children or grandchildren." By this point, Mom's voice was cracking and tears had formed in her eyes. "They actually thought I would give up Christmas with my grandchildren. I told them I couldn't do it. Then, I got up and left. I could tell they were upset with me."

I was unbelievably proud of Mom for standing up for herself and not going ahead with the procedure. I couldn't help but feel a little uneasy that she got herself in this position in the first place. I definitely needed to be more involved with her care as I was really starting to worry about her.

I soon got my parents settled in the family room and then went upstairs to get on the computer. I needed to find out what type of thyroid procedure involved iodine.

Fifteen minutes later, I had my answer. The procedure was apparently called radioactive iodine therapy. It was typically used to treat an overactive thyroid or hyperthyroidism which could be caused by Grave's disease. When the iodine capsule was swallowed, the thyroid gland would absorb the iodine. The radiation it gave out would ultimately destroy the cells in the thyroid.

I was very confused. I had thought from my mother's earlier emails that her condition was hypothyroidism. The iodine treatment was clearly for hyperthyroidism. Those were two completely opposite conditions. My mother routinely saw her endocrinologist every three months. On her next visit, I definitely needed to accompany her and try to get to the bottom of this.

I was slowly coming to the realization that my parents were no longer able to tend to their health issues on their own. I could no longer simply ask my parents what the results of a doctor's visit were. From now on, I would inevitably have to go with them. Both of my parents strongly needed an advocate for them and I had to become that person.

After lunch, I coaxed Dad into going outside and walking around the house. Then, we moved a plastic chair onto the front stoop for him to leisurely sit in and enjoy the sunshine. He absolutely loved it. For years, he had sat out in front of his home on their wrought iron bench, his customary spot. As people would drive in and out of the subdivision, Dad was always there to greet them, apparently becoming a neighborhood fixture. He looked unbelievably happy to once again be back outside.

The new schedule was working out wonderfully. Today marked the fourth day that we had actively used it and Dad was doing so much better. Getting to this point had certainly been tough. I still had some outstanding questions for his doctors, but I now had a much better handle on it. My daily routine was to go over early every morning and prepare Dad's medications, with a different set of pills to be given at three different times of the day. I also monitored his blood sugar, fixed their meals and did other miscellaneous tasks, usually not returning home until mid-afternoon. I called my mom every evening to verify she had given Dad his evening meds. I hoped as he got stronger, I could reclaim some of that time. I hadn't run in three weeks and I missed it terribly.

The bottom line was that Dad trusted me implicitly and felt a certain security when I was there. I think I had made a positive difference in nursing him back to health. With each passing day, he got better and I got better at taking care of him. My Dad had always been there for me. Now, it was my turn.

Saturday, December 25, 2010

I slowly opened my eyes to the sound of silence, taking a few moments to get my bearings. It was Christmas! I leisurely woke up today without the aid of an alarm, feeling unbelievably refreshed. Yesterday, I had carefully packaged up all of Dad's pills for today and labeled them. I had given Mom detailed instructions on when they were to be dispensed. She had repeatedly assured me that she'd be able to handle things. It was important to her that I spend today at home with my family. I had to admit that it did feel wonderful!

Last night, we had planned on having a Christmas Eve get-together at my house. When I previously spoke to my parents about it, they both agreed that they'd prefer staying at home. So, Monica and I had prepared the food and brought the party to them. I had returned home earlier in the day to do my cooking. We all eagerly met at Mom and Dad's at 5 p.m. Between the spinach & artichoke dip, pigs in a blanket, shrimp ring, cocktail smokies, chicken nuggets, vegetable and sandwich trays, cake, fudge and nuts, the kitchen counter top was completely covered, with an abundance to eat. It had turned out to be a very special night with Mom and Dad really enjoying themselves.

As I quietly made my way into the living room this morning, I found Shawn sitting in the green recliner. I was convinced that no matter how old he was, he would always be the first up on Christmas morning. No one got more excited than he did. Riley was faithfully lying beside him on the floor and started wagging her tail as soon as she saw me. "Good morning," I said to the both of them.

The weather forecast predicted snow later, so we would be picking Mom and Dad up. I put a pot of coffee on and then sat down to enjoy the peacefulness of the moment. Before long, Preston and Chris joined us. Randy would be the last to get up, as was the norm.

I poured him his first cup of coffee and we soon began our annual gift ritual. The longstanding tradition in our home was that everyone took a turn and opened one present at a time. One person was designated to be Santa and that was usually Shawn. Randy was always the camera man. When it was his turn, someone else would temporarily take over. We inevitably had to include Riley as well. She could usually be heard in the past video recordings whining. I always gave her a rawhide bone to keep her occupied and out of the living room.

After all of the presents were opened, I put some sweet rolls in the oven. I then called my parents and Mom let me know that she had decided to drive them over herself. "Be careful, Mom," I said. "Just take your time."

An hour later, they safely pulled up in the driveway. We had already brought their Christmas presents over last night, currently positioned in front of the tree waiting to be opened. Mom had always done the shopping for the both of them. For years, I remember Dad making comments about him wanting to do some holiday shopping himself, but Mom's response was invariably that she went to great lengths to make sure she spent the same amount on all of her children. If he started doing his own shopping, then she would have to ensure that he was also spending the same amount on all of the children. It was much easier for her to take care of everything herself.

For the past two years, Dad had furtively decided to do something on his own. He would drive over the week before Christmas and give us a special card, always making sure to tell us that it was supposed to be a secret. I knew that he did the same for Bob. There would be a check inside of the card from Dad's account for $500.00. It was his kind way of saying thanks for all that we had done throughout the year. It made him feel good to be able to do this. He was so incredibly generous. I truly believed he would do absolutely anything in the world for us.

As Mom and Dad carefully made their way up the stairs, we all gathered to kiss them hello, with Riley insisting on standing at the front of the line. I made them both some coffee and served them some sweet rolls. Soon after, we opened the remaining presents. We then ended up watching *A Christmas Story* as we did every year during the 24-hour marathon.

At about 4 that afternoon, Mom and Dad suddenly decided to leave. I tried to talk them into staying for dinner, but they really wanted to get home. They were a little nervous about being on the road in case it started snowing. Again, Mom would drive them. "Call me when you get home, okay?" I asked.

Dad appeared very calm today and seemed to thoroughly enjoy the time with his family. However, I could definitely sense that he was getting tired. He very much wanted to get back to the comfort of his own home and I didn't blame him. As I watched them slowly drive off, it felt like so many past times. My parents seemed to have gained some of their independence back today.

About five minutes later, the phone rang. "We made it," said Mom. I explicitly reminded her to give Dad his pills before he went to bed.

Today was a major milestone for all of us. My parents had successfully managed to take care of themselves for the day. I was grateful they had insisted that I take the day off from coming over. Until today, I hadn't realized how much I needed to be at home with my family, having missed so much of their lives this past month. I felt confident that just five miles away, my parents were safe and sound in the warmth of their home and that they too were enjoying the peacefulness of this special day.

October, 1949

I was leisurely walking past the veranda in the hallway at Miami Edison High. I happened to look down to the floor below. That is when I unexpectedly saw him. He was sitting on a bench with a group of his friends, actually talking to a couple of girls. I will never forget it. He had a yellow leisure suit on and he looked so incredibly handsome. I closely watched him, but he never looked up. I would have given absolutely anything to have met him.

He was a rising senior when I started the 10th grade. Even though he was two years ahead of me in school, I still knew of him. He was so popular. He played basketball and was involved in the Key club. I had tried on so many occasions to get his attention, undeniably having a major crush on him. Unfortunately, he didn't even know I existed back then.

June, 1956

Mother had asked me to drive my younger brother, Ronnie, to his baseball game. He currently played in the American Legion League. It actually was the first time in years that I had seen him play. After graduating from Miami Edison High School in 1952, I had gone on to college at the University of Florida where I got my Bachelor's degree in Education. A young teacher at a school nearby was going on maternity leave, so I graciously filled in for her and taught a third grade class in Jacksonville before returning home to Miami to teach.

I cautiously made my way up to the top row of the bleacher, glad I had worn flats. It would be a great view. As I looked around, I suddenly saw him. I absolutely couldn't believe he was here, my heart racing uncontrollably. I remembered so many times back in high school when I desperately wanted to meet him. Unfortunately, I never had the chance.

I knew from friends that after he graduated from high school in 1950, he had enlisted in the Air Force where he trained on airplane engines, always very mechanically oriented. He even owned a little coupe that he had fixed up. It was so cute. He had always been exceptionally good at fixing cars. After his military training, he was promptly stationed in Okinawa during the Korean War. He had successfully finished his tour of duty and was now back in Miami.

Chester contentedly sat on the bottom row of the bleachers with his younger brother, Ronnie. He was here to watch Shelby, his other brother, play baseball. Both of our brothers were coincidentally on opposing teams.

The game was extremely exciting, but I had a hard time concentrating. I secretly watched him from behind as he talked and laughed.

After the game, I waited anxiously for my brother. I noticed that Chester was waiting for his brother, as well. I decided that it was now or never. I started stepping down the steep bleacher rows. Somehow, coming down was much scarier than going up, even with my flats, as there were no rails. "Oh Lord," I said, "I better be careful. I'm going to break my neck."

He abruptly looked up at me. Before I knew what had happened, he *had put both of his hands under my arms and carefully picked me up. He then gently set me on the ground. I could not have asked for the situation to be handled any more perfectly. He then started walking with me.*

In no time, we were at my car. We ended up talking for quite awhile. Then, it miraculously happened. "Do you want to go out with me Wednesday night?" he asked.

Wednesday night was a whole two nights later. I felt unbelievably giddy and bold. "What is wrong with tomorrow night?" I asked smiling.

"I already have a date tomorrow night," he responded.

"Well, break it," I said. We both laughed.

"I can't do that," he genuinely replied.

Even though I desperately wanted him to break his date, a part of me was glad he didn't. It said so much more about his character. I knew then that he was a true gentleman. So, I gladly gave him my phone number.

September 7, 1956

Three short months after our first date, my ultimate wish came true. I married the man of my dreams and the love of my life. Upon announcing our engagement to our parents only three weeks after our first date, none of them expressed any worry. No one considered it a rash decision, least of all Chester or me. We absolutely wouldn't have listened anyway. We were deeply in love.

September 7, 2006

Today, we joyously celebrated our 50th wedding anniversary. From the very first time that we laid eyes on one another, it had truly been love at first sight. I saw my husband for the first time while in high school in

1949. I knew back then that he was definitely the one. Chester saw me for the first time at that fateful baseball game in 1956. He also fell in love at first sight. We had been together ever since that special first date on that Wednesday night so long ago.

Sunday, December 26, 2010

He slowly ran his fingers through his hair, so evident that it bothered him. It was getting so long, a lot longer than he normally liked. He unfortunately hadn't gone to a barber in a couple of months. Dad had asked Randy yesterday if he would mind giving him a haircut, knowing that Randy had been cutting Preston's hair for awhile now. As we leisurely drove to my parents' home early this morning, I carefully held the trimmer in my lap.

Randy thoughtfully set up a chair in the kitchen for Dad. He then went to the basement and got one of Dad's barber capes. "Are you ready, Chester?" Randy asked.

"You better believe it, Ran," Dad replied.

"How short do you want it?" inquired Randy.

"How about we use a number two all over," responded Dad. He had finally got his nerve up and decided he was ready for all of his hair to be cut off.

Randy gently trimmed his hair as Dad sat perfectly still, looking so content. Being a barber himself, Dad wouldn't allow many people to cut his hair. He trusted Randy completely.

I thought back about all of the times after my dad had moved here from Pensacola that he spent searching for a good barber. I honestly didn't think there was a shop around that Dad hadn't tried.

One day, he was casually driving around looking to get a haircut. He suddenly ran across a little shop in a strip mall called Montel's Barbershop. He had somehow missed this one and was only too happy to give it a try. He carefully parked his red truck and proceeded to go inside. A small sign in the window said they specialized in fades, twists and cornrows, but Dad didn't pay much attention to it. As soon as he opened the front door, an African American gentlemen said "Well, hello sir".

Dad smiled and said "Hello. Do you think I can get a trim?"

"You sure can," the man answered. "Give me about five minutes." He then kindly offered Dad something to drink.

As Dad slowly took a seat, he couldn't help but notice that he was the only white person in the shop. It may have made other people uncomfortable and they may have even left at that point, but not Dad.

As he attentively looked around, he noticed that every one of the barbers currently had a customer in their chair, apparently doing excellent business. As only a former barber would do, Dad methodically surveyed the set up and compared it to his previous shops. He was thoroughly impressed.

A few minutes later, he was happily seated in one of the barber chairs and was on his way to getting that much needed trim. Dad and the barber exchanged many pleasantries. He didn't however tell him that he, too, had been in the business.

Dad ended up walking out of that shop that day with a haircut that he was very pleased with. Whether he had unintentionally provided a chuckle for the remaining customers or employees after he left, we would never know. What I did know was that it hadn't mattered to Dad that he was the only white man in the room. It apparently hadn't mattered to the barber that cut his hair either. Dad wasn't at all concerned with whether or not they had experience cutting hair of his texture. It was simply a man walking into a barber shop to get a haircut. Nothing else mattered. Others may have found this humorous, but it truly didn't faze my dad.

I continued to watch Randy and my dad from the other room, always amazed at the closeness between the two. I felt a certain warmth inside of me that I always experienced when I observed them together.

Randy then got Dad's electric razor from his upstairs bathroom. Dad was deservedly going to get the complete treatment. To anyone watching him, he looked like the picture of happiness. By the time Randy took the cape off of Dad, he honestly looked like a different man. His hair had surprisingly turned completely white since the heart surgery. He had routinely colored it at one time, but that was no longer a priority for him.

Randy soon handed Dad the handheld mirror. As he carefully looked in it, he smiled. "Ah yes, you did good, Ran," he said. "Thank you, Bud.

What do I owe you?" They both laughed.

Later that afternoon, Bob brought Dad's new dog back to him. He had previously taken Barron back to his home after Dad unexpectedly went into the hospital. Now, it was time to return him.

Earlier in the day, he had given Barron a bath so that everything would be perfect for his arrival. Dad was unquestionably a dog person and always would be. I absolutely knew that Barron was going to be good for him. Mom had also felt the same way as she had even gone out earlier this week and bought him his very own dog bed.

As Bob and Andrew came in the front door, Barron excitedly ran ahead. He spotted Dad and immediately started wagging his little tail. It was hard to tell who was more excited. "Hey there, little guy," said Dad lovingly. Barron then jumped up on Dad's lap. It was as if the two of them had been together forever.

Randy and I eventually said our goodbyes and then drove home. I couldn't help but feel happy over how the day had gone. So much progress had been made today towards getting Dad's life back to normal. I honestly hadn't felt this hopeful in awhile.

Monday, December 27, 2010

It seemed that with every passing day, my father's health was greatly improving, but my mother's was worsening. I was rapidly becoming very alarmed. During one of our conversations today, I had mentioned something about the hospital stay when Dad had his heart surgery. My mother looked at me questioningly like she didn't know what I was talking about. "Mom, you spent over a week in the hospital with Dad," I stated. "Don't you remember?"

"I just can't seem to recall it right now," she replied. I was feeling very troubled. It was as if she had woken up and her short term memory had been erased. The recent hospital stay was surprisingly just a little over a week ago.

"Mom, have you been taking your medications lately?" I asked.

"I'm pretty sure I have," she responded.

"Can you show me where your pills are?" I asked. It had never dawned on me that I needed to be monitoring Mom's medications, as well as Dad's.

She obligingly showed me a small container on the kitchen counter with several assorted pill bottles. I also found a pill box that didn't appear very organized. Immediately to the side of the plastic container was a cardboard blister pack that contained numerous large, white pills. I quickly gathered all of them together and headed upstairs to get on the computer to do some research. "I'll be back in a minute," I said.

After a short while, I returned downstairs. "Mom, what are these pills?" I asked, holding up the blister pack.

"They're for a clinical study that I've been doing," she replied.

"Do you know what the pills actually are?" I questioned.

"No, honey," she responded.

"Who is conducting the study?" I asked. "I need to call them and find out what these pills are that you're taking."

"They won't tell you," Mom said. "It would invalidate the whole study." This revealing news left me very uneasy. I then began to remember that awhile back Mom had mentioned participating in a clinical study. They were actually going to pay her for her involvement. I distinctly recalled her saying that Dad had not wanted her to do it, but she still went ahead anyway.

"How do you know it's safe?" I asked.

"I've been doing it for awhile and haven't had any problems so far," she replied. Something about this clearly didn't feel good. Unfortunately at this point, I had nothing concrete to base that fear on.

I carefully loaded her pill organizer with her morning medicine. She was taking Avalide and Atenolol for high blood pressure, Estradiol, aspirin and six pills from the blister pack, which were broken up into three different times of the day. She also took Simvastatin at night before she went to bed. That bottle would remain upstairs in her bathroom. She occasionally mentioned that she took several supplements, but I never could find any. I would definitely get her a multi-vitamin appropriate for her age the next time I went shopping.

I had some explicit concerns about some of her pills. For now, I would just ensure she was taking everything that was prescribed to her. I had absolutely no way of knowing if Mom had been taking all of her medications on a regular basis or not. She had unfortunately experienced a lot of additional stress during the past couple of months. I truly hoped that as things settled down, she would eventually start to improve. At least with me taking over her medications, I would know that any problems she experienced were not from neglecting her medicine.

Tuesday, December 28, 2010

"Dad, do you want to change into one of your tank tops?" I asked jokingly. I had been relentlessly teasing him all morning about his upcoming therapy session, or weightlifting session as I referred to it. The first time had evoked an inquisitive look from him. After I repeatedly assured him it was just some minor physical therapy, he had laughed every time thereafter.

The therapist was a young man named Mark who I had spoken to on the phone last week when the appointment was originally made. I was very impressed with him and hoped that Dad would ultimately feel the same way.

As I invited Mark inside, it became obvious that he was even nicer in person. He was exceptionally polite and had such a gentle tone to his voice. It would end up having an incredibly calming effect on Dad. I knew then that Dad was going to respond well to him.

The initial therapy session lasted about thirty minutes. Mark started by diligently checking Dad's vitals and recording them in his 3-ring binder. He additionally had several questions for me regarding his current medications and blood sugar readings. I quickly made a list of them for Mark to include in his file.

After the preliminary paperwork was complete, Mark had Dad sit up straight in the recliner and do several leg exercises. Then, he gradually had him stand and do a couple of arm exercises, which were very similar to the ones that we had previously practiced. Dad unsurprisingly moved very slow and cautiously. Mark followed his lead and went at the same leisurely pace, never pushing him. He eventually got Dad to slowly walk around the downstairs level.

The plan was for Mark to come out two times every week. In time, they would work up to an hour long session. Today's meeting had gone better than expected. Dad had originally been a little nervous about someone coming into his home to work with him. The session today had really put his mind to rest. Mark always addressed Dad as Mr. Lee. Everything he said was followed by Sir. I knew Dad well enough to know that manners and politeness went a long way with him. His huge smile was evidence that he was happy with his new therapist.

Thursday, December 30, 2010

As he slowly stood up, his face grimaced in pain. His hand was currently pressed against the right side of his lower abdomen. I could tell immediately that something was wrong. After taking only a few steps, it apparently became too much for him and he began complaining about the area. "How long has it been hurting?" I asked.

"Maybe a couple of days, Pootie," he said.

"Do you remember if you did something to strain it?" I asked.

"Not that I recall," he responded.

Later that day, I quietly talked to Mom in the family room while Dad had gone upstairs to take a nap. "Your father went down in the basement a couple of days ago," she said. "I could hear him down there. I'm not sure what he was doing."

I then decided to go down to the basement myself. I intentionally turned all of the lights on and entered the back room where his many workbenches were set up. I quickly noticed that one of the riding lawn mowers was moved a couple of feet, its right tire flat. I strenuously tried to push it, but it was very difficult for me to move. I could only imagine how hard it would have been for Dad.

Dad and I had previously talked several times about him going into the basement. Even while he was in the hospital, all he could talk about was coming home and returning to his beloved yard work. He couldn't wait for the weather to warm up so he could get back to doing what he loved so much. The doctor had repeatedly told us that he wasn't supposed to lift anything over 25 pounds for the first month after his surgery. Every time he talked about doing some work, I would reiterate the doctor's instructions.

I knew my dad was getting highly impatient. I had a bad feeling that his current pain was a result of him trying to organize things in the basement. No matter how much I wanted to, I unfortunately could not watch out for my daddy 24/7. I suddenly felt very torn. I knew that once he woke up, we would inevitably have to have another talk.

Friday, December 31, 2010

A few days back, Mom was busily sitting at the computer in the bonus room. While she was working, she thought she heard the truck engine. A minute later, she looked out the window and surprisingly saw my dad walking through the front yard, coming from the driveway in front of the house. He didn't have any shoes on, only his socks. He had apparently moved the truck from the basement driveway around to the garage driveway.

I had inadvertently noticed for several days now that every time I came over, the truck was in a different location. One day it would be outside of the basement and the next day, it would be outside of the garage. On one particular occasion, the truck was parked so close to the basement door that it was actually resting on it. When I went into the basement to check on it, I noticed that one of the vertical support braces on the garage door was broken. The handle was also damaged. I worried endlessly about what would happen one day when instead of my dad just moving the truck, he accidentally continued out of the subdivision.

Today, I had an uncomfortable talk with Dad about the driving. "Daddy, if you're worried about the truck, I can move it for you," I said. "That isn't a problem at all. It's just not a good idea for you to be driving at this point. You're still recuperating." Dad just sat there quietly nodding his head. I felt absolutely terrible, like I had scolded a child. This was my 79-year old father. When had the roles been reversed?

We agreed that it wasn't good for the truck to just sit idly in the driveway. So, the immediate plan was that I would drive it whenever I had to run errands from their house. I would also obligingly move the truck for my dad any time he wanted. I truly hoped that the issue of driving was now resolved.

Later that afternoon, Mark showed up promptly for Dad's physical therapy session. "Hello, Mr. Lee," he said. "How are you doing today?"

"I'm doing just fine, partner," Daddy replied. Then, Mark politely extended his hand to Dad and they firmly shook. There was absolutely no doubt about it. I was in the presence of two gentlemen.

The therapy again lasted about thirty minutes, Dad still not up to a full hour just yet. We were explicitly reminded to practice our exercises daily until his next session on Monday.

After Mark left, Dad informed me that his abdomen was still hurting him. "Was it hurting while you were doing the physical therapy?" I asked.

"Just a little," he said. "I think I aggravated it." It was hard to know whether he had pulled something earlier in the week when he was in the basement or whether the therapy was causing it. Or, maybe it was the persistent driving that he had apparently been doing every day. One thing was for sure, he needed looking after and Mom didn't seem to be able to keep up with him, at least not in her current state. I gave him some over-the-counter pain medicine and then made him some lunch.

An hour later, I noticed that he had fallen asleep on the couch. The peaceful look on his face clearly told me that the pain had once again subsided.

Monday, January 3, 2011

Her current health was weighing heavily on me as she didn't seem to be getting any better. I was worried sick for my mother. I had been consistently monitoring her medications for a week now, but still saw no difference in her. Her current medicine raised some definite red flags. First of all, she was taking two different pills for high blood pressure that were dispensed by two different doctors. What if one of the doctors invariably didn't know what the other doctor had prescribed? That could be extremely dangerous. Mom had been having dizzy spells for over a month now. While researching her prescriptions, I had found a list of the symptoms associated with taking too much blood pressure medicine. She clearly seemed to be having several of them.

The second issue I had was with the blister pack. It really had me uneasy as there was no identifying information on it anywhere. I couldn't even be sure of what she was taking.

"Mom, something is not right," I said. Between having no appetite, losing a substantial amount of weight, always looking tired, not shaking her cold and starting to lose her short term memory, I knew inside that Mom was not well. "How can we be sure that these pills aren't part of the problem if we don't even know what they are? You have no business taking part in this type of study at your age and especially not with everything else that is going on right now. Did they know what other medications you were taking?"

"Yes, they had me fill out a form before they ever accepted me into the study," she responded.

I had concentrated all of my effort on my dad and my mom was literally falling apart before my very eyes. I knew that I should probably take her to the doctor, but taking care of dad was taking all of my time right now. Until I could do that, I had to make a judgment call. She had lost so much weight and I was very concerned that the dosage for her high blood pressure medication was too strong for her. One was prescribed by her primary doctor and the other one was prescribed by her endocrinologist. I knew emphatically that her endocrinologist based all of his prescriptions on blood tests. So, I strategically decided to have her continue taking the blood pressure medicine from him. I also stopped her from taking any more pills from the blind study.

I carefully took the medications that I had temporarily stopped and bagged them up, filling her plastic pill box with the remaining medicine. I'd have to watch her very closely this week. I prayed that she would soon start showing some signs of improvement.

Wednesday, January 5, 2011

The phone rang unexpectedly just as I finished up with the dishes, her voice sounding grim. She soon gave me the disturbing news that Dad had slipped in his bathroom and fell. Luckily, she had heard him and immediately called us. Even more lucky was that Dad had not hit his head on anything when he accidentally fell to the floor.

He was completely fine when I left earlier this afternoon. All of his blood sugar readings were consistently within normal range. He had routinely taken his medicine this morning and eaten two good meals today, his spirits great. Absolutely nothing had indicated there were any problems.

I quickly called Bob's cell phone and he was already on his way over to their home. He promised to call me back once he saw Dad.

When he eventually got there, Dad was still lying on his back in the master bathroom, his lifeless eyes rolled back in his head. Bob quickly knelt beside him and tried intensely to arouse him. A couple of minutes later, he finally came out of it. "How are you feeling, Dad?" Bob asked.

"A little dizzy," Dad responded softly. Bob then dialed 911. While they were waiting, he slowly helped get Dad back into his bed.

The paramedics soon arrived and carefully checked Dad's vitals. His blood pressure was dangerously low.

"Do you want to go to the hospital, Dad?" Bob inquired.

"I think that'd be a good idea," said Dad.

The paramedics gently put Dad on the stretcher and moved him downstairs. After loading him into the ambulance, they quickly drove Dad to the hospital. The plan was for Mom to stay home with Barron. She was not doing well and another hospital stay might actually push her over the edge. Bob and I would have to take care of Dad by ourselves this time.

On his way out, Bob called me and gave me the bleak update. I lovingly kissed my family good night and then quickly left to meet my brother at the emergency room.

We checked in at the desk and began the customary wait. Before long, they called us back. We were taken through what seemed like a maze until we finally arrived at Dad's room.

He was fully awake and seemed to be coherent. "Hey Daddy," I said. "You really scared us tonight."

"I don't know what happened, Pootie," Dad said. "I got up to go to the bathroom and on the way back, I got a little lightheaded. The next thing I know, I'm on the floor."

The attendant on duty soon came into the room and routinely asked what had happened. Bob filled him in on the details while I gave him the list of Dad's current medicine. We also told him of Dad's recent surgeries. The decision to keep Dad overnight was a given.

The orderly thoughtfully brought Dad a warm blanket and covered him with it before dimming the lights. Dad was currently in a very calm state. As I turned the volume on the television down, a football game was actively in progress. "Who is your favorite football team, Mr. Lee?" asked the attendant.

"The Miami Dolphins, of course," replied Dad. The attendant laughed, doing a good job at making Dad feel completely at ease. He even had him chuckling out loud a couple of times.

The emergency room was unusually crowded tonight as flu season was in high gear. The attendant furtively let us know that the ER was currently flooded with people that didn't have insurance, but knew how to work the system. They could easily come to the emergency room for non-life threatening ailments and not be turned away. We were also told that, as a result, no beds were available for Dad to be moved to. My dad who willingly paid for his insurance would be the one that suffered.

His current room in the ER was very small and had nowhere for us to lie down. "Why don't you both go on home," said Dad. "You won't be comfortable in here." He deeply wanted us to get a good night's sleep and knew that it wouldn't happen in this room.

Before long, Dad fell asleep. Bob and I decided to take Dad's advice and go home, planning to return first thing in the morning. Hopefully, Dad would still be asleep when we arrived.

I called Mom when I got home to tell her Dad's condition. I also wanted to see how she was doing. She was actually lying in bed when I called. The dog had previously been walked and she had already taken her evening meds. She was ready to call it a day.

Tonight certainly didn't end the way I would have envisioned it earlier in the day. Circumstances simply existed beyond our control. It was definitely not the perfect situation, but it was what we were dealing with. Sometimes, all you could do was what you thought best and then prayed that everything else would somehow fall into place. That was exactly what I was relying on tonight.

Thursday, January 6, 2011

Chris was still sound asleep as I quietly walked into his dark room. I knelt beside his bed and gently rested my head in the crook of his neck, so thankful that he still loved the act of snuggling as much as I did. I then tenderly kissed his cheek and whispered "I love you" in his ear before I left.

Randy had planned on taking Chris to school this morning so that I could get to the hospital early. Unfortunately, it wasn't early enough. By the time I got there, Dad had unexpectedly already moved into a private room. As I walked in, it became very apparent that things had escalated since last night. Dad was extremely upset. The nurse was busy trying to get his meds together. He was sitting upright in his bed with his breakfast tray in front of him, unwilling to eat any of it.

"That looks really good, Dad," I said, eyeing his breakfast.

"I can't eat that," he stated adamantly. "You know that's not what I eat for breakfast." His demeanor clearly indicated that he was getting more upset, so I decided to leave this issue alone.

The nurse was having a hard time getting Dad to take his potassium. The pills were very big and she hadn't split them in two. I knew from experience that he couldn't swallow them whole. "I usually have to break them up when I give them to him at home," I said.

"I don't have a pill cutter on me," the nurse said. "Why don't we put them in his applesauce and soften them up that way?"

It seemed like a good idea. As she handed me the two potassium tablets, I carefully placed them into the applesauce container. I then got a spoon to try and break them up.

A little while later, Bob walked in the door. Dad was still visibly upset.

85

Bob also tried coaxing Dad to eat his breakfast, but he wanted absolutely no part of it. I then defeatedly rolled the steel cart with the uneaten food to the side of his bed.

After about thirty minutes, Dad began to calm down. I did successfully manage to get him to eat the applesauce with his potassium hidden in it. The breakfast tray would be taken away untouched.

Bob and I stayed with Dad all morning and continuously watched television. I managed to find an old western on one of the channels. While Bob was still there, I decided to take a necessary trip to Buford and check on Mom. I got her medicine laid out for the day and made sure she was alright. She had yet to eat breakfast, so I made her some cereal with peaches on top. I gently kissed her and then headed back to the hospital.

By lunchtime, Dad was apparently famished. He ate this meal, unlike the last, in its entirety. Dad generously offered us part of his dessert and I accepted it. Not so much because I was hungry, but more to keep Dad content.

After a couple of hours, Bob left to go back to work, his job conveniently right across the street from the hospital. I stayed the rest of the day with Dad. Randy picked Chris up and worked from home that afternoon so that I could remain by my dad's side.

When the doctor came by later in the day, Dad was in extremely good spirits. The physician informed us that Dad's blood pressure medicine was a little too strong and needed to be adjusted. They cautiously wanted to keep Dad for one more day just to be on the safe side.

That evening, Bob came back to the hospital after first going home to get a change of clothes. A long couch was conveniently positioned in front of the window. The nurse soon brought in some extra bedding. That would inevitably be Bob's bed for tonight.

Except for the early morning episode, Dad had had a good day, remaining calm and content the entire time. I was totally convinced that our staying with him made all the difference in the world.

A couple of hours later, someone came by and mysteriously left a sandwich tray in the room. He offered no explanation, but simply placed the tray on the metal rolling cart next to Dad. Dad had already eaten dinner earlier, so he really wasn't interested. It worked out great though because Bob had actually not eaten yet. We never found out if the staff had made a mistake or whether someone was kindly looking out for my brother. By the time the food cart rolled around again, the tray was completely empty.

Friday, January 7, 2011

As I cautiously picked up my cell phone, I noticed there weren't any missed calls, my home phone never ringing either. I hoped that was a good sign. I had felt comfortable knowing that Dad wasn't alone last night. I knew that if anything critical had happened, Bob would have definitely let me know. As I quickly drove the familiar roads back to the hospital, I was amazed at how many other people were doing the same.

Bob needed to shower before work and I wanted to be there with Dad. We were slowly learning how critical it was to Dad's well-being that a family member stay with him around the clock when he was in a hospital. It helped tremendously to stave off any anxiety attacks. We knew only too well that once it began, it could take a substantial amount of time to completely calm him down. It was much easier to try to prevent it from ever happening in the first place.

After Bob left for work, Dad's breakfast was wheeled in. I had carefully placed his breakfast order the day before, knowing it needed to be cereal with fruit on top. I secretly watched Dad as I got his food ready, definitely improving since yesterday. He was apparently hungry and ready to eat.

After breakfast, I tried to find one of Dad's favorite judge shows. There was certainly no shortage of them during the day. A single cup of coffee sat on the tray. I added sugar and cream to it just the way Dad liked it. I had gone down the hall to a break room earlier to get myself some coffee. Now it was time to relax and enjoy this time with my dad.

Around lunchtime, the cardiologist came into the room. I talked to her extensively about Dad's current medicine. She felt he was indeed taking too much medication for his high blood pressure. Dad was currently taking three different prescriptions for the same ailment. Frankly, this had always concerned me. I had hoped that after the heart surgery, he could possibly reduce the number of pills he was taking.

The doctor felt that his blood pressure medication had caused the dizziness which may in turn have caused him to fall in the bathroom. Through testing, they determined that Dad's blood pressure lying down was different from his blood pressure standing up. Normally, there would only be minor variations with changes in the position. His was of concern. The bottom line was he was unquestionably taking too much medication. Since his heart surgery, his heart and arteries had improved so much that he no longer needed the same dosages as before.

The doctor changed his dosage of Carvedilol from 25 mg. to 12.5 mg. She also changed the prescription for Caduet which was a combination pill that contained both Amlodipine for high blood pressure and Atorvastatin for high cholesterol. The current dosage was Amlodipine 10mg./Atorvastatin 40 mg. Since the long term goal was to remove the Amlodipine completely, the doctor decided to get rid of the Caduet altogether. She would replace it with two separate prescriptions, Amlodipine 5 mg. and Lipitor 40 mg. She left the Lisinopril at the same dosage.

A month ago, I would have felt in over my head, but now I was so familiar with all of Dad's meds that I understood the doctor's instructions completely. I was actually able to participate in the conversation. I glanced at Dad as I continued talking to the doctor and he had such a contented look on his face, leaving me with a high level of confidence that Dad's meds were in good hands.

The funny thing was that Dad had an appointment to see his cardiologist yesterday. I had to call and cancel it after the unfortunate accident. Had he not fallen and actually made it to the appointment, his doctor would probably have reduced his meds much the same way that this doctor just did. The whole hospital episode could have been completely avoided. Dad missed it by one day. I truly believed that everything happened for a reason even when we couldn't see it.

I also brought up my deep concern about the Risperdal. Dad was put on this drug when he had his heart surgery to control his aggression. Since then, I had researched it extensively. Risperdal in an elderly patient with dementia could alarmingly carry a lot of risks. It could cause heart failure, pneumonia or even sudden death. It was also not approved by the

FDA for people suffering from dementia. I was very concerned that his doctors had used it to treat him. If my father was truly suffering from this condition, it could be very dangerous for him to continue taking this medicine.

The doctor said that it was fine to take him off of this drug, but it had to be done gradually. He was currently taking 1 mg. The doctor instructed me to give him .5 mg. for three days. Then, I could safely remove it completely.

At about 1 p.m., Dad was discharged from the hospital. I securely buckled him in my car and drove him home. He was in such a good mood. "It turned out to be a beautiful day, didn't it?" I asked.

"It sure did, Pootie," he responded. "It's a little chilly, but it feels good inside the car. You know how I love being outside in the warm sunshine." On the drive home, I fully explained to Dad that some of his medications had changed.

When we got to my parents' home, I carried Dad's things and slowly walked him inside. Mom was happily there to greet us at the front door.

After I got them completely situated, I explained that I would be back later that evening. I needed to pick Shawn and Chris up from school and I wanted to visit with them for a little bit. It would also give my parents a chance to spend some time together. After all, they hadn't seen each other in two days.

I left my boys at 3:15 p.m. and headed straight to Walmart to get Dad's new prescriptions. It literally took about an hour to get them filled. As I was busily checking out, my cell phone rang, the eeriness of the ringtone startling me. I knew invariably it was my parents calling. I looked at the time and it was 4:45. I had my hands completely full and couldn't answer it at that moment, so I let it roll over to voice mail. I then hurried to my car.

As soon as I got in, I got my cell phone out and quickly checked my mail. It was my mother. "Vanessa, when you get this, please call us back. Your father needs to talk with you." I could clearly sense that something was terribly wrong as her voice was quivering.

Then unbeknownst to my parents, the message continued. "That is not what I want to hear," stated Dad slowly. I could hear him speaking in the background.

"She isn't answering, Chester," Mom said. "I don't know what you want me to do." Then, I heard her slowly place the phone down. She thought she had hung it up, but she had only set it down. I didn't know whether that was intentional or not.

The next voice I heard was my dad. The voicemail had unexpectedly recorded what happened next at my parents' house. "I am going to hit you harder than you have ever been hit before," he exclaimed in a voice that was almost unrecognizable. My dad was threatening my mom.

"If you do, I'm going to call the police," she responded. "I can't live like this any longer."

"Get downstairs now!" Dad ordered. He wasn't yelling, but was talking slow and calmly. He was very much in control.

I could hear my mother crying. "Chester, let go of my arm," she cried. "You're hurting me." Then, the message abruptly ended. I felt sick to my stomach. I had absolutely never heard anything so ugly. The voice in the message was clearly my father, but it was in no way the man I knew to be my dad. Never in my entire life had I heard him talk like that.

My heart began racing faster than it ever had. Never before had I felt the type of panic that was rising in me at that very moment. I had no idea what was currently happening at their home, but I imagined the worst. I had to get to my mother in time. As I sped to my parents' house, traffic seemed to stand still. I didn't remember the actual streets as I rapidly passed by them. All I knew was that time was of the essence.

While I hastily drove back, I called my brother at work and frantically told him what had happened. "I'm leaving right now," he said.

"Please hurry," I pleaded.

I had absolutely no idea what I would find when I got there. A million thoughts were going through my head on that short ride back to their home. My dad had suddenly snapped. Mom had repeatedly told me for years that he was sometimes mean to her and I could never believe it of my dad. A part of me always thought that she was partly to blame. Dad had never treated anyone else that way. I just assumed it had to be my mom.

As I swiftly drove the remaining mile, I felt very confused. I had just seen them a few hours earlier and everything was seemingly fine. Now all hell was breaking loose. What had happened? It was an absolute nightmare.

I quickly pulled up in their driveway. I couldn't even remember getting there. Dad eventually answered the door, not looking like himself. Not a single word was said to me, his expression completely stone-faced. It was almost as if he was looking right through me. He was definitely a different person. Something had clearly happened to him since I had last seen him.

He turned and slowly walked back to the family room. He was leaning forward as he walked and looked so unbelievably aged. I realized at that point that however he was treating me had nothing to do with the voice mail. He still had absolutely no idea that the incident had been recorded.

I silently followed him into the family room. I then looked at Mom as she was sitting in the loveseat, clearly distraught. "Did he hit you, Mom?" I asked.

"No," she replied. I closely examined her arms and then I absolutely lost it.

I looked sternly at my dad, feeling the intense anger growing inside of me. "I just checked my phone messages," I said. "I heard what happened upstairs. You told Mom you were going to hit her harder than she had ever been hit before." My voice was rising with every word. "For years, I have taken your side. Every time Mom called to tell me you were being mean to her, I always questioned her because I knew my daddy could never have done the things she was accusing you of. I defended you and now I find out that it was you. She's been telling the truth all along, but I didn't believe her."

By now, I was screaming at the top of my lungs. I felt certain the neighbors could hear me, but I didn't care. Dad was just sitting there. I had no idea what was going through his head.

"What happened?" I yelled. "I dropped you off and everything was great. You were happy that you were finally home. Four hours later, everything has completely changed."

"You were supposed to be coming back with my medicine," he responded.

"Dad, I told you that I would be back later this evening," I said. "You don't remember that? I said that I had to pick up the boys from school and take them home. You don't take your evening meds until later at night anyway. So, why couldn't you have waited?" Dad continued looking at me, not moving a muscle.

"There is absolutely no excuse for what I heard on that message," I shouted. "It made my skin crawl. Do you want me to play it for you?"

"I don't know anything about a message," he replied.

"Well, I have it all right in here," I said, holding my phone up to him.

"I don't want to hear a thing from you," he stated.

"When I first listened to that message, I was in shock, absolute shock," I yelled. "I still can't believe that this has happened. How could you have said that to her? How could you have fucking threatened her like that?"

Then, there was complete silence. I just stared at him and he stared right back at me. His blue eyes looked glazed and his pupils were as small as pinpoints. "I feel like I don't even know you," I said.

I had never talked to anyone like this, especially not my father. We all had our breaking points and I had obviously hit mine when I heard the contemptible message. I cursed at him relentlessly for what seemed like an eternity. He said things back to me. Of course, they paled in comparison to my angry words. I was enraged. I felt so unbelievably betrayed and had no control over what I was saying. It was as if I was talking to a complete stranger. During most of my rampage, Dad just sat there quietly staring at me.

"Well, you aren't going to have the chance to hit her again," I said heatedly. "Mom, I want you to go upstairs and pack some clothes. Get your medicine and any bathroom supplies that you need."

Mom got up and quickly left the room. As she walked up the stairs, Dad furiously yelled up to her. "Shirley! If you leave this house, don't you come back!" Then, he angrily looked at me. "You either!"

"Don't worry," I said. "I won't be back."

The scene that was playing out was incredibly vile, this person I was looking at a stranger. He probably thought the exact same about me. It felt like I was living out a scene in a horror movie. What was happening could not be my life.

Mom soon came back downstairs and silently got her medication from the kitchen counter. Meanwhile, Dad was unsuccessfully trying to use his key on the front door lock. He eventually turned and took Barron upstairs to his bedroom. I escorted Mom out the front door and securely locked the deadbolt from the outside.

We dismally sat in the driveway until Bob got there, after which I let him listen to my voicemail. He didn't say a word, but it was written all over his face. It was a look of shock and anger and sadness, all in one. He soon went inside to make sure Dad was okay. He expectedly found him upstairs with the dog. Bob got him settled in his bed and then came back out. Mom would come home with me.

Both of my dad's brothers were already in town for the weekend, flying in earlier in the day. Bob stopped at their motel to let them know what had shockingly happened. It was not at all what they had envisioned for this weekend.

An hour later, I got Mom situated in Chris' room. She seemed to be doing okay. I wearily looked at her and my heart broke. I never imagined the incredible strength that this woman before me possessed. She had undoubtedly dealt with so much for so long and most of the time, kept it quiet. I knew that she had hidden things from us. I'm sure part of it was to protect my father whom she loved dearly, but I'm also sure that part of it was to protect her children, as well. The sad thing was I never totally believed her until now.

Later that night, Bob went back to their house. He called me and I carefully walked him through which pills Dad needed to take before bed. I asked him to bring the container of medicine back to me so that I could more easily prepare tomorrow's pills from my home. Bob gave him his evening meds as instructed. Dad looked so unbelievably distraught. As incredibly hard as the day was for me, it had probably been much worse for him. Bob eventually turned the lights off and locked the front door. Dad ultimately went to sleep with his dog, alone for the night.

Bob stopped by on his way home and gave me the small crate containing Dad's medications. I asked him how Dad was doing. "He didn't say too much," said Bob. "I honestly don't know how he is feeling, but he was calm when I left." Bob was especially quiet, also.

Even though I was still so angry, he was my father and I was worried. I didn't want anything to happen to him. I was thankful that Bob was able to handle the situation calmly.

Today had been devastating. In some ways, it was the worst day of my life. It had taken an incredible toll on all of us. Things did not end well between my dad and me. I wasn't sure that we would ever be able to repair the serious damage that had occurred today. Would things between us ever be the same again? Tears streamed down my face as I closed my eyes to pray.

Saturday, January 8, 2011

As I quietly peered in the bedroom door, I saw her sleeping soundly, giving me some comfort on a day when I desperately needed it. I quickly made my way into the kitchen and prepared all of Dad's medications first thing. Bob stopped by to pick them up a short while later on his way over to Dad's. My Uncle Ronnie and Uncle Shelby were also planning on spending the day with him. Knowing that my dad wouldn't be alone today helped somewhat to ease my distress.

After breakfast, Mom and I sat on the couch in the living room, urgently needing to talk about yesterday. It had been gnawing at me ever since. "I didn't sleep at all last night," I said. "I couldn't stop thinking about all the times in the past when you called me or came over after one of your fights with Dad. A part of me had doubts about what you were telling me. You were talking about my father. I'm so sorry for not doing more about it sooner. I can't imagine what you've been going through." Mom didn't say a word.

"Is this the first time since his heart surgery that this has happened?" I asked. She slowly shook her head no. I definitely wasn't prepared for that answer. "When was the last time?"

"Maybe a week ago," she replied. "I can't remember exactly when it happened." I was completely shocked. I had consistently gone to my parents' house every single day since Dad had come home from the hospital, except for Christmas. I never saw him get the least bit upset, nor did I see any warning signs. On the contrary, he looked extremely happy every day.

It seemed to be the same story that I had regularly heard for years. Dad was fine during the day. Sometime in the late afternoon, occasionally after dinner, something would unexpectedly set him off and he would lose control. All I could think of was Sundowner's.

As I stared at my precious mother, I thought back about some of the issues that existed between my parents, especially during the past year. I had assumed they were just petty arguments, nothing more. I never had a clue at the extent of what was happening at my parents' home. I never had any idea about the immense level of stress that Mom had been under. Or maybe I did and was just in denial.

Later that afternoon, my uncles went to see my dad. They had stopped at a restaurant and kindly filled up some take out boxes for Dad so he would have something to eat. They had also brought him a smoothie, which he always loved. Unfortunately, he didn't have much of an appetite. Most of the food went into the refrigerator for later.

My dad had the most loving brothers that anyone could ever ask for. They had always been very close, but in the past several years, that bond had strengthened considerably. Early in 2004, my uncles had made the significant decision to fly up to Atlanta to see Dad. At that point in Dad's life, he no longer liked to travel long distances. His brothers knew that in order to see him, they would inevitably have to make the trip. And they had. Every two to three months like clockwork, my uncles would devotedly come to visit Dad. They had continued that unique tradition to this very day.

Some cousins of Dad's also lived in Georgia. They had all grown up together and were very close. Two specific cousins were Johnny and Jeanneen. The five of them would get together on every visit, always having something special planned for Dad. Sometimes, they would make a day out of going somewhere locally that held fond memories for them. On one visit, they took Dad to Lakewood where he was born, his childhood home actually still intact.

No matter where they went, they came back with endless stories of happiness and so much laughter, always bringing a spark to Dad's eyes. In some ways, it was like they were still young kids growing up, no one aging at all. Distance and time had done nothing to change that, still as incredibly close as ever. These were very special times for Dad and I would forever be grateful to them for the selfless way they looked after him.

As they watched television in the family room, Dad just sat in his recliner quietly, looking like his world had ended. His brothers had definitely never seen him like this before. An hour later, Bob despairingly came through the front door. The four of them would spend the afternoon together, with only three of them talking.

I had spent the entire day thinking about what had transpired yesterday. I couldn't go see my dad yet as it was just too soon. I was still so angry. I was also deeply ashamed of how I had talked to him. No matter what had occurred, he was still my father.

I honestly didn't know what was happening, but I did know that something was very wrong with my dad. He would have never acted this way normally. He'd always been a kind and loving man, completely devoted to his family. We were his entire life. I didn't know if he just suddenly snapped or if it had to do with all of the drugs that had gone into his system during the past couple of months. Could they have in some way been responsible? If he was sick, was the disease getting worse? Was this episode evidence that he could no longer hide it from us? From everything that I had read about dementia and Sundowner's Syndrome, it sounded all too familiar, especially the violent events. I had so many questions and very few answers.

I knew that Dad ultimately needed to be tested. I just didn't know the best way to get it to happen. Mom had already informed his doctor about her suspicions of Alzheimer's. I was not convinced that the doctor had actually believed her. She had even gone to an appointment with Dad. On that particular day, the doctor had administered a test to Dad that was supposed to evaluate him for Alzheimer's. It was called the Mini-Mental State Examination or MMSE for short, also known as the Folstein test. One part of the test was to have Dad repeat three items. A few minutes later, the doctor asked him to once again repeat the three items. Dad unfortunately couldn't remember them. I never found out the actual results of that test. I did know that no further testing had occurred afterwards.

The bottom line was that Dad invariably needed much more extensive testing. What he needed ultimately went far beyond this doctor's expertise. The best option would clearly be for him to see a neurologist or a geriatric psychiatrist. He needed a complete mental evaluation by someone that was very familiar with disorders common in the elderly. I knew that the ideal situation would be to have him admitted into a geropsychiatric unit where he would receive a full mental assessment, in addition to having all of his current medications evaluated which could actually be part of the cause. At this point though, that would be a lot to ask of Dad and I honestly couldn't see that happening. Having him tested on an outpatient basis was probably more attainable. I was just hopeful that Dad would cooperate and agree to whatever testing needed to be done.

Another possibility would be to talk with Dad's cardiologist. He was especially familiar with his medical history and his aggressive behavior surrounding his heart surgery. In addition, they had done a CT scan on him before the operation to make sure he hadn't had a stroke. Dad already had an upcoming appointment with him. It would be an ideal time to mention this episode.

A million thoughts were reeling in my head, so much to think through. I felt overwhelmed and still wasn't sure where to turn. I had reached out to my sister-in-law, Vicki, who had a degree in nursing and she had given me a lot of the information that I needed. Now, we just had to make some hard decisions.

Later that evening, Bob went back to Buford to give Dad his evening meds. He also tested his blood sugar which looked good. Dad appeared very tired and ready to go to sleep, so Bob got him situated in his bed and turned the lights off before saying goodbye. My dad was once again alone with his dog and his thoughts.

Sunday, January 9, 2011

I could hear the loud, rumbling sound of a car engine outside and realized that my day had officially begun. It seemed like sleep had only come a couple of hours ago. I felt terrible inside as I awoke with knots in my stomach, feeling both mad and heartbroken at the same time. Both of my uncles and Bob had caringly spent the past two days with Dad. I, however, was still not ready to face him, partly due to anger and partly over regret. I was deeply upset over how I reacted and just couldn't seem to shake the dreadful feeling inside. I only prayed that Dad couldn't remember what I had said to him. The tears had been falling uncontrollably for two days straight. It felt like I had lost my father.

Mom was doing considerably better. She had her appetite back and I no longer had to force her to eat. On the contrary, she willingly ate every meal, even snacked in between. She was comfortably sleeping throughout the night and no longer looked tired. I didn't know if it was the change in medications or removing her from a stressful environment. I slowly realized that she had lived in hell for so many years and I never knew the half of it.

The predicted snow storm for tonight was very serious. The unwavering decision was made that Bob would take Dad home with him. It wouldn't be safe for him to remain by himself in their home. If God forbid an emergency occurred, it was questionable whether an ambulance would even be able to reach him.

As Bob was packing some miscellaneous items for Dad, he also retrieved some necessary things that Mom had forgotten. I felt very strange knowing that Mom would be in our home and just a couple of houses down, Dad would be in Bob's home. Nothing like this had ever happened to them. They had been totally separated for their own safety.

Later that night, I got an unexpected call from Bob, sounding flustered. When it came time for Dad to get ready for bed, he started getting anxious, insistently wanting to go home and sleep in his own bed. Bob had generously offered Dad the use of the master bedroom. Regardless of the set up, it just didn't feel like home to him. Bob soon handed the phone to Dad so I could talk to him. "Dad, you can't go back home right now," I said. "You have to stay at Bob's."

"I just want to go home and sleep in my own bed," he replied.

"We are in the middle of an ice storm," I stated. "They say that the roads are not going to be passable. It would be risky for you to be there alone, Dad. What if the power went out? What if there was an accident and no one could get to you? It would be too dangerous." I sensed that Dad was growing restless and there was already enough tension between us. I knew it was critical that he calm down before it escalated any further. "Does that make sense, Dad?"

"Alright," he said, sounding defeated. I knew he wasn't happy about this, but at least he wasn't arguing with me.

"Bob is going to take care of you, Dad," I continued. "You'll be okay there." As I warily hung up the phone, I hoped that I had made a difference in calming Dad down and that he would actually get a good night's sleep. Inside, I felt somewhat dubious.

Later that evening, I thought once again about the critical dilemma facing our family. We were still trying desperately to figure out what to do. The only good thing about the ice storm was it had given us some additional time to think things through. Dad clearly needed to be tested and I hoped that he would do it voluntarily. I knew that even if he did, it would take considerable time. What did we do until that point? When the Sundowner's kicked in, it caused him to completely lose control. What happened during one of those episodes could be extremely dangerous. I couldn't in good conscience allow Mom to return to that.

I truly believed that everything happened for a reason. The chance of my mom calling me and instead of hanging up the phone, accidentally setting it down so that everything that happened next would be recorded in a voicemail was very slim. What were the odds that it would happen on the very day that my dad's brothers were coming to town? In addition, all of this happened on the cusp of a major winter storm that would totally isolate us for many days. I truly believed that God was in control of this situation. And as devastating as it was, He had a plan.

Monday, January 10, 2011

As a child, I learned to carefully weigh every word before letting it out of my mouth. Spoken words could never be forgotten. When I was 7 years old, I swam on the Hialeah Seahorses swim team at Milander Park. One Saturday morning, I excitedly attended a swim meet. One of my events that day was a relay race. Unfortunately, my team didn't do that well. After the race, I was lying on my blue towel, feeling down. A little girl walked up to me, looked me directly in the eyes and said "It was because of you that we lost the race." Then just as quickly as she had walked up to me, she walked away. I felt both shocked and hurt, her words stinging deeply. To this day, I couldn't remember what the event was or even what the little girl looked like. I actually remembered very little of that day, but I would never ever forget her scarring words.

Once something was said, it unfortunately could never ever be taken back. Living with that type of regret was painful. No words had ever rung truer to my ears than those, losing my temper in the most tumultuous way. Never once in my entire life had I ever raised my voice to my daddy, nor him to me. I had certainly never said anything remotely ugly to him. We had always treated each other with the utmost respect, with nothing but loving and kind words between us. In a moment of sheer hysteria, I allowed my anger to come out in the most profane way. I was protecting my mother. At the time, I reacted in the only way I knew how. I knew my words struck hard as I had fully intended them to. I could never erase the image of my father as I said them to him. For the rest of my life, I would have to somehow live with this.

Earlier, I had called Bob to find out how Dad was doing. "He's sitting on the couch with the recliner up," he said. "Barron is in his lap. The television is on, but I don't think he's watching it. He seems like he's in a daze." I thought this would probably be a good time to come over.

All of the schools in Gwinnett County, as well as most other counties, were cancelled today. The roads were completely iced over and very dangerous. Everyone was urged to stay put.

As I cautiously made my way to Bob's, I found that the roads were indeed treacherous. I had to be very careful just walking across the street. As I nervously stepped inside, I saw my father. My first impression was that he looked like the gentle and loving man that I had always known as my daddy. I slowly came over and sat next to him on the couch. "Hi Daddy," I said.

"Hi Pootie," he responded. I smiled lovingly at him and he gently took my hand in his.

"How are you doing?" I asked, always amazed at how handsome he could look, even in the worst of times.

"Well, I've been better," he replied. "I'm just doing a lot of thinking."

"Do you remember what happened the other day?" I questioned. He slowly nodded his head yes.

"Daddy, I said some things to you that I shouldn't have. I am so sorry," I said. Tears filled my eyes as I looked at this precious man sitting next to me. I had honestly never seen him look as vulnerable as he did right now. "I didn't know how to handle the situation. I lost my temper and let my anger get the best of me." He squeezed my hand tightly. "Can you forgive me?"

"You don't need to apologize," he replied. "You were just defending your mother. I understand. That's exactly how I would want you to act if you thought your mother was in danger, even if it was from me." The intense pain from those last words tugged at my heart, no longer able to hold back my emotions. Dad lovingly handed me a tissue from the table. "Pootie, I said some things that I also regret. I'm sorry."

I wiped my eyes as best as I could. "I just wish that I had handled it differently," I said. "I don't know if that would have even been possible, but I wish I had tried harder." I paused a few seconds and looked inquisitively at him. "Do you remember everything that I said?"

He smiled at me. "Do you mean dropping the f-bomb?" he asked.

I laughed. "I guess you do remember," I said grinning. "Were you surprised?"

"Well, you were upset and you are my daughter," he responded. His smile and his heartfelt words helped to melt my tension. For this, I was truly grateful.

I sat there wondering how I would possibly approach my next question. "Daddy, do you remember how everything started?" I asked.

"Not really," he said. "I don't remember much of what happened before you came to the door." I tenderly laid my head on his shoulder knowing that the conversation was over. I was right. That had clearly not been my dad in the voicemail. He had absolutely no memory of the altercation.

For the first time in days, I felt a ray of hope and tremendous relief. My dad and I talked for the first time since the terrible fight. It was eating away at me. We both genuinely apologized to each other and had a very honest conversation. Before this incident, we were always so close. I wanted nothing more than to forever put this nightmare behind us.

My dad looked and sounded like he had hit rock bottom, the time away from home pure agony for him. He had a lot of time to reflect. I didn't think he completely understood or remembered what happened. The only thing that he wanted was to be given a second chance, the thought of losing his family absolutely tearing him apart. I tried to visualize things through his eyes. "Without my family, I'm nothing," he said. I truly believed that he meant those words from the bottom of his heart.

When I got back home, Mom anxiously wanted to know how the visit went. In some ways, I felt like I was watching two school age kids that had crushes on each other and couldn't stand to be apart. This situation was ripping my heart out. Here were two people that unconditionally loved each other so much. She was willing to hide her hell to protect the man she loved. He didn't want to live his life without her in it. I didn't know what to do, but I did know that the critical decision looming over our heads would be pivotal in their relationship. It had the potential to forever change the course of their lives.

Wednesday, January 12, 2011

As I gazed out my kitchen window, the roads were completely deserted, with absolutely no signs of life outside. It was day four of the ice storm and all schools in the area were still closed, our entire city shut down. We had definitely made the right decision in not allowing my dad to stay at home by himself.

When I visited him today, he was comfortably lying in Bob's bed. I slowly walked into the room and gently sat on the mattress beside him. His demeanor was very much like the previous time I had seen him, very calm and reflective. "Hey honey. How's your mother doing?" he asked.

"She's doing well, Dad," I replied. "She's eating well and actually looks better than she has in quite awhile."

"So what is going to happen?" he asked. I wanted more than anything to be able to give him the right answer, but unfortunately I still didn't know what that was.

"I don't know, Daddy," I said. "I just don't know yet."

"All I want is another chance," he pleaded. "I promise that it will never happen again. These past few days have been the most miserable days in my entire life. I know what's important to me and I don't want to lose it." I peered into his blue eyes and saw the genuineness of my father, wanting so much to believe him. I just wasn't sure if what we were dealing with was bigger than either of us knew. I definitely wasn't sure it was as easy to control as he thought. I hoped I was wrong. I later walked back home feeling completely torn.

After leaving the hospital on Friday, I had given Dad .5 mg. of Risperdal for three days. He had been off of it completely since Monday. I had previously read that one of the side effects of this drug was confusion. Prior to the heart surgery, I never saw any confusion. There was forgetfulness, which was normal at his age, but there was no confusion. I hoped that getting the Risperdal out of his system was the right move and that we'd soon notice some improvements.

The hospital also had him taking 50 mg. of Sertraline for depression. I had noticed awhile back that the prescription from his primary doctor had been increased a month prior to surgery to 100 mg. I accordingly increased his amount up to 75 mg. for a couple of days and then 100 mg. He had now been on the correct dosage since Sunday.

Physically, his heart was doing great. Mentally, he was really suffering. I think all of the drugs that he received while in the hospital had done extensive damage to him. He had undergone anesthesia three times in one month. In addition, they had given him morphine and other narcotics to control his severe pain and aggression. It seemed like every time he was administered drugs, a little less of him came back, never to be the same afterwards. We unfortunately lost a little bit more of him with each procedure. I wasn't sure if he would ever totally recover from them.

Both of my parents had freely expressed to me that they wanted to go home. I didn't want to inadvertently put my mother in harm's way. I knew that Dad wouldn't want anything to happen to her either. I had talked openly to him about getting a mental evaluation done and he had agreed to it, willing to do whatever it took to get his life back to normal.

I desperately wanted both of my parents to be comfortable and happy during their remaining time. At this point, we still didn't know what to do. I had turned it over to the Lord and would listen to my heart. I knew

He had the answer even if we couldn't see it.

Monday, August 13, 2001

I had somehow forgotten how chaotic school mornings could be. As I lovingly watched the boys scurrying to get ready, I was soon reminded of so many similar times in the past. Today was the first day of school, the boys so excited about seeing their friends again. Preston was in the 4th grade and Shawn was in the 2nd. This would be my second year staying at home with them. Never once had I regretted putting my career on hold.

The boys were considerably lucky to have spent all of their elementary years at the same school, K.E. Taylor Elementary. They had the routine down pat. As I slowly pulled up in front of the school, I casually looked their way. They apparently knew the drill as both of them leaned in and gently kissed me on the cheek. "Have a great first day, guys," I said. "I love you both."

I longingly watched them walk through the doors and realized that it never got any easier. The first day of school was always the hardest day of the year for me. After spending the entire summer with them, I hated that our special time together was ending.

Today was indeed an emotional day for many reasons. My parents were busily packing up their belongings at this very moment. The movers had been there since 7 a.m., loading two trucks. By this evening, all of their worldly belongings would be completely packed up.

I had been begging my parents to move to Atlanta for years. Actually, it began early in 1984 after we first moved here. About a year ago, they finally acquiesced and made the long-awaited decision to relocate. Two of their children, Bob and I, currently lived here along with our families, which included five grandchildren. They had eventually made the decision for the sole purpose of living near their loved ones.

I was absolutely beside myself. They had previously purchased a home in Buford on one of their visits. The next year was busily spent trying to sell their home in Pensacola and preparing for retirement. Dad had officially sold his business, John's Barber Shop. Mom had put in her early request to retire from NARDAC at the Navy Base. And now today, it was finally happening. It was a very exciting day indeed. By this time tomorrow, they would already be on the road to their new home and the next chapter in their lives.

At 11:30, I had lunch with my close friend, Donna, unanimously deciding to meet at our favorite Chinese restaurant. Not only was the food delicious, it was also cheap. After having eaten so many lunches there, we had become especially fond of one of the waiters. Whenever we ate there, we always looked for him to serve us. He would tease us relentlessly. No matter what mood we were in, he always managed to put a smile on our faces.

His big thing was to fill our doggy boxes with extra goodies. We never knew what he was ultimately going to add. It might have been an extra egg roll. Or it might have been an extra helping of our current lunch order, so that it would conveniently make another complete meal. Regardless, it was always a pleasant surprise when I would open the plastic container at home in the evening.

Later that day, I eagerly picked Preston and Shawn up from school. They both needed some additional items, so we stopped at the office supply store on the way home. It seemed that no matter how thorough I tried to be in getting them ready for school, something was inevitably missed.

We soon made it home and they headed straight to the kitchen cabinet for a snack. The best news was that no homework had been assigned for either of them. I knew this freedom probably wouldn't last the rest of the week, so we were going to thoroughly enjoy it today.

Not long after that, I heard the garage door opening. Randy was apparently home from work. I went to our bedroom and immediately noticed the light on the answering machine flashing. I heard an unfamiliar voice as I played the recorded message. She asked that we call my sister-in-law, Vicki, in New Orleans, as soon as possible. I grabbed a pen and a pad and carefully jotted the number down. I then dialed it about the same time that Randy came into the bedroom.

Instead of saying hello, an unfamiliar voice immediately said "Is this

Vanessa?" After I replied yes, she handed the phone to Vicki. I could never have prepared myself for what I heard next. Vicki reluctantly got on the phone and painfully spoke. "Vanessa, Curtis is dead!"

It took a few seconds for what she said to actually register. When it finally did, it hit me unbelievably hard. I felt like the room was spinning around me and I was frozen in that one spot. "Nooooooo! Nooooooo!" I carelessly let go of the phone and dropped to my knees. My heart had been pierced.

I could still hear her voice, small and muffled, as the phone lied on the floor. "Vanessa, is there someone with you right now?" she asked. Her voice had sounded strange, like it was hoarse from crying. Randy quickly picked the phone up and started talking. I could hear his voice, but nothing he said made sense. I sat on the floor crying uncontrollably, the hurtful sounds coming out louder and louder with every passing second. My beloved brother was gone, the pain inside killing me.

I remembered Preston and Shawn coming into the room and watching the painful situation unfold. As I needed to be by myself, I slowly made my way into the corner bedroom and sat in the rocking chair, the same rocking chair that I had spent so many joyous hours in with my children. I just cried and cried.

Sometime later, Randy came in and held me. I was having a hard time breathing. He tenderly caressed my back to comfort me. I just couldn't grasp what was happening. It was all too much for me to process at one time. And I absolutely couldn't stop crying, the intense pain excruciating.

"Someone needs to call my parents," I uttered. I couldn't think of anything in the world that could be harder than having to tell a mother and father that their child was dead. I couldn't do it. I despondently looked at Randy. "Can you call them?"

A couple of minutes later, I heard Randy on the phone. "Shirley, this is Randy," he said. His voice sounded so gentle as he broke the heart wrenching news to them about their firstborn son. "Something bad has happened. It's Curtis. He passed away today."

I couldn't begin to imagine the anguish that my parents were feeling in their home at that very moment. Not only could I not talk to them, but I couldn't hold them or mourn with them either. We had lost one of our precious family members and we were all far apart, separated by so many miles.

It soon dawned on me that we also needed to contact my younger brother, Bob. His best friend's father had recently passed away and Bob was currently on his way back from the funeral. Randy fortunately got a message to him to stop by on his way in before he went home. The last thing he wanted to do was to have to tell him the crushing news over the phone and for Bob to have to drive after that.

Hours later, I was despairingly lying on my bed. I don't remember if we had eaten dinner or not. Randy was my rock and he had lovingly taken over for me. I was crying silently for my precious brother, Curtis. Bob sadly walked in and I sat up. He immediately came to my side and we hugged each other tightly. No one else in the world could have possibly understood my agony in that moment or shared it with me like Bob. It was specifically reserved for a brother and a sister who would never see their older brother again. The rest of the world ceased to exist at that point in time. We didn't say anything. The deep pain we were sharing inside needed no words.

I went to bed that night completely in shock. I still couldn't believe it. Curtis was only 42 years old. He hadn't been sick. In fact, he had just gone on vacation the week before with his family. Everything was good. He had gone to sleep the night before like normal. Then at around 1 p.m., his youngest son, Trevor, had surprisingly noticed that his work van was still outside. He went into his bedroom and found Curtis still in the bed, unable to awaken him. It was too late. He had already passed away in his sleep. The look on his face was one of incredible peacefulness.

I began to cry once again. Randy rolled over and gently held me. "I just can't believe he's gone," I said. "I'll never ever be able to spend time with him again. I'll never get to tell him how much I love him, or how much I've always loved him. I didn't even get a chance to say goodbye." With that, I closed my weary eyes, the pain reaching into depths unknown inside of me. I never knew a person could hurt so much. What began as one of the best days in my life had turned into the worst. At some point in the middle of the night, I finally fell asleep.

Tuesday, August 14, 2001

I was in a stupor as I carefully dialed the number, Mom solemnly answering on the third ring. They were about to get on the road. Dad would be driving the U-Haul to Atlanta and Mom would be following him in one of their cars. They had previously brought their other vehicles up months earlier. The movers had already left in their large truck. "How are you doing, Mom?" I asked.

"I'm numb," she replied. "Neither one of us slept that well. I'm trying not to think about it too much and just do what I have to do. We have a long trip ahead of us today and I won't make it if I don't stay strong."

I wasn't so sure she'd be able to put her feelings on hold so easily. For her sake, I definitely hoped I was wrong. "Please be careful," I said. "If it gets to be too much, just pull over and take a break. Don't push yourselves." I paused to give her a chance to speak, but she remained silent. "We'll be waiting for you. Call us if you need anything. I love you and Daddy."

I had tried so hard to be strong for them, but as soon as I laid the phone down, my strong composure broke and the tears once again began to fall. As hard as this was for me, it was nothing compared to the living hell that they must be going through. I then slowly bowed my head and prayed that God would comfort them and give them the necessary strength to get them to Atlanta safely. I couldn't begin to fully comprehend the agony and sorrow that they were feeling while still having to put on a brave face and make the long drive to their new home. They would each be alone all day in their respective vehicles, alone with their endless thoughts and their pain.

I'll never know how they managed to drive for more than six hours feeling such heartache, but they miraculously did. I truly believed that to lose a child was the worst pain that anyone could ever endure. I knew that my parents were strong, but what I saw today was clearly on a different scale. I witnessed the most incredible fortitude in my parents that I had ever seen. It was a strength that I had never known existed. I felt moved beyond words and so unbelievably proud of them both. I could only hope that faced with the same adversity, I would manage as well.

Later that afternoon, I talked to Vicki on the phone, explaining the current situation with my parents. The timing of everything couldn't have been worse. It was unfortunately too late to change their moving plans. Everything had already been put into motion.

At that very moment, my parents were on the road. We expected them in a few hours. We would plan on unpacking everything tomorrow. Hopefully, they'd be able to find appropriate clothes to wear. I knew that it was a lot to ask, but we desperately needed the funeral to be delayed, if at all possible.

Thursday, August 16, 2001

As the garage door slowly came down, I closed my eyes and performed one last mental check. The decision was made for everyone to meet at my parents' new home in Buford at 7 a.m. We would drive two cars, our truck and one of my parents' cars. Bob would ride with my parents and Preston and Shawn would ride with us.

Before long, we reluctantly set off on our six hour drive to New Orleans. An hour into the trip, we decided to stop for breakfast. We needed to eat before continuing on. While we waited on our food, the boys joked with their Grandpa. Even though the circumstances of their first time spent together after the move was not what I had envisioned, it was still good to see them laugh. That would be our only major stop on our drive. It would inevitably be a long day.

Many hours later, we began to hit the outskirts of New Orleans. The prevailing feeling was one of incredible sadness. I had previously been to this city several times, every one of them to see Curtis. This would forever be his city. Now, it felt completely different. It was so difficult to drive through it knowing I would never see him here again. I would never experience it the same way, with my brother. I slowly leaned my head against the window and once again, began to cry. I wanted so much for this hurt to subside.

After checking into our motel, we drove to Curtis and Vicki's home. All of the past memories that I held of Curtis and this dwelling came flooding back. Vicki was holding up as well as could be expected. While everyone else was busy talking, I freely made my way into the kitchen. I then moved into the bar area and the family room. As I sorrowfully looked around, I saw Curtis everywhere.

Not long afterwards, we left for the funeral home. Before the viewing officially began, I had a unique chance to see my brother for the first time. As he lied in front of me, I carefully examined every inch of his face. I struggled to remember the last time we had seen each other. None of this seemed real to me. I knew this was my brother, but it wasn't an image that I could readily accept. A part of me expected him to open his eyes at any moment and say "Hey Pootie", but he never did.

Once the viewing started, Vicki faithfully stood next to Curtis, occasionally rubbing his forehead. Her devotion was as strong in death as it had been in life. They had been happily married for 21 years and had two beautiful children together. They were the love of each other's lives.

Mom, Dad, Bob and I all stood next to Vicki. People soon began to come in to pay their last respects. Before I knew it, a long line had formed. Most of the people that I met that night were strangers to me, but they all shared one thing in common. Curtis had touched them deeply in some special way. They each had a different and equally powerful story. I was getting a glimpse into the incredible life of my brother that I had not been a part of.

As exhausted as I was, I somehow got strength from all of the people standing selflessly before me. An hour into the viewing, the extensive line had now begun to stretch out the front door. Traffic in front of the funeral home had rapidly become an issue. Eventually, they enlisted the help of a policeman to direct traffic out front. I had never in my life seen anything like it. They also had to bring out a second signature book after the first one astonishingly filled up.

There seemed to be no end to the wonderful people and special memories that they were giving to me and my family, lasting for hours. As incredibly proud as I had always been of Curtis while he was living, it was here in his death that I was most impressed. I had been moved to tears. Most people lived their entire lives without ever affecting this many people. In his short life of 42 years, he had not only deeply touched these people; he had forever changed their lives. They couldn't praise him enough. How many people could say that?

A couple of hours into the visitation, I noticed that Dad was exhaustingly sitting on a bench in the foyer. Preston and Shawn were seated next to him. He was no doubt living through the worst time of his life and it had taken a serious toll on him. He then looked up and saw me. I slowly smiled at my dad, hoping he would feel my love for him. He smiled back.

I learned the most valuable lesson of my life tonight. Life was truly short and it came with no guarantees. One day when you least expected it, it could be taken from you in an instant. You should never live it expecting a tomorrow because it may not come. Live every day as if it was your last. Just as was the case with my brother, it might be.

I wished that I had taken the time to visit Curtis more, to call him on the phone more. I wished that I had made it to one of his spectacular fireworks displays. I would always regret not having seen one. Most of all, I wished I had told him that I loved him more.

Friday, August 17, 2001

I stood back against the wall as I prepared for what was about to happen. This morning would be the last viewing of Curtis before his eulogy. Seeing his beautiful face for the last time was not something I could have ever anticipated. I watched as Preston and Shawn stood next to the casket to say their goodbyes, watching him so intently. I was thankful that despite the many miles between us, my children were blessed to have spent time with Curtis and gotten to know him in the past. Through different visits, we had spent time at Stone Mountain Park and Six Flags, to name a couple of places. I was so grateful for those special memories.

We had also gone to Dave & Buster's during one of their visits. On this particular night, one memory will forever stand out. Preston was eight years old. He was excited about a game located against the back wall called The Strongman Game. Preston was diligently trying to collect enough tickets to get a prize. He approached Curtis and earnestly asked him if he would play a game for him. Of course, Curtis obliged. I watched Preston lead Curtis over to the particular game, his eyes lighting up when he saw what game it was. Preston wanted his uncle to use his muscles to win him some tickets. How perfect was that? Curtis nonchalantly played it off. I think inside though, he was on cloud nine. He took the mallet and vigorously hit the puck three different times. Every time, he hit it with such force that the puck rose high enough to easily hit the bell. He inevitably won the most tickets possible. Preston had no idea, but I think he had made Curtis' day. It gave me the sweetest, most precious memory of my older brother and oldest son together. I would always hold it near and dear to my heart.

As the visitation neared its end, it was eventually my turn. Knowing that this would be the very last time I would ever see Curtis' face here on Earth was almost too much to bear. I sadly began to cry, feeling the intensity from deep within. I could soon feel my legs start to buckle. Randy could feel it, too. He firmly held me up and we slowly made our way over to Curtis. I bent down and gently kissed his cheek. I truly hoped he was looking down on us at that very moment and knew how much we all dearly loved him. Our lives would never be the same without him.

Several people compassionately spoke at his service, the words heartfelt and touching. As I quietly sat and listened to such powerful testimonies, I couldn't shake the underlying question that I had asked for days now. Why? Why did you choose to take him from us, God? I had always known that Curtis was a good person with an incredible heart, but until last night, I hadn't known the half of it. He dedicated his life to generously helping others. This world that we lived in was such a better place with him in it. Why then? Why did you take him from us when he was doing such good work here?

And then it hit me. Maybe I had been looking at it all wrong. Maybe it was because of all the good things he had done for others. Perhaps the selfless way he lived his life was the reason you brought him home when you did, God. I had no doubt that Heaven was a much better place with him in it.

As the last person to speak took his seat, the song "Wind Beneath My

Wings" by Bette Midler began playing, so appropriately. I thought about the incredible difference that Curtis had made in so many lives as was evident by last night's showing. He truly was a hero to so many.

Soon afterwards, a limousine pulled up outside. Vicki, Chad and Trevor got inside, with my parents following them. Bob and I then squeezed into the last two seats. We would all fittingly ride together to the cemetery with everyone else following. As we made the final drive to the mausoleum, I slowly glanced at all of their precious faces. Surrounding me were the people that Curtis loved the most. He had no doubt touched the people in this car the deepest.

Arriving a short time later, we made our way inside the somber building, with the casket soon following. It was then placed in the appropriate opening in the wall. One by one, people walked up and dropped a single flower on top of it. I soon did the same. In some ways, I felt removed from the scene, like I was participating but it really wasn't happening to me. I was going through the motions, but emotionally, I felt drained and empty.

As we drove away from his final resting place, I felt an incredible emptiness inside. Today, we said goodbye to Curtis. Tomorrow, we would make the long trip back home and somehow try to put the pieces of our lives back together. How were we ever going to fill this void that Curtis had left? Inside, I knew the dreaded answer. We couldn't. It would forever remain devoid.

Thursday, January 13, 2011

My home felt like one of complete desolation, easily portraying the setting for a scary mystery. The roads were still icy and the schools had now been closed for four days straight. Everybody was starting to get cabin fever. Shawn had desperately wanted to get out and run for days. He'd be having track tryouts soon and really needed the practice. We were all hoping that we'd actually be able to get out tomorrow.

Today was Curtis' birthday. He would have been 52 years old. The last ten years had been so difficult without him. He left a considerable void that had never been filled. Not a day had gone by that I hadn't thought about him in some way. I missed him terribly. Mostly, I missed knowing that if I needed to talk to him, he was only a phone call away.

Faced with our current dilemma, I repeatedly asked myself what Curtis would have done. I wished so much that I could turn to him now. The only saving grace was that he didn't have to live through this hardship and watch what was happening to his parents.

I had constantly thought about the current situation for almost a week now. I had discussed it at length with Bob and Randy. Mom and I had also talked about it every day. Our family had gone through so much already. The last thing I wanted to do was break them up any further.

I had had several heart-to-heart conversations with my dad. He had spent the entire week experiencing what life without his family would ultimately feel like. Sometimes you had to hit rock bottom in order to pull yourself back up. I truly believed that nothing was more important to him than getting his life back. And I believed in my dad. He desperately wanted a second chance and Mom was willing to give it to her. She missed Dad so much and he missed her as well.

Assuming that the ice cleared up tomorrow, Mom and Dad would be returning home together. I would make every effort to ensure that the critical plans to get my dad tested were carried out. We would all have to vigilantly keep our eyes open from now on, denial no longer an option. I prayed that we had made the right decision.

Friday, January 14, 2011

The feeling of freedom was palpable in the air. The sun was out in full force and the roads were once again alive with cars, as a lot of the ice had already melted. Coming and going as we pleased was a luxury we hadn't experienced in days. The boys had been out of school and Randy had worked from home the entire week. We were finally able to get out of the house and it felt wonderful. We made a quick run to the grocery store to get some milk and orange juice for my parents. I wanted their homecoming to be perfect.

Randy and I were originally planning on driving Mom and Dad home sometime after lunch. We still had several things to get done before then. That morning, I got an unexpected phone call from Monica. Dad was very restless and was pacing. She was diligently trying to work from home, but was having a difficult time with all of Dad's interruptions. Bob had already gone back to work, so I had her put Dad on the phone in hopes of calming him down.

An hour later, we relented to go ahead and drive my parents' home. Dad had unfortunately remained anxious despite my phone call. I was brutally honest with both of my parents. My dad knew that if another violent outburst occurred, he would have to come live with us. I had urged my mom to be completely honest about the behavior from now on. The crucial decision for her to return was contingent on that promise. I felt like I was on pins and needles. This was where faith ultimately came into play.

The drive over went very smoothly. We didn't run into any icy patches. As we slowly pulled into the driveway, I noticed that it was completely covered in ice. We had to be very careful getting my parents inside as all of the walkways were dangerous. Even the few stairs leading up to the front door were covered. While I got them settled inside, Randy helpfully cleared the walkways, at least the areas that they might hit going to the mailbox.

I packaged my parents' evening meds in small containers and labeled them. Meanwhile, Randy went through the entire house and made sure that no pipes had accidentally burst. He also made sure the basement was secure. Both thermostats were adjusted and within five minutes, the house was once again comfortable.

Once everything was in order, we reluctantly decided it was time to leave my parents alone. I lovingly kissed them both goodbye, but refrained from saying the obvious. Instead, I said "I love you" as I looked both of them square in the eyes. Everything else had already been said at this point.

Later that day, I made a vital appointment with Dad's primary physician for the 25th of this month. I wanted to get the testing underway. This would undoubtedly be the first step of many.

After dinner, I nervously called my parents. I knew that I had to eventually let them be and not check on them constantly. This time, however, was necessary. Mom answered the phone, sounding completely at ease. I could clearly hear the television on in the background as they were apparently watching it together. "Everything is going fine, Vanessa," she said. "Don't worry." This was definitely music to my ears. I then let out a deep sigh, hoping to sleep better tonight than I had all week.

Saturday, January 15, 2011

Chris quickly climbed into the backseat after running back into the house to grab his jacket, his warm-nature always amazing me. If it was left up to him, I had no doubt he'd be in shorts today. The three of us soon loaded up into the truck and drove to my parents' home early this morning. I had felt extremely nervous ever since we had dropped them off yesterday.

As we leisurely sat in the family room, everything seemed to be going fine, both of my parents in good spirits. I soon gave them their morning meds and checked my dad's blood sugar. I really wanted to get them back to the routine we had followed before the storm had hit.

I looked over at Dad and noticed the gray stubble on his face. He had casually mentioned yesterday that he was beginning to feel very unkempt, so Randy had planned on giving him a shave first thing. He had Dad carefully sit on a stool in the kitchen. His expression gave nothing away, but I knew inside, he was beaming.

When Randy finished, he set the electric razor on the kitchen counter. Dad appreciatively smiled at him. "Thank you, Ran," he said. "You always do a good job." Dad hadn't yet seen the actual results, but it didn't matter. He had complete faith in Randy. The shave had indeed done wonders. Not only did Dad look great afterwards, but it had put him in such a good mood.

After lunch, Mom compiled a small list of items that they needed. We decided to take Dad's truck to the store as it hadn't been run in over a week. It was currently parked in the driveway outside the basement door, the area still very icy. I cautiously looked down and watched Randy from the deck as he tried to back it out. The icy cement was very slippery and caused the tires to spin repeatedly. He eventually had to steer the truck onto the grass in order to get traction and back it out. I was thankful that Dad had not attempted the same maneuver.

Upon later returning to the truck in the Walmart parking lot, we happened to look at the license plate and noticed that the registration sticker was missing. It must have accidentally fallen off at some point. We were lucky that no one had been pulled over.

Once we got back to the house, we checked the license plate on Mom's car. Her registration sticker was actually there, but it had expired. The renewal date was December 2nd, which was over a month past due.

I carefully searched Dad's desk for the vehicle registration bills that should have come months ago, unable to find the light blue envelopes anywhere. I decided to take my chances and go to the tax office in person to explain the situation. Luckily, the office was open all day on Saturday. I had Mom get her checkbook and brought her with me. The Pacifica needed an emissions test, but we were able to go ahead and pay the ad valorem taxes on the truck. We unfortunately had to also pay a late penalty.

Once we got back, Randy and Mom took her car to get the emissions tested, stopping by the tag office afterwards and successfully paying the taxes and fine on it. They would now be set for another year.

As soon as they returned, Randy attempted to put the new decals on the vehicles. He surprisingly found that the previous sticker on the Pacifica wouldn't come off. In addition, glue residue was visible on the truck's license plate where the sticker should have been. When Dad had put them on the previous year, he had gotten confused. Instead of peeling the sticker off the white backing, he had mistakenly glued both of them on the license plate together. Now, they were securely stuck.

It took Randy an hour to clean the glue off and remove the old decal, eventually coming off in pieces. The adhesive that was used was very strong. They had probably been affixed using super glue.

Dad had routinely placed these decals on his vehicles his entire adult life. For some reason, he had forgotten how to do it in December. This confusion would actually have occurred over a year ago. Randy had called me outside to tell me what he'd found. We just stared at each other. Was this what getting old was all about or was my dad dealing with much more? We were finding out that Dad was forgetting a lot more than we realized, and it had been going on for quite some time.

As we drove home, the concerned feeling over what we had uncovered increased. It seemed that every time we turned around, we were finding something else that my parents could no longer manage on their own. We certainly didn't mind the work. They had always been there for us and now it was our turn to reciprocate. I was more concerned over the severity of what we would find next. The penalty for today's mishap was a simple monetary fine. Would the next incident be as minor? Would we catch it in time or as similar to what happened today, would we find out after the fact that something critical had been missed? We would have to be very vigilant from now on.

Monday, January 17, 2011

As I pulled into the crowded parking lot at the elementary school, I looked over at Chris. "Are you sure school isn't cancelled today, Mom?" he asked, clearly grasping at straws.

I laughed at his comment. "Nice try," I replied. "Yes, school is open today." Chris would have been thrilled with another day off. I gently kissed him on the cheek. "I'll pick you up this afternoon, sweetie." He waved to me as he slowly made his way into the building. I had to admit that I would definitely miss him today. I had easily gotten accustomed to being with him every day since his school had closed for the storm.

After dropping Chris off, I quickly headed over to my parents' home. I wanted to be able to get all of our morning routine out of the way and have some time for Dad to relax a little before his appointment at 11:00.

At 10:30, I drove Dad to the cardiologist office. The doctor from his last hospital visit had informed me that he needed to be scheduled for a CHEM-7 blood test which would be used to check Dad's metabolism. The visit today was simply to have his blood drawn. I also made a follow-up appointment in two weeks to talk about the results. It would be at that meeting that I would discuss Dad's behavior and additional testing.

While sitting on the couch later that afternoon, the phone rang. I watched Mom as she answered it. Based on her side of the conversation, it apparently had something to do with the blind study that she was involved in. She politely informed the person that her daughter had taken her off of the pills and that she actually hadn't taken them in a couple of weeks. I had a sinking feeling that the news was not going over well, Mom's expression visibly indicating the conversation was turning unpleasant. I then mouthed the words "Do you want me to talk to them?"

She gratefully handed me the phone, looking very relieved. "Hi, this is Shirley Lee's daughter," I said. "My name is Vanessa Luther."

The woman on the other end was clearly upset, wasting no time with greetings. "Mrs. Lee was part of a study that had been going on for awhile," she informed me. "She can't just stop taking the pills midway through the test. It would invalidate everything we've done so far."

"My mother was not doing well," I stated. "Her health was in serious condition. I had no idea what the pills were that she was taking and I was told that no one would release that information to me. I had no choice but to have her stop taking them."

"Your mother signed up for this study on her own," she said. "She was evaluated and determined to be a good candidate." I didn't seem to be getting through to this person.

"My mother is 76 years old," I replied. "She already takes several different medications. She was in no position to be a part of this study. I'm sorry, but I had to make a judgment call and do what was best for her."

"We should have been notified," she said. I took a deep breath. This woman was not letting up and I was starting to lose my patience.

"Well, I would have, but I had no idea who was running the study," I responded. I could hear my voice rising as Mom stared at me. "Nothing on the blister packs identified who was conducting it. Everything was very secretive. Mom couldn't even remember who it was with. I had no way to get in touch with you." This woman's persistence had now pushed me over the edge. Not once had she expressed the slightest interest in my mother's health. Her only concern was the damn study.

"Well, you'll need to bring all of the remaining pills back to us," she said curtly. "Your mother will have to sign some papers formally withdrawing her from this study."

Before she hung up the phone, I managed to find out who this woman worked for and got directions to their office. The conversation had ended very abruptly. She was clearly upset, but it was no excuse to be so rude. Her impolite response hadn't changed my position in the least. My mother had needed an advocate and I had done what I thought was best at the time. I still stood by my decision.

Tuesday, January 18, 2011

As I determinedly walked through my parents' home this morning, my mission was clear cut, find every single blind study pill in the house. The number of blister packs that I actually collected had surprised me, seemingly everywhere. I still had yet to find out what they were, but I wanted them gone.

My mother specifically wanted to return them to the office on her own. I had her explicitly tell me the roads she was planning on driving to get there. It ended up being the same route that I would have taken. She seemed to be back to her normal self, so I had no problem with it. I really didn't feel like having a run-in with the woman I spoke to yesterday.

Mom briefly came into the family room and kissed us goodbye. As she was walking into the garage, I said "Don't forget to turn your phone on. I need to be able to get in touch with you if there is an emergency." With that, she promptly left.

I then made Dad breakfast. The sun was out and the shades were wide open. It was a beautiful day. The outside temperature was low, but from inside the house, it was perfect.

After breakfast, Dad and I relaxed in the family room with our coffee. He asked how the boys were doing and I told him all of the latest news. It was so nice to just sit around casually and talk freely with my dad.

Before long, he nervously looked at me and smiled. I could read that look so well. I knew exactly what he was thinking. "When do you think your mother will get back?" he asked.

"It'll take a little while, Dad," I responded. "It is an hour round trip from here. She'll probably be getting back in about half an hour. Don't worry. It's a straight shot. She'll be fine." I was truly not worried and tried to convince Dad of the same.

I then turned the television on to keep him calm, knowing that any distraction would help. I soon found an older rerun of *Law & Order*, a show that would normally have piqued his interest. In no time at all, he was giving me that look again. I was really not concerned about Mom. I also hesitated to call her because I wanted her to focus on her driving and not on answering her cell phone. I knew, however, that it would go a long way in calming Dad, so I quickly dialed her cell phone. Immediately, I got the standard message indicating that the phone was not currently on. Now, I was equally concerned, too.

Mom had a bad habit of not turning her cell phone on. She always had it with her and frequently called me from it when she was out. It was usually from a store that was having a sale, wanting to know if I was interested in an item. Occasionally, she would call me from a doctor's office. After she was done talking on it, she would immediately turn it off again. Sometimes I would call her right back after having just talked with her and couldn't reach her. It was so frustrating.

I had repeatedly explained to her that the phone had a dual purpose. It wasn't just for her to use. I also needed to be able to get in touch with her. As often happened, Mom would be out running errands. Hours later, Dad would call me because he was worried. I'd try to call Mom so I could let him know where she was and invariably her phone would be turned off. These situations could easily have been avoided, but they never were.

Not long afterwards, I gladly heard the garage door open. I then looked at Dad. "See," I said. "I told you she'd make it back fine." Inside, I felt very relieved. I would definitely have to talk to her about turning her phone off, just not in front of my dad.

As Mom walked into the kitchen, I asked her "So, how did it go?"

"It went fine," she replied. "I gave her the bag of pills and signed the forms. It was fairly straightforward."

"How was the woman?" I asked, trying to hide my smile.

"Actually, she was fine," Mom said. "She seemed to have calmed down quite a bit since yesterday. I think you got to her." We both laughed.

After lunch, Mark came by for a physical therapy session. It would be the first one since the ice storm. Dad had surprisingly not complained to me about his abdomen in over a week. I hoped that with the additional rest he got the previous week, his injury had healed.

Mark ended up staying for the full hour, although it seemed as though half of it was spent talking. His wife was anxiously expecting their second child and he was so excited. Dad really enjoyed his company and Mark seemed to feel the same. I considered it great therapy for Dad for many reasons.

Friday, January 21, 2011

My heart skipped a beat as I heard the eerie ringtone that I had set up for my parents, the sound of it actually very appropriate. It was to the point now that whenever I heard the scary tone, I'd get a pit in the bottom of my stomach, usually signifying that something was wrong. This morning, Mom called to find out when I would be arriving at their house. Dad was already dressed and waiting for today's doctor appointment and it wasn't for hours.

Earlier in the week, I had made the unfortunate mistake of telling my dad about the upcoming visit. Every day since, he had persistently asked me about it. His concept of time seemed to be a little off which caused him to get very anxious.

When I arrived at my parents' home, Dad was indeed ready. I realized at that moment that I definitely had to change the method I used for letting my dad know about future appointments. From now on, I would tell him about it the actual day of the visit. I'd make sure I got to his house early enough for him to get ready. Telling him ahead of time only seemed to create unnecessary tension.

After lunch, I drove Dad to his appointment with his endocrinologist, Dr. Jorge Martinez. This particular doctor monitored Dad's diabetes and cholesterol. Some scheduling issues had unexpectedly arisen with the doctor and after waiting for a short while, the physician assistant came into the room. I was fine with seeing her as I really didn't think it was a good idea to keep Dad waiting too long.

We carefully went through his current medications and I gave her the new additions. I also told her about his heart surgery the previous month. She then checked his blood sugar, in addition to his blood pressure. Everything looked good.

She politely asked Dad how he was doing and he mentioned to her that he was having a pain in his lower abdomen. She then had him lie back on the table to examine him. The offending area that Dad pointed to was tender to the touch. Her professional opinion was that he had a floating hernia. The assistant instructed me to give Dad ibuprofen to help with the pain. If it got any worse, he might actually need an operation. We really needed to address it with his regular doctor.

While Dad was lying on the table, the assistant wanted to look at his feet. She gently took his shoes and socks off and began to poke different points on each of Dad's soles to make sure that he could feel them. One of the serious risks for a diabetic was that of nerve damage which, in turn, could cause a person to be unable to feel their feet. That unfortunately opened up the door to dangerous sores or ulcers developing without the person knowing it. They could get infected and become very risky. In addition, with poor blood circulation, any sores or infections that were present might not heal properly. Since the feet could be especially hard for an elderly person to reach, the P.A. felt it was a good practice to have them regularly checked at each appointment. I was extremely impressed with her.

Dad's feet ended up having several rough calluses on them and were in dire need of a trim. She recommended making Dad an appointment with a foot specialist. I'd definitely find one as soon as we got home.

The assistant then routinely asked me several questions about Dad's blood sugar readings. How often did I take it? What was the average reading? She then gave me a blank form and asked that I record all of his readings for the next month.

The appointment had gone very well. None of Dad's prescriptions from this doctor were changed. He simply got new refills. It was added proof that Dad was becoming more stable every day.

Sunday, January 23, 2011

Chris and I were sitting at the bar in the kitchen, busily doing homework, when I received the disturbing phone call. Mom quickly informed me that the paramedics were currently at their home and were getting ready to take Dad to the emergency room. Earlier, he was having intense pains in his lower abdomen and asked Mom to call 911.

They had carefully loaded Dad on the stretcher and he was now in the back of the emergency vehicle. Mom would ride to the hospital in the front with the driver. I told her I would leave immediately to meet them at the ER.

Randy had heard me while I spoke on the phone and knew that something was definitely wrong. I soon relayed the alarming news. Then, I lovingly kissed my family good night. I probably wouldn't see them again until the next morning.

On the drive to the hospital, I hurriedly called Bob to let him know about Dad. It seemed pointless for him to come to the hospital, too. I promised to keep him apprised of Dad's condition.

Not long after that, I arrived at the ER, soon to be taken back to Dad's room. "Hey Daddy," I said, as I gently kissed him on the cheek. He seemed very relaxed. "How are you feeling?"

"Those pains that I was having came back earlier at the house," he replied. Dad actually hadn't mentioned the pain since Friday at the doctor's office. It unpredictably seemed to come and go. He might complain about it one day and then not bring it up again until several days later. I had truly hoped that the problem had gone away for good. "Right now, I'm feeling okay. It's not hurting anymore."

According to Mom, the pain had suddenly stopped not long after getting to the hospital. It seemed that whenever Dad was lying down, the pain would eventually subside. A part of me wondered if the reason we were here had more to do with the anxiety of not knowing than the actual pain it was causing. The ER always seemed to calm Dad down, as long as the visit was short. Maybe he just needed the reassurance from the doctor.

Dad was already dressed in a hospital gown and calmly lying in the bed. I had him lift the blue gown up and show me exactly where the pain was. The spot he pointed to was on the right side. It felt like a small lump and was a little pink. "Does it hurt when I apply pressure?" I asked while lightly pushing down on the area.

"Not too much, Pootie," he answered. Before long, an orderly came in and swiftly wheeled Dad away. The doctor on duty had ordered an ultrasound, which would take about fifteen minutes.

About an hour later, the physician came in to examine Dad. According to the ultrasound results, Dad clearly had two inguinal hernias, one on each side. He had probably had them since birth. The doctor firmly applied pressure to the spot on the right and was actually able to push the bulge back through the abdominal lining. He then mentioned that we could do the same thing at home.

I curiously asked the doctor what would cause the lump to break through the lining in the first place. He told me the most common reason was lifting a heavy object.

The doctor felt that the hernias were fine at this point and that emergency surgery wasn't necessary. If they got worse, we would definitely need to contact a specialist. He then supplied us with the names of two doctors.

Dad was eventually discharged at 12:15 a.m. I managed to get them home by 1. We were all extremely exhausted. I got them safely settled inside and then headed home myself.

I thought about what the doctor had said regarding the heavy lifting. I had previously suspected that the injury was from Dad moving the riding lawn mower. It was very likely that I was right. Only time would tell whether the pain would completely subside or not. I truly hoped that another surgical procedure was not in my dad's future.

Monday, January 24, 2011

Sometimes the familiar drive to my parents' home seemed almost non-existent. I was deep in thought today as I travelled the customary roads. I couldn't remember how many red lights I had to stop at or how many cars were on the road. It seemed that no sooner had I pulled out of my driveway than I saw the red brick of their house. As I casually walked inside, Dad smiled at me, seemingly doing much better this morning. Hearing firsthand from the doctor last night that everything was okay had carried a lot of weight. He didn't seem quite so anxious about the hernias today.

After breakfast, I asked Dad if he wanted to sit outside for a little bit. "I would love that, Pootie," he said. I then moved his plastic chair outside on the front stoop. I cautiously stood by him for a minute and then left him to enjoy the sunshine.

As Dad was peacefully sitting out front, I began straightening up the family room. I soon ran across the crossword puzzle book that I had bought Dad when he first came home from the heart surgery. I curiously opened it up and saw that only one word was filled in on the first puzzle. I then flipped through the other pages and all of the remaining puzzles were blank. There was a time when he would have easily completed all of the puzzles by now. Dad was a true crossword aficionado.

He also loved to read anything by Louis L'Amour or Lewis Grizzard. Dad didn't seem to have any interest in reading anymore, not even the daily newspaper. I had bought Dad a copy of *The Purpose Driven Life* awhile back, thinking that he would really enjoy it. It remained unread on top of his dresser. Unfortunately, I couldn't remember the last time I saw him pick up something to read.

He did still watch television. His favorites were anything with Clint Eastwood, *Gunsmoke* and *Law & Order*. He used to watch them for hours. Now, he usually fell asleep during the middle of a program. They just couldn't seem to hold his attention for the entire show anymore.

I had solemnly accepted that this was the way things were now. I didn't know if it was just part of the normal aging process or not. I truly hoped that as Dad got stronger, he eventually would be able to return to doing some of the things he loved the most. Only time would tell. I understood that as people got older, things sometimes changed. This might very well be my new dad.

After about ten minutes, Dad decided to come back inside. I fixed him a glass of iced tea as he sat in his recliner. "So, what are you going to do later?" he asked.

"I'm going to pick Chris up at 3," I replied. "Shawn has tryouts after school for the Track & Field team. This will be his second year. I'm not too worried though. I know he'll do great." Shawn was a very determined person. I had absolutely no doubt that he would make the team.

"Oh, I agree with you on that," Dad said. I knew that he truly felt the same way.

I suddenly remembered a time at the end of Shawn's 8th grade school year when Dad was especially proud of him. An award ceremony had been held at Creekland Middle School. As it was nearing the end of the presentation, a few awards still had yet to be handed out. The first was for perfect attendance for all three years of middle school, with only one student actually accomplishing this. As one of the teachers called Shawn's name out and respectfully handed him his trophy, the audience began clapping, a few of them even whistling. It was a tremendous accomplishment. As the joyous applause started to wane, Shawn took a few steps off of the platform to return to his seat. The announcer suddenly said "Shawn, hold up a minute. Can you come back up on the stage?"

Shawn slowly turned around and stepped back up on the platform as the teacher eagerly continued. "Shawn has also managed to get straight A's for his entire time here at Creekland." He then handed Shawn his second trophy. With that, everyone in the audience stood up and again started clapping and whistling for him, the entire faculty on stage standing as well. Not a single person in the whole room was seated. As I lovingly watched him on stage looking so humble, I had never been so proud of him. Tears filled my eyes. This was his special moment and he deserved every bit of it.

Dad smiled at Shawn. "You did great, Shawnee," said Dad. I had no doubt that he was just as proud as I was.

After lunch, I heard a startling knock at the front door. Dad had another physical therapy session scheduled. It was unfortunately too late to cancel it after last night. I hoped that Dad would be able to get some exercise in anyway.

The unfamiliar gentleman introduced himself as Mark's replacement for the week. Mark's wife was actually in labor at that very moment. They were having a baby.

I explained that Dad had a hernia that was causing him some pain. The therapist decided to concentrate more on the walking. He carefully took Dad's vitals and then, they headed outside. I watched as they slowly walked along the street in front of the house. It was the farthest that Dad had walked since the surgery.

The session had only lasted about thirty minutes. Afterwards, the new therapist shook Dad's hand. "Have a great day, Mr. Lee," he said. I didn't think that anyone could measure up to Mark, but this guy was right up there with him. Dad was batting two for two with physical therapists.

Tuesday, January 25, 2011

A couple of days ago, we were happily eating lunch together, having a casual conversation. It was something we did almost every day. Out of the blue, he had asked me a question about his hernias. I hadn't thought twice about answering him honestly, mentioning that we would be seeing Dr. Linske in a couple of days. In an effort to calm him down, I had brought the appointment up, but it had backfired on me. Dad had been extremely anxious about it ever since. Sometimes, it was a no-win situation.

At about 10:00, I drove Dad to his appointment. Dr. Marcus Linske was Dad's primary physician and had been for years, his main office conveniently only a few miles away. We ended up arriving early, but it worked out though, since I had lots of necessary paperwork to fill out. Before I had finished, we were called back to an exam room.

In no time, Dr. Linske came in. I introduced myself as he promptly sat down, wasting no time in getting down to business. I informed him of Dad's recent heart surgery. He then asked me about his current medications and I carefully went over the list with him. "Is he still taking Aricept?" the doctor asked.

"No," I replied. Even though I had seen a bottle of it in Dad's bathroom, it was not on the list of meds from the hospital after his heart surgery. I knew nothing about this drug and had not taken it upon myself to start him back on it again.

After the doctor had updated his list, I mentioned my concern over my dad's weight loss. He recommended that I give him a specific supplement. It just so happened that I had already researched this item prior to the appointment. What I had found was that it was not recommended for people with diabetes. I didn't say so during the visit, but I wasn't about to give it to my dad.

I also mentioned that my dad was experiencing high levels of anxiety. Without looking up, he wrote out a prescription for Lorazepam. "They call it the hip drug," he casually said.

"Why is that?" I asked.

"It can cause dizziness," he replied. "Since so many elderly people fall and break their hip when they are on it, it has become known as this." He said it so matter-of-factly. I just stared at him in disbelief. There was absolutely no way that I would put my dad on this drug either. All I could think about was him accidentally falling down the stairs.

At this point in the visit, the doctor listened to Dad's heart. I communicated to him that Dad was diagnosed with two inguinal hernias and that one of them had been bothering him for a couple of weeks. He gently examined the area, but at the moment, it wasn't bothering Dad. It also wasn't bulging outward. Dr. Linske basically said what we had already been told, that we needed to keep an eye on it.

As the visit came to a close, he handed me a small stack of papers that had the new prescription, some refills and a note with a doctor's name on it. The name read Dr. Kenneth D. Franklin. Next to his name was written Geriatric Psychiatrist and his phone number. This particular doctor hadn't been discussed during the exam. Was he referring us because of the anxiety that I had mentioned? Or was this based on my mother's earlier letter to the doctor suspecting my dad of having Alzheimer's? For whatever reason, the doctor had felt compelled to give me this man's contact information.

During the entire time that we were there, the doctor had only smiled at us once. That was when he stood up to leave. He wasn't the least bit personable, seemingly more concerned with updating his records than looking either one of us in the eye. In addition, some of his recommendations left me very skeptical. I was not impressed at all. He had definitely lost some credibility with me.

Later that day, I looked over the paperwork from the doctor's visit. I had no plans to start my dad on either one of his suggestions as I wasn't convinced that they might not make things worse. The new prescription for Lorazepam would remain unfilled.

As I curiously looked at the other note with the psychiatrist's name and number on it, I thought about the testing that still needed to be done with my dad. I googled Dr. Franklin and was very impressed with what I found. I then dialed his phone number. I briefly spoke with a woman and expressed my desire to have my dad come in for some testing. Unfortunately, Dr. Franklin was currently booked out for several months, so they added Dad to his waiting list.

While I sat at the computer, I also researched Aricept, which was a very common drug used to slow down the progression of dementia caused by Alzheimer's disease. I was now very confused. Why had the doctor previously put my Dad on this drug? Had he already diagnosed him with Alzheimer's? If so, why hadn't he insisted that Dad start taking it again when he asked me about it today? He never once mentioned anything to me about Alzheimer's when I brought up Dad's anxiety. At this point, I still wasn't quite ready to add it to Dad's current medications.

Physically, my dad was doing very well. Mentally, he was having some serious issues. I hoped to get him to a more steady point where he continued to get stronger every day. Right now, some new medications could possibly help with his anxiety and memory, but I was a little hesitant to introduce anything else until his current meds were more stable.

Friday, January 28, 2011

While he was casually relaxing in his recliner after breakfast, I knelt in front of him on the carpet. I slowly held up the bottle of lotion and smiled, his grin clearly one of anticipation. He knew what was coming. Yesterday, I had taken Dad to see a podiatrist. He had several calluses that needed to be looked at, in addition to a trim. The doctor had been very gentle in caring for Dad's feet. At the end of the visit, he gave me a tube of Kerasal and said it needed to be rubbed on Dad's feet twice a day.

As I gently took Dad's shoes and socks off, he looked at me so lovingly. I proceeded to slowly rub the lotion into his feet, knowing he truly appreciated how I took care of him. I decided that it was the perfect opportunity to bring up something that was bothering me.

"Dad, Randy and I were talking about the truck," I said. "It really needs to be driven more often. Until you are at the point where you can drive, we thought it would be a good idea to bring it over to our house." I paused to get his reaction as I had really been nervous about approaching this issue with Dad. I knew that it was a sensitive subject. He didn't say anything, so I continued on.

"We could park it in our driveway and Randy could drive it to work a couple of days a week just to keep the engine in good shape," I said. "Once you're ready, we could bring it back to you. That way, you wouldn't have to keep moving it from one driveway to the other. It would take some stress off of you. Anyway, just think about it and let us know." Dad nodded his head and smiled. I wasn't sure what he was thinking at the moment.

Early this evening, Randy went to Athens to pick up Preston, deciding to come home this weekend instead of next. I was beyond happy at this news. The timing couldn't have been more perfect. A lot had happened in the past few weeks and I really needed a weekend of laughs and hugs with my family.

While I patiently waited on them to return, I sat down for a minute in the living room. It was the first time all day that I had a chance to relax. I began to think about everything that had transpired over the past couple of months.

Sometimes in life, we were faced with things that we hadn't had a chance to prepare for. We did the best that we could during such stressful times. It was so hard though. I felt like I had aged so much in the last two months. My mom was doing much better now. Dad was steadily improving, at least physically. My parents were both very appreciative of everything I had done. Randy and Bob helped out a lot, but the brunt had definitely fallen on my shoulders. On top of everything, I wasn't taking care of myself. It had unfortunately been weeks since I had jogged. I was starting to feel like things were slowly slipping away from me.

I had watched a segment awhile back on the news about the sandwich generation which was a term that someone had coined to describe people that cared for their aging parents while also raising their own children. They were squeezed in between caring for members of two different generations, the group growing larger every day. There had never really been a time in history where we had been faced with this as much as we were today. Our parents were living so much longer than ever before. It could be a very stressful and demanding position to be in as I was finding out. I clearly knew that I had to make some changes if I was going to continue down this path as caregiver. Tomorrow, I would take the first step towards this. Tomorrow, I would start running again.

Monday, January 31, 2011

I remembered seeing all of my dad's medications for the first time back in December, feeling astounded that he was taking so many. I was also concerned with the interaction between each of them. Today, I hoped to simplify his medicine. Dad had an important doctor's appointment with his cardiologist later. I had secretly told Mom about it a couple of days ago. I didn't want Dad to get anxious, so I had intentionally refrained from telling him. The plan was for Mom to make sure that Dad was up and dressed by the time I got there.

Earlier today, I heard the eeriness of my parents' ringtone. "Your father is still in bed," Mom said. "He won't get up. I've told him that you are coming over to take him somewhere and he says that he isn't getting out of bed."

"Can you put him on the phone, Mom?" I asked. I could hear her slowly walking up the stairs and handing Dad the phone.

"Hello," said Dad.

"Daddy, I need you to get up and get dressed," I stated. "You have an appointment this morning with Dr. Kadam. He's your cardiologist."

"I really don't feel like getting out of bed," he said. "I'm tired, Pootie."

"You need to get up, Daddy," I pressed. "This appointment is very important. The doctor is going to change your blood pressure medications today. I really don't want to put this off. The sooner we get your meds straightened out, the better." I waited a few seconds, hearing nothing but silence. "Daddy, we really need to go." I knew I had to be forceful. "I'll be there in fifteen minutes. You need to be dressed, Dad." We said our goodbyes and I hung up the phone. I truly hoped that he would be waiting for me when I got there.

As I later walked in the front door, I happily saw my dad in the breakfast area. He was not only dressed, but he was actually eating some breakfast. I felt a tremendous relief. On the outside, I lovingly smiled at him. On the inside, I worried because I knew that something must have happened, his behavior this morning not normal for him. I would definitely need to talk to my mom about it later today.

On the drive over, I pointed out several different landmarks that Dad was familiar with. We passed Chris' elementary school, the road to my house and the spot where his favorite Hardee's resided before the construction on 316 had begun. He had calmed down quite a bit and was looking out the window enjoying the ride.

After arriving at the doctor's office, we sat in the waiting room and I routinely filled out Dad's paperwork. The room was huge and had televisions at several key spots on the wall. Dad soon found one that interested him. Thankfully, it helped to pass the time.

Not long after I turned in the necessary forms, we were called back. Dad's appointment was with Dr. Siddharth Kadam. Dad had already seen several other doctors in this practice. They were very familiar with his history.

While patiently waiting for the doctor in the exam room, Dad and I talked. "Pootie, I was thinking about what you mentioned before about you all keeping my truck at your house and Randy driving it to work every now and then," he said. "I think that would be a good idea."

As I stared at my father, I was stunned, not expecting this in the least. I wasn't even sure if Dad had remembered our earlier conversation, much less deciding to take us up on our offer. "Dad, I'm so glad you made that decision," I said. "I think it's a good one." I was pleasantly surprised. I thought he might have viewed it as losing some of his independence, but he genuinely seemed happy with his choice. Maybe it would truly be one less weight on his shoulders. I lovingly smiled at him as at that very moment, everything was looking better.

The doctor soon came into the room. He was very personable as he asked Dad how he was doing. There was something about a doctor with a beard that made him easier to relate to, almost as if he suddenly became more down-to-earth. We then discussed Dad's current medications. Once his list was successfully updated, he began to listen to Dad's heart, seemingly happy with everything he heard.

Since Dad was doing so well, the doctor decided once again to change his blood pressure meds. The Carvedilol would be changed from 12.5 mg. to 6.25 mg. The Lisinopril would be changed from 40 mg. to 20 mg. The Amlodipine would be removed completely. This was a major step in getting my dad's medications more stable. His blood pressure meds were finally reduced from three prescriptions down to two. I had looked forward to this moment ever since the heart surgery.

The doctor also mentioned that the results of the CHEM-7 test looked fine. He was extremely happy with Dad's progress. It was at that point that I decided to address the anxiety issue. So as not to catch him off guard, I had told Dad earlier that I needed to talk to the doctor about this. I knew that I had to be very delicate as it upset him whenever others talked about him and treated him like he wasn't even there. "How long does it take for the drugs that were used in the heart surgery to be completely out of his body?" I asked.

"It sometimes takes several months to totally recover from the type of procedure that your father had," the doctor replied. "It was major surgery."

"There have been times since the surgery, and even some before, that Dad has acted out in a way that was completely opposite of his normal behavior," I cautiously said. I looked at Dad and he seemed to be okay with the conversation, so I continued. "Sometimes, it was in ways that I had never seen him act, almost like he was a stranger."

"Well, everyone is different," the doctor said, "but, it can take a long time to completely get back to normal."

I also mentioned that we wanted to have some testing done on Dad, reminding him of the CT scan that was done in the hospital. "Unfortunately, that isn't really our area of expertise," he said. "I would recommend a neurologist or a geriatric psychiatrist." At least I then knew we were on the right track, having already contacted the latter.

I then asked Dr. Kadam about Dad taking Aricept. He actually thought it was a good idea. Now that his blood pressure meds were more stable, I also thought it might be the opportune time. I truly hoped the change in meds would make a difference in Dad, especially the anxiety.

At one point during the exam, I found myself staring at Dad, seeming so frail and innocent. It absolutely broke my heart. Some days, it was so hard. I knew he had had some bad episodes, but that wasn't my dad. He would never act like that normally. Regardless of some of the ugly scenes that had played out, he was still a good man. He had always been such a doting and loving father to me. I could never have asked for a better dad. I just wanted him to be happy during his remaining time. He definitely deserved that.

Later that day, Dad was leisurely watching television and fell asleep on the couch. I took that opportunity to talk to Mom upstairs. "Why was Dad so upset this morning?" I asked.

"He didn't get a lot of sleep," she replied. "He had been up since around 3 a.m."

"How do you know that?" I questioned. "Were you up at that time?"

She looked at me apprehensively and didn't say a word, realizing that she had slipped. She was reluctant to say anything, but I pressed on. "What happened last night, Mom?" I asked.

"He has a bad habit of getting up in the middle of the night," Mom said. "He'll go to the bathroom and then, he gets cold. He tries to adjust the thermostat. He'll get confused and then turn my bedroom light on. He demands that I get out of the bed and set it for him."

"Mom, do you get up and do it?" I asked.

"I do," she answered. "It stops him from getting more upset."

"Have these incidents ever turned violent?" I inquired, bracing myself for the answer.

"If I don't get up, he'll sometimes threaten me," she reluctantly said. "One time, he made good on it and pulled me out of the bed by my hair. I know now that I have to get up, no matter how tired I am."

"No wonder you're always so exhausted, Mom," I said. "Why didn't you tell me?"

"He told me not to tell you or Bob," she replied. I sat there completely stunned. Nothing had changed. I looked at my mother and wondered at what point she would ever tell me about Dad's behavior. How bad would it need to get in order for her to finally say something?

"How long has this been happening, Mom?" I asked.

"Ever since we came back home," she responded. The words stung. How could that be? He had promised me. They both had.

I thought about what the cardiologist had said about it possibly taking months for Dad to return to normal. I knew undoubtedly that Dad's normal did not include combative behavior. Would the change in meds help him? Was it possible to get my dad back to the way he was before? Was this the new normal for my dad? Or was a disease slowly taking more of him every single day?

When Dad eventually woke from his nap, he looked refreshed. "Hey Pootie," he said. "How long was I out?"

"Only about an hour," I responded. "You must have been really tired." He nodded his head in assent.

"Dad, I'm going to raise the temperature on the thermostat upstairs so that it's a little warmer," I said. I hoped beyond hope that this would keep Dad comfortably warm all night.

Before I left to pick up Chris from school, I carefully packaged Dad's evening meds, including his first dose of Aricept. The doctor recommended he take 5 mg. I hoped that this drug would be as promising with Dad as it was with so many others. We needed a miracle.

Tuesday, February 1, 2011

I peacefully stood outside the door watching Riley run around in the backyard. Every few steps, she'd look back up to make sure I was still there. I'd then call her name and she'd tilt her head at an angle in that precious way she always did. I absolutely couldn't imagine our lives without her. As she turned around to look at me once again, I heard my parents' ringtone. Mom had called to tell me that Dad's hernia was really bothering him.

"Chris' class is going to a book fair this morning," I said. "I promised him that I would meet him there. After that, I'll stop at the store and try to find something to help with Dad's pain."

I managed to successfully locate a medical supply store a few miles away. They actually had a couple of hernia support belts to help ease the pain. I carefully selected the one I thought would be best for Dad. I truly hoped it would work.

A little while later, I arrived at my parents' home. Dad was quietly sitting in his favorite recliner in the family room. I showed him the hernia belt and he seemed open-minded about trying it. He removed his pants and I gently adjusted the belt on him. It had special pads that would rest on each side where the bulges were located. The idea was that the pressure from the padding would help to alleviate the pain. Since they were removable, I only used the one on the right side. I then gave Dad some ibuprofen, after which he decided to go upstairs and rest for awhile. It seemed that whenever Dad was lying down, the pain would inexplicably subside.

While Dad was napping, Mom said she wanted to talk to me. "Something happened a couple of days ago that I wanted to tell you about," she said.

"Okay," I replied. I had urged my mom to tell me whenever anything crucial happened. This felt like progress. She now had my undivided attention.

"It was after dinner one evening," she continued. "Your father had asked me if I would lie in bed with him and watch some television. I told him I would." She paused to take a sip of her coffee. "While we were lying down, he told me that he wanted me to form a pact with him."

"What kind of pact?" I asked, starting to feel very concerned.

"The pact would be that if either one of us got to a point where we knew we were going to die, we would agree to die together," she responded. My heart absolutely sank. Dad clearly knew that something wasn't right, which was probably what prompted him to do this. I knew he was terrified of dying. Mostly though, he was scared of being without Mom. He didn't want to go without her by his side. I began thinking about how much my dad loved my mom. It really scared me. The thought of losing both of my parents was unbearable.

"Promise me you would never ever do anything to take your own life," I pleaded to Mom.

"I wouldn't, Vanessa," she replied. "I told your father that it was crazy talk. He wasn't going anywhere." I truly hoped that the subject would never come up again.

Before leaving that afternoon, I again included Aricept in Dad's evening meds. It would be his second dose. Possibly after the third dose, we would begin to see a recognizable change.

Later that night, I got an unexpected call from Mom. Dad's hernia was still causing him a lot of discomfort, making him very irritable. Mom was giving him ibuprofen every six hours, but it didn't seem to be enough. She also had some acetaminophen on hand, so I told her to give him a dose of it. She could alternate between the two as long as each specific drug was not given more often than the package indicated. I instructed her to write down the medication and time whenever she gave Dad something for pain to make sure she wasn't giving him too much.

I absolutely hated that my dad was in pain, but I felt terrified at the thought of another operation. I knew that the anesthesia required would take a little more of him away from us. I was beginning to wonder if we really had a choice.

Wednesday, February 2, 2011

The severe strain in her voice was apparent, the situation not going well. Dad was still in unbearable pain this morning. I had set up a schedule that Mom could follow that allowed Dad to receive the maximum amount of over-the-counter pain medicine, alternating between ibuprofen and acetaminophen. He had his last dose two hours ago and wasn't due for anything else for another couple of hours. She was slowly running out of options.

At one point this morning, Dad came downstairs and decided defiantly to take matters into his own hands. He began carelessly going through the medications on the counter, complaining all the while about how Mom was administering them. As she tried to stop him, he became more agitated. Eventually, Mom had to hide them in the closet as Dad was beginning to get out of control.

When I arrived, I had him sit down and get off of his feet, hoping that would help. "Daddy, Mom is trying to take care of you," I said. "It doesn't do anybody any good when you get ugly with her. She is only doing what I have asked her to do. You can't take pain medicine every hour. If you aren't due for it, you need to get off your feet. That seems to relieve some of the pressure." I paused to give him a chance to respond, but he remained silent. "We have a situation right now. I'm not sure what to do. The easiest thing would be to schedule a hernia procedure, but that would involve you going under anesthesia again. Every time you get drugs in your system, you're never the same afterwards. You're still not completely recovered from the heart surgery. I was hoping to get you back to normal before you underwent any more operations. Does that make sense?"

"Yes," he replied, "but I'm still in pain."

"I know you are, Daddy," I said. "We need to find a way to manage the pain better." I could sense him getting more upset.

As we continued our conversation, he became very short with his answers. Something just didn't seem right. I soon convinced him to lie back in the recliner for awhile, hoping the pain medicine would hurry up and do its job. We desperately needed Dad to calm down.

Earlier in the week, a friend of my parents gave me the name of a woman that did in-home care, coming highly recommended. I had previously contacted her and she was very interested. Unfortunately, she could only work during the day. I was already here during the day. Even though it could have helped me out, it wasn't what I was looking for. Ideally, I wanted someone to be here during the night. I seriously worried about my mom and dad being alone during that time, which seemed to be when the Sundowner's kicked in. I was still trying to decide what to do.

Dad had heard us talking about it and brought it up to Mom this morning. He was adamant that he wouldn't feel comfortable with a stranger coming into the house and he let her know this. Dad was very much against the idea.

This afternoon, I had to leave early to pick Chris up from school as it was an early release day. I also had a conference scheduled with his teacher at 1:00. I didn't feel comfortable leaving my parents, but I had no choice. I carefully packaged Dad's evening meds. Tonight would be his third dose of Aricept. I was watching Dad's behavior very closely. If it was going to cause a change in Dad, there was a good chance that it would surface tomorrow.

At 8:15 p.m., I got an alarming call from Mom, sounding so exasperated. She was giving Dad his pain medicine around the clock. Unfortunately, he wasn't due for anything for awhile. While she was standing at the sink, Dad had angrily walked into the kitchen looking for the medication. He asked her to give him the pill bottles, but she had refused. The unrelenting pain was making Dad very irritable.

At my request, she put him on the phone. "Pootie, why are you all doing this to me?" he asked. I could already tell that this wasn't going to end well.

"Daddy, we're trying to take care of you," I replied. "It could be dangerous if you took too much pain medicine."

"She hasn't given me anything," he complained.

"She has, Daddy," I said. "It may not seem like it, but she has. You have to be patient. Do you have your hernia belt on?" I needed to change the subject to help calm him down.

"Yes," he answered, "but, it's not helping any."

"Why don't you try lying down on your side and get some sleep?" I offered. "That always seems to make the pain go away." I then heard muffled sounds, apparently handing the phone back to Mom without so much as a goodbye.

As I lied in bed that night, I felt like I was nearing the end of my rope. I wasn't prepared for the way Dad had talked to me on the phone. Maybe I was too sensitive, but he had never talked to me like that before. If his behavior was caused by the pain, then we had no choice but to have the hernia operated on. He seemed to be steadily getting worse. I needed to talk to Bob and Randy about going forward with the procedure. Sometimes in life, the hard decisions came down to the lesser of two evils.

Thursday, February 3, 2011

I seemed invariably to catch every red light while driving the familiar roads. As I sat through my third one, I could feel the knots in my stomach beginning to form, knowing that things weren't well. I had already received my morning call with the eerie ringtone. I slowly braced myself for what I was about to encounter.

After nervously entering their house, I tried to act as if nothing was wrong and went about my normal routine. I checked Dad's blood sugar and then gave him his morning meds. He was very quiet and seemed distracted. I then made him a bowl of cereal with peaches on top which was one of his favorite breakfasts. Normally, he would have eaten it quickly.

I carefully watched Dad as he stared intently at the bowl of cereal, beginning to get visibly upset. I then looked at the table and noticed that his dentures were sitting next to his orange juice. "Daddy, you need to put your teeth in," I said. He just looked at me unwaveringly, his eyes so cold.

Before long, he picked up his bowl of cereal and stood up. He also grabbed his teeth as he determinedly started walking towards the stairs. This was clearly an accident waiting to happen. "Daddy, why don't you let me have the bowl of cereal?" I asked. I managed to get it and place it back on the table, but he continued upstairs. I then worriedly looked at Mom. "Has he been like this ever since he got up?" She nodded her head yes.

Several minutes later, Dad came back downstairs. He was now carrying a glass that had sat on his nightstand, along with his house key wrist band and a pencil. His teeth were now inside the glass. He was moving so slowly as he methodically set the items down on the breakfast area table. I didn't know what was happening to him, but I began to get scared.

"Dad, why don't you eat some breakfast?" I said. "I'll help you get your teeth in." He looked at me and began to say something, but then shook his head in disgust, as if he had changed his mind. He got up again and headed back upstairs.

My mind was running in a million different directions. Dad's behavior was very irrational. I soon noticed that a pattern had developed. Dad would go upstairs and ten minutes later, he would invariably come back down with his arms full, usually with an additional item he had picked up from his bedroom. He also seemed a little unstable on his feet. His constant going up and down the stairs made me feel very nervous.

As Dad once again came back into the room, I noticed how incredibly thin he looked. He was dressed in a white thermal shirt and thermal underwear, almost looking emaciated. When had he lost so much weight?

Before long, Dad moved to the breakfast area and once again sat down at the table. He just stared at us, as if he were willing us to say something. No matter how I responded, he found a way to argue with me. If Mom happened to say something, it was even worse. He was so combative. I honestly didn't know what to do. With every word that was said, I hoped it would be the one to finally settle him down. Unfortunately, things were just getting worse. The contention had now gone on for more than thirty minutes. It didn't seem like it was close to ending.

Dad was clearly not himself. He had a glazed look in his eyes and his pupils were very small. Unfortunately, I had seen this side of the disease on more than one occasion during the past month. I knew all too well that once it happened, it usually took a substantial amount of time or a major act to bring him out of it. When he finally did return, it was quite possible he'd have absolutely no memory of what had happened at all.

I felt very overwhelmed and desperately needed some help. I wanted for Randy to be here as I felt confident that Dad would have listened to him. Unfortunately, he was at work and I vowed not to bother him. Mom had also called Bob, but he too was busy at the moment. We would somehow have to handle this crisis on our own.

Dad's words weren't making any sense. When I tried to respond honestly to them, it only made him more upset. I soon realized that the only thing he wanted to hear were words of agreement, regardless of whether it was the truth or not. Was it right to lie to him just to get him to calm down? It went against my basic human nature. What if he remembered the lies later? How would I explain them? If someone verbally attacked you, the normal thing to do was defend yourself. Unfortunately, that was only adding fuel to this fire. I felt like I was clearly in over my head.

I had to dig deep to remain calm and bite my tongue. "Do you want a can of Glucerna?" I asked. He just looked at me. "You always liked them before." He still said nothing, so I took this as my cue to get one. I carefully placed it in front of him on the table and opened it. He completely ignored it.

He then picked up the bowl of cereal once again as he slid the chair back. I worried that he was going to drop it. As I tried to take it from him, he smacked my hand, looking enraged. Never in my life had he laid a finger on me. My heart was racing uncontrollably. I could tolerate the mean words, but the violence escalated things to an unacceptable level. "Don't ever hit me again," I said sternly. Maybe this wasn't the right thing to say, but I needed to know what I was dealing with. I needed to know if he would back down.

"I'll do whatever the hell I want," he exclaimed. "This is my house."

"That doesn't give you the right to put your hands on someone," I said.

"If you don't like it, then leave," he said angrily. "You're not doing anything here anyway."

The ugliness of the situation soon gripped me and before I knew it, I was arguing with him. "If you lay a hand on either one of us again, I'll call the police." I hoped beyond hope that this would bring him out of it.

Unfortunately, he wasn't the least bit afraid. "I don't give a shit," he said. I stared into the intense eyes of a stranger. Mom stood in the kitchen a few feet away not saying a word, but taking every bit of the horrible scene in.

"What has happened to you?" I asked. "I don't feel like I know you anymore. All we're trying to do is take care of you, Dad."

"You two don't do a damn thing for me," he argued.

With that, I reached my breaking point. "Are you kidding me?" I asked, my voice rising. "I have sacrificed everything for you. I come over here every day to take care of you. I take you to all of your appointments. I take care of your medicine. There isn't any more of me to give." I struggled to catch my breath. "I haven't spent any quality time with my family in months. You know Chris, my 7-year old? That little boy desperately needs his mother. He's having trouble in school with his writing. He needs my help, but I haven't been there for him like I should have. Do you know why?" I just stared at him waiting for him to say something. I had never in my life felt so unappreciated.

"I haven't been able to help him because I have spent every minute taking care of you," I continued. "I have done everything humanly possible to be there for you. And you sit there and say I don't do anything for you." As I stood there in the middle of the breakfast area, I lost my composure, the tears finally breaking through. I bowed my head and just stood there crying uncontrollably. Never before had I felt so alone.

Dad soon came and stood directly in front of me. I had no idea what he was about to do, but it didn't matter anyways. I had no energy left to be scared. I looked up at his face bracing myself for what would inevitably happen next. And then, right before my eyes, my dad came back to me. His eyes softened and even through the tears, I could see that it was my daddy. Watching his daughter go through such agonizing pain had touched something deep inside of him and brought him back. He tenderly put his arms around me and I leaned into him, continuing to cry deeply in his shoulder for what seemed an eternity.

"I'm so sorry, Pootie," he said. It had absolutely crushed my dad to see me like that. "You're a good daughter. I don't want you to neglect your family anymore." His voice was so gentle and his words so loving. We stood in the breakfast area and hugged each other tightly. Nothing else in the entire world mattered at that moment.

Not long afterwards, he sat down and drank his shake. When he was done, he went upstairs to take a nap. After about five minutes had passed, I went up to see him. He was quietly lying in bed and was completely calm. I saw absolutely no sign of the man I had seen just fifteen minutes earlier. I had never before witnessed anything like it.

My father looked so unbelievably sad, like he knew something bad had happened between us but he didn't know exactly what it was. The look of shame on his face broke my heart. I knew that it hadn't been him. He was currently looking at me with the most beautiful, loving eyes. He apologized once more and promised that it would never happen again.

"I love you, Daddy," I said.

"I love you, too," he replied back. I then gently kissed him on the cheek. We talked for about twenty minutes, the conversation between us flowing effortlessly. It was our chance to say what was necessary in order for us to move forward.

"I have to pick Chris up from school," I then said. "It's another early release day. Are you going to be okay?"

"I'll be fine," he replied. "I'm just going to stay here in bed and take a nap. You go do what you need to do." I smiled at him as I hesitantly walked away.

Before I left, I had a necessary talk with Mom, wanting more than anything for Dad to remain calm the rest of the day. We both agreed that it would be a good idea for her to stay in his bed tonight and watch television with him, letting him pick whatever show he wanted. I hoped that her company would do wonders for him.

As I carefully packaged Dad's evening meds, I thought about his erratic behavior the past couple of days. Something was clearly different with him. I had never seen such a drastic change in his demeanor. All I could think of was the Aricept. It unquestionably had to be the cause. I wasn't going to give it to him anymore. Now, I just had to wait until it got out of his system to see if I was right.

Today had been an absolute nightmare. I didn't want us to ever have to live through anything like it again. Next time, it might not end as well. I knew that it was probably not entirely over yet. I just hoped that today was the worst that we'd have to endure. I began to feel scared and helpless and overwhelmed. So much of what we were dealing with was out of our control. Why was this happening? I prayed that the Lord would give my dad a break. He desperately needed one.

Friday, February 4, 2011

I quietly leaned against the kitchen counter while Chris took a bite of his pancake. As I watched him eat, I was so thankful that the crisis going on all around him had yet to take his innocence away, still the happy child he'd always been. The serene moment was soon interrupted as my cell phone rang. I had developed such a hatred for the ringtone that played, but I knew that changing it wouldn't make a difference. The news would undoubtedly still be the same. This time, Mom called to let me know that Dad was not in a good mood. He had gotten mad at her last night and apparently, it had carried over into today.

I had suspected that the Aricept was the problem. If I was right, then I knew that it would still be in Dad's system and we would unfortunately be in for another tumultuous day. The thought of what was awaiting me made me cringe inside.

As I later opened their front door, I saw my dad slowly coming down the stairs. "Hi Daddy," I said timidly. It was immediately evident that he was not himself. I then went into the kitchen and proceeded with my normal morning routine.

Before I made Dad's breakfast, I went into the family room and sat down on the loveseat. He apparently wanted to talk and I wanted to be there for him. He soon came and sat next to me. "So, did everything go okay last night?" I asked. I already knew the answer, but I needed Dad to feel like he could open up to me.

"No, it didn't," he replied. "Your mother brought the newspaper in the bed with us. She had her nose in it the whole time. All I wanted was for her to watch television with me. She couldn't do it."

I tried to be impartial. I could honestly see both sides. "Daddy, you know how Mom is," I said. "She likes to be doing something while she watches a program." I had measured my words so carefully so as not to upset him any further. Unfortunately, Dad didn't like my response.

"Pootie," he began. Before he could finish, he gave me that disgusted look that told me he felt it wasn't worth it to continue. He then started to get up off of the loveseat. He had wanted me to side with him, but I wasn't going to get in the middle of it.

"Wait, Dad," I said. "Please don't get upset. I know it meant a lot to you. I'm sorry it didn't work out."

"All I wanted was for her to pay attention to me," he said. "Was that too much to ask?"

"No, Dad, it wasn't," I replied. "That's just the way Mom is. Try not to take it personally." I smiled at him, before proceeding honestly. "I just think you're making too much of it."

"I knew it was useless talking about this," he said. I could already see where this was going. It was clearly a no-win situation, right back to exactly where we were yesterday. Regardless of what I said, Dad wanted to argue with me. I didn't want to go through this today. Dad attempted to get up once again, only this time, I didn't stop him. I had the most miserable feeling inside and was truly dreading this day.

Dad soon began the same pacing routine that he had engaged in yesterday. He just couldn't sit still, so I tried to stay out of his way, determined not to break down like yesterday. This behavior was not my father. It was a combination of the drugs and the disease doing this to him. I had to keep reminding myself of this.

I tried to carry out my normal routine and stay as busy as I could which would also mean ignoring all of the remarks meant to start an argument. I got a can of Glucerna out of the fridge without even bothering to ask, knowing that even the slightest of words might set Dad off. I opened the can and set it on the table where he normally sat. He looked at me in a challenging way, but I turned my head and refused to make eye contact, not having the strength to go down that road again.

Unfortunately, today had ended up being another disaster. As hard as I tried, there had been some regrettable arguments. I wanted so badly to just fast forward until tomorrow or the next day when no signs of the Aricept remained in Dad. I knew that we needed to do whatever we could to get through the day, but it was so difficult at times. I had walked on eggshells all day. It had been crucial that I disconnected my emotions and treated this strictly as a caregiver-patient situation. Eventually though, I had reached my limits.

Later that day as I arrived home with Chris, I let him play a video game. Dad's hernia was obviously still bothering him. The last ER doctor had given me the number of a physician that performed hernia procedures. I went ahead and scheduled an appointment with him on Tuesday for Dad to be evaluated. It couldn't wait any longer.

I then called Dr. Franklin's office, trying to keep my composure while explaining to the woman on the other end of the line the dire situation we were in. It was truly an emergency. After patiently listening, she agreed to make an exception for Dad and try to get him in earlier. She'd call me back to let me know when this would be. For the first time in two days, I felt a small ray of hope.

May, 1980

After the spring semester had ended, I found myself letting loose. I had just finished my first year of college and was starting to go down a wild path. It seemed as though every night was spent going out with my friends and invariably coming home late which didn't go over well at home. Two of my best friends had moved in with each other and were currently renting a house a few miles away. One day, I made the painful decision to leave.

Nobody was home at the time. Both Mom and Dad were working and Bob was in school. I hurriedly packed my clothes and some necessities. Then, I patiently waited for Bob to come home.

Before long, I saw him walking through the field near the entrance to our subdivision. When he walked up to the door, I met him and told him I was leaving. I would never forget the somber look on his face, staring at me in shock. "Why?" he asked. That was all he could say, the pain in his eyes so evident.

"I just need to leave for a few days," I replied. "I'm tired of fighting all the time with Mom." I paused to let the news sink in. "I promise I'll see you soon." I sadly hugged him goodbye and then left. He was utterly devastated.

That night, my mother called my dad to break the grim news to him. At the time, he was working on an oil rig in Texas. A neighbor of ours was a manager on the rig and had offered Dad the job. Times were hard for us and he desperately needed the work. He would routinely work two weeks out and one week in. The drive was long and the work was hard, but he did what he needed to do in order to financially provide for his family.

Dad happened to be out on the oil rig on the day that I moved out. The news had left him heartbroken and terrified. His daughter had suddenly left the security of their home and he had no idea where she was. Being so many miles away, he couldn't have done anything about it anyway. He felt completely powerless. It was very hard on all of my family when I left, but more so for my dad.

I ended up moving into the rental house with my girlfriends. It was a four bedroom home, so it was really not an imposition. I would simply take one of the unused bedrooms.

One of the girls was dating a guy that worked on a construction crew. They were currently working on a nearby hospital. The work crew happened to frequent a pool hall called Crazy Caleb's, a small hole in the wall that was located on an unpaved corner lot completely by itself.

A few days soon turned into a few weeks and before I knew it, I was living on my own. I had officially moved out. I knew that I needed a job if I was to continue down this path. Caleb, the owner of the pool hall, soon offered me a position. Since I was spending so much time there anyway, I decided to take him up on it and work the night shift. The bar closed at 2 a.m. Since I didn't have a car, one of my girlfriends would drive me to and from work.

Across the street from the pool hall was a pizza place named Geno's. A young man worked there, fresh out of high school. He would come to the pool hall after his shift ended. His name was Randy.

Sunday, June 15, 1980

One night, my dad came to the bar looking for me, pulling into the unpaved parking lot in his wood paneled station wagon. Caleb's wasn't a fancy establishment by any means and I'm sure my dad looked very out of place, but it didn't matter to him. He had but one mission that night. His daughter was going through a rough time and he was going to do whatever it took to help her safely find her way back home.

As it turned out, I wasn't there when he arrived, actually having the night off. Still, it was common for me to stop in even when I wasn't working. For some inexplicable reason, I didn't that night. It might have been a blessing.

The next day, one of the regulars at the bar mentioned that a man had come in the night before looking for me. I asked him to describe this person. The man was wearing jeans and a flannel shirt. The clincher was when he told me what he was driving. I was stunned. He had come looking for me. My daddy had actually come looking for me.

He had never frequented Caleb's before and had no way of knowing what kind of place it was, nor what he would find when he entered it. Had I actually been there, it may not have ended well. But, as it turned out, his act had touched me deeply. He may not have accomplished what he had ultimately set out to do, but his visit meant more than he would ever know. It was probably the most loving thing he had ever done for me in my life. I truly had the best father in the world. I only hoped he knew it.

Later that night, I thought about my family. I was going through a difficult time and I just wasn't ready to come home. They were in such turmoil over this. Just last week, my mother had driven my younger brother over to the rental house because he wanted so much to see his sister. He genuinely missed me. I felt moved beyond words over my family's concern for me.

July, 1980

It felt like a lifetime had been squeezed into the past three months. The young man that frequently came into Caleb's after his shift across the street ended had asked me to marry him. We had only known each other for two months, but I absolutely knew he was the one. I was deeply in love, probably one of the few people that could honestly say they met the love of their life in a bar.

We had made so many plans for our future together. Next June, I would marry the man that forever changed my life. I would be nineteen years old and Randy would be twenty. I had also decided to move back home and start back to college in the fall. Randy had been so good for me. It certainly hadn't happened overnight, but he never gave up. I had settled down so much because of him.

I openly talked to my mom today and told her about our plans. She had graciously invited us over for dinner. She didn't say so, but I think it was a celebration. My dad had brought back shrimp from the rig awhile back. Tonight, Mom would fry them up, along with fries and hush puppies. She also had green beans and a salad. Everything was delicious!

My family met Randy for the first time at this dinner, the bond instantaneous. I watched their faces as they slowly got to know him. There was such an ease in their manners, almost as if they had known each other all of their lives. They were beyond happy. I knew they would grow to love Randy as much as I did. Inside, I knew the reason for their incredible joy. Randy had done what they had not been able to do. He had safely brought their daughter back home. For this, my parents would forever be grateful to him.

Sunday, February 6, 2011

My nerves were on edge all morning, thankful that the drive over was a smooth one. I held my breath as I strode up the walkway towards the front door, staring at the crepe myrtles looking so bare. I hadn't received a phone call this morning, so I felt extremely hopeful. As I cautiously walked inside, Dad looked up from his recliner and I smiled at him. He then smiled back and said "Hey Pootie" at which point I began to breathe again. My dad was back. I then bent down and gently kissed his cheek.

He seemed to be doing so much better and was finally returning to his old self. The Aricept was slowly coming out of his system. I knew that it was a common drug for his condition, but I would never give it to him again. It had caused an absolute nightmare. My hope was that he wouldn't remember any of the resulting episodes.

"Hey Chester," Randy said. He held out his hand to shake and Dad happily reciprocated.

"Hey Ran," said Dad. He was in such a good mood. It was the best thing in the world to see him this way.

After breakfast, we all leisurely sat in the family room and relaxed. Barron hopped up on Dad's lap as he always did. "Dad, do you still want us to take your truck back to our house?" I asked. A lot had happened since we had initially discussed this and I needed to make sure he was still on board with the plan.

"Yes," he replied. "I think that would be the best thing. It needs to be driven more and I just can't do it right now."

"I'll take good care of it for you, Chester," said Randy. "Don't worry about a thing." Dad smiled at Randy, as if to say he had complete trust in him looking after his beloved vehicle.

Not long after we drove Dad's truck home, Randy decided to clean it as it hadn't been washed in months. Randy generously spent hours doting over Dad's truck. After he washed it, he put some wax on it. Then, he vacuumed out the inside, actually finding some cobwebs in the cab.

As I looked out the window and watched him work so diligently, I wondered how many son-in-laws did this type of thing. I didn't think too many. Ever since the first time they had met, they had shared a special love. It had only grown with time.

Tuesday, February 8, 2011

He always liked sitting in the front seat where he'd have a better view. His smile, as he stared out the front window, clearly indicated he was soaking up every bit of scenery, so many places holding special memories. It had such a calming effect on him. I had explained to Dad earlier that we would be meeting at 1:00 with Dr. David Parker, the hernia doctor referred to us at the last emergency room visit.

We were routinely brought back to an exam room not long after we arrived. After carefully describing the symptoms, Dad showed Dr. Parker the area that was bothering him. It was actually bulging a little at the moment. The doctor then had us move to his office in the next room.

The evaluation had been very quick as there was no doubt in the doctor's mind. Dad did indeed have a hernia. "What kind of timeframe are we looking at?" I asked. "Is it critical that it be operated on immediately?"

"You really don't want to wait too long," the doctor replied. "The sooner it's repaired, the better. There is a risk of strangulation if it's left untreated. It could eventually cut off the blood supply to the intestine." He paused and looked at each one of us. "There is also a danger of obstruction. When a part of the bowel herniates, it can cause the bowel contents to be blocked by the obstruction. Both conditions can be fatal." The doctor's expression visibly indicated how serious the matter was.

"My dad had triple bypass surgery in December," I said. "He also had two other procedures within a month of that. I'm concerned about the anesthesia. Dad is very sensitive to drugs." I looked at Dad to see if he wanted to add anything, knowing how important it was for him to feel like he was a part of the conversation, especially when it concerned him. He didn't say a word, so I continued. "It always takes him so long to recover when he is put under. He still isn't completely over the last surgery."

"This is a relatively quick procedure," the doctor stated. "He would only be under for about an hour. I don't think it would be long enough to be concerned about." Dad remained very quiet during the meeting.

Dr. Parker then drew a very simplistic picture on a piece of paper to help explain what was going on inside of Dad. I wondered if the procedure might help Dad in more ways than the obvious. If he wasn't in such pain, then maybe he would be calmer.

The doctor then left the room to check his schedule. He also wanted to give us some time to discuss our options. "What do you think, Dad?" I asked.

"Well, I like this doctor," he responded. "I think I should have it done." Dad apparently trusted the doctor and felt comfortable with him, even though he had just met him. Mostly, I think he just wanted the pain gone.

When the doctor returned, we promptly told him of our decision, all of us agreeing it needed to be done as soon as possible. A pre-op appointment at the hospital was scheduled for next Monday with the actual procedure occurring the following Wednesday.

He gave me all of the necessary instructions and explained that I would have to obtain a pre-op evaluation letter from Dad's cardiologist stating he was physically able to have the operation. I was instructed to stop giving Dad aspirin as of today. He could continue it again after the surgery. A substantial amount of paperwork also needed to be completed before Monday.

I was glad the procedure wasn't scheduled until next week. It actually worked out better for me as I had a busy week ahead. A Track & Field meeting for Shawn's high school was scheduled for tonight at 7:00. Tomorrow, Chris had a routine dental appointment at 2:50, which necessitated checking him out of school early. I already felt exhausted and the week had only just begun.

I had recently been doing a lot of thinking about Dad's situation. He had a combination of good days and bad days. On the good days, I was filled with hope that together, we could beat this thing. Unfortunately, the bad days seemed to overshadow the good. I began to wonder how much longer we could continue like we were. Was this disease bigger than any of us could handle? I tried to weigh our options, but there didn't seem to be many. If Dad got to be too much for Mom, I would have no choice but to separate them.

One option would be to bring Dad to my house. I honestly wasn't sure how well that would work nowadays. With my children, I was always on the run. I was usually at home in the mornings, but the afternoons and evenings were typically very busy. A lot of my time was spent at cross country and track events where I did a lot of walking following the runners. I didn't think that would bode well with Dad. The alternative would be to leave him alone and I definitely didn't like that idea.

The alarming thought of Dad being around the boys during one of his sundowning episodes also left me very concerned. They adored their Grandpa and to see him in one of those states would be devastating to them. He wouldn't have wanted that either. I had to find a way to take care of my dad without disrupting their lives at the same time.

Another option would be for my dad to remain in his home. I would simply continue to come over every day and take care of him. He'd be by himself in the evenings though and I wasn't sure he could manage alone anymore. I had looked into hiring someone to provide in-home care during the time that I wasn't there. Unfortunately, the cost to have someone there around the clock was outrageous.

The only other option that I could think of would be to find a home for him. The thought of that absolutely broke my heart. I wasn't ready for that tough decision to be made. I also knew that his Sundowner's would be an issue as a lot of homes would be leery of that type of aggressive behavior.

There was clearly no good answer. Things weren't supposed to have worked out like this. My father lived his entire life being such a good man. He was completely devoted to taking care of his family and had always worked so hard. This was supposed to be the time in his life when he could sit back and relax. This vile disease that was taking him away from us was never meant to be a part of the plan.

Thursday, February 10, 2011

She was busy in the kitchen as he sat down at the table, making sure to put his plate in the microwave at the last minute to get it piping hot. That was how he liked it. She soon brought everything to the table and sat down to join him. As he stared at her, it became obvious that something was terribly wrong. He had seemed completely fine earlier in the day, nothing out of the ordinary occurring.

When Bob had gone over last night to visit, he was a little nervous over Dad's behavior. He was short with his answers and just didn't seem like himself. He had also snapped at Mom a couple of times. It was enough of a concern for Bob to mention it to me.

Now, Dad was very agitated. Mom had made them both a tossed salad to go along with their meal. Normally, Dad loved to eat salads, but for some reason tonight was different. While they were seated at the breakfast area table, my Uncle Ronnie, Dad's brother, called. Mom tried to hand the phone to Dad, but he refused to talk. While she tried to explain the situation to my uncle, Dad got up and took his salad bowl over to the sink. He then dumped it into the trash.

As soon as Mom hung the phone up, she said "You didn't have to throw it away, Chester. I would have eaten it."　Dad said nothing in response. They remained at the table for a little while longer. Mom managed to eat her dinner, while Dad ate very little of his.

Afterwards, Mom cleaned the kitchen while Dad sat in the family room watching television. She then put the trash can and the recycle bins out on the curb.

Not long after that, Dad walked into the kitchen. "Why did you put the trash can out?" he asked angrily.

"The trash truck comes on Friday now," she replied.

"They most certainly do not, Shirley," he stated, his voice getting louder. "You are lying. Go out and bring them back up to the house."

"I'm not lying, Chester," she said. "I've been putting the trash out on Thursday nights for awhile now."

"You're going to get them now!" he demanded. With that, he pulled her out the kitchen door by her arm. He quickly pressed the button for the garage door and continued to drag Mom out to the curb. Once there, he yelled at the top of his lungs for her to do what he said. She had no choice but to bring the trash can and recycle bins back up to the house. No neighbors came out to assist even though they had to have heard the commotion.

Not long after that, Dad forced Mom to come into his bedroom where he made her sit on the bed and watch television with him. A little while later, Bob called to see how they were doing as he was still a little apprehensive from the previous night. When Mom answered the phone, her voice clearly indicated that something was terribly wrong. He drove over immediately.

When he walked upstairs into Dad's bedroom, Dad had that crazed look on his face. Mom looked terrified. "You are not going to use my mom as your personal punching bag!" Bob said angrily. He then told Mom to quickly grab her things. They soon left.

On the way back, he called me to let me know that Mom was on her way over to stay with me, briefly letting me know what had happened. In just a few minutes, they pulled up in the driveway. Mom was shaken up, but otherwise seemed okay. They came into the garage and then revealed what had happened in detail.

I knew that my mom was now safe, but I worried about my dad. It sounded like he was having a severe Sundowner's episode. I was scared to go over and talk to him, not knowing whether he was thinking clearly or not. I was also concerned that there were guns in the house. I felt the best thing might just be to leave him by himself until this incident had passed. I didn't want to make it worse.

The three of us continued to talk, but unfortunately couldn't come up with a good solution. After Bob left, I continued to worry about my dad. I then asked Randy if he would ride over to their house to check on him, having come up with the best plan I could under the circumstances. I told Randy that if the lights were on and it looked like Dad was still up, he was not to go inside, but to call me instead. I knew that it could be dangerous inside and we might have to make a hard decision. I desperately hoped that the lights would be out.

As Randy slowly drove by their house, it was completely dark, appearing that Dad had indeed gone to bed. I felt a certain amount of relief at this news. Assuming that Dad was already asleep, we both felt he would most likely be alright for the night. It was not a good situation, but I didn't know what else to do. I prayed that he would stay in bed until morning.

Friday, February 11, 2011

It was still dark outside when I opened my eyes, feeling like I hadn't slept a wink. All I could think about was whether he was safe or not. I absolutely hated our predicament and honestly had no idea what to do. I felt both nervous and scared at the same time.

Knowing that I needed to be strong, I dialed my parents' phone number a short while later. No one answered. I waited a few more minutes and then tried the number again. After three rings, Dad answered the phone. "Oh thank goodness, Pootie," he said, so happy to hear my voice. I felt the exact same way. My dad was okay. It was such a tremendous relief.

"Are you alright, Dad?" I asked.

"No, not really," he replied. "I need you to come over, Pootie." He sounded calm, but something was definitely wrong. I wasn't sure what I would find when I arrived.

"Okay," I said. "Mom and I will be over in a little bit. Daddy, I want you to stay inside the house." He agreed that he would before eventually hanging up the phone.

Fifteen minutes later, Mom and I nervously pulled up in the driveway, the garage door already open. Before we could get out of the car, Dad swiftly walked up carrying a butter knife and a can of Glucerna. He had tried to open it, but was unsuccessful.

I slowly walked Dad back inside the house. There in the kitchen sink, I found a roll of biscuits that was punctured with a knife, dough bulging out the side. I then had Dad sit down at the table and I got him a shake, as well as his meds.

As he sat at the breakfast area table, he appeared calm. I saw no visible signs that anything bad had happened last night. I took the opportunity to talk to him about something that had really bothered me. "Daddy, I need to talk to you about something," I said. He slowly nodded his head okay. At that point, I continued. "I'm concerned about the guns that are in the house. If, God forbid, they were ever used in the heat of the moment, we would never forgive ourselves." Again, he nodded. "Would it be okay if I had Bob keep them at his house? It would make me feel so much better."

"That'd be fine," he said calmly, actually agreeing with me. I felt like a tremendous weight had just been lifted off of my shoulders.

I then made Dad some coffee and he sat in the family room with Mom. They very much needed some time alone to talk. While Dad was distracted, I quickly retrieved all of the guns from upstairs and put them in the trunk of my car. I would give them to Bob later this evening.

Mom and I stayed with Dad all day. He remained completely calm the entire time. He seemed receptive to talking, so we discussed the current situation. I was brutally honest with him. I knew that he wanted Mom to come back home, but he didn't seem to be able to control his anger when the Sundowner's kicked in. Things could absolutely not continue the way they had been anymore.

There really was no good solution. For the time being, I would bring Mom over each day and we would spend all morning and afternoon with Dad. In the afternoon, we would leave to pick my boys up from school. Once they were situated at home, we would return and I'd then make my parents dinner. After Dad got his evening meds and was in bed, Mom and I would leave.

The proposed plan would be very demanding of us, especially me. It meant that my children would have to manage without me for awhile. Randy would have to take care of dinner, homework, extra activities and everything else that was on my plate, in addition to his fulltime job. We would try it for a couple of days to see if it was even remotely possible. As I listened to myself explaining this to Dad, I realized how poor of a plan it really was. It was going to be extremely difficult. I was at a loss for how we were going to make it work, but I couldn't think of a better option.

I wanted so much to take care of my dad, but it just wasn't that simple. Both Bob and I had children that we needed to think about. Dad's behavior was getting more violent every day. It was hard enough for me to endure it, but I didn't want the boys to witness something that they might not be able to get past. The thought of bringing Dad home with me and him having a meltdown left me terrified. Inside, I knew it would just be a matter of time.

As the afternoon eventually approached, we needed to pick the boys up from school. "Daddy, I want you to stay inside the house," I said. "You can watch television or take a nap. Barron will keep you company. We'll come back later to make you dinner." He seemed fine with this plan.

At a little after 3:00 p.m., we dropped Shawn and Chris off at home. Mom was very tired and decided to stay with them. I made a quick run to Athens to get Preston. He had already planned on coming home this weekend and I had promised that I would pick him up at 4:00.

At dinnertime, Mom and I returned to take care of Dad. When we got there, we walked around the main level and he was nowhere to be found. I quickly became alarmed. As I rushed upstairs, I could hear his shower running. "Are you okay, Dad?" I yelled into the bathroom.

"I'm fine, Pootie," he said. "I'll be out in a minute."

After getting dinner started, I packaged up Dad's evening meds. He soon came downstairs and looked so much better than he had earlier. He was in a good mood and smelled wonderful. Dad had always worn cologne. Being one of those women that loved it when a person walked by and their wonderful scent lingered, I appreciated this effort so much. "You smell so good, Daddy," I said, as he smiled at me.

Before long, I served Mom and Dad their dinner. I had already arranged for Randy to pick up pizza for the boys. I hoped that I'd get to spend some time with them this weekend as I really missed them.

Dad soon tired and decided to go to bed early. He apparently hadn't slept well the night before either. After I tucked him in, I gently kissed him good night and pet Barron on the head. Mom then did the same.

As we made our way downstairs, we turned all the lights off and locked the deadbolt lock in the front door. Even though Dad had seemed calm today, the thought of leaving my parents alone still frightened me. Mom and I would return as promised in the morning.

That night, I met Bob and carefully gave him all of the guns in my car. I had desperately wanted to remove them from my parents' home for awhile, but didn't know how to approach the subject. I would definitely rest much easier tonight knowing they were out of the house.

Saturday, February 12, 2011

The familiar ride over was a quiet one, both of us lost in thought about what we would inevitably find. We had intentionally gotten up early this morning and quickly returned to their home. I had again worried incessantly about him all night. As soon as we opened the front door, we surprisingly saw him standing in the hallway, looking very haggard. He was dressed, but only had one white sock on, a small bruise visible on top of his bare foot. When I asked him what happened, he said that he fell in the hall upstairs. I was immediately alarmed.

It was a serious wake-up call for me. Dad had made it through the night, but only by the grace of God. He clearly couldn't stay by himself anymore. What if he had fallen down the stairs? By the time we would have found him, it might have been too late. The plan that I had wouldn't work as Dad definitely needed someone with him at all times. I was so thankful that nothing too serious had happened to him last night.

While Dad was upstairs brushing his teeth, I openly talked to Mom. She had already expressed to me that she wanted to stay with Dad. Even though it was not a good situation, I didn't feel like we had a choice. I still worried about Mom being alone with Dad, but I worried even more about Dad being alone without Mom. We finally decided to give it another try. It certainly was not ideal, but it might have been the best option we had. Mom would remain at home with Dad and we would check on them throughout the day and night. I called Bob to tell him the latest developments. He wasn't happy about them, but also realized we had no choice.

Later that night when I called Mom, she mentioned that Larry, the neighbor from across the street, had talked to her when she had gone to the mailbox late that afternoon. During the time period yesterday when I had asked Dad to remain inside, he had actually left the house and gone over to Larry's. He was looking for us.

My stomach sank after hearing this. A million things could have happened to him. What if he had locked himself out of the house? What if someone had gotten into the house? And my worst fear, what if he had wandered off? This disturbing news only reinforced what I already knew. For Dad's own safety, he could no longer be left alone.

I later sat down at the computer and decided to do some research. It seemed that every week, a startling story aired on the news about someone with dementia suddenly going missing. What I read was shocking! It said that six out of ten people with Alzheimer's disease would eventually wander off and become lost. I knew how dangerous this could be. I didn't want for my father to become another statistic.

Wednesday, February 16, 2011

Several cars were on the road even though it was still dark outside. It seemed as though this town never slept. As I drove my usual route, I tensely thought about everything that needed to happen today for the hernia surgery. I had taken Dad to his pre-op appointment at Parkland General Hospital on Monday. After completing all of the necessary paperwork online, Dad was officially registered for the procedure. His vitals were carefully checked and everything looked good. The doctor had given me a complete list of pills that Dad could take before the surgery. Once again, I had strongly expressed my concerns about the anesthesia after which the doctor had made some notes in Dad's chart reflecting this. I had helped Mom make a detailed schedule for everything that needed to happen prior to the procedure. Even though I had to call and remind her several times, she had done a good job getting Dad ready.

He had showered the night before with the Betasept solution that we were given. For some reason, he chose to bathe in the hall bath which had a shower curtain instead of his shower with the glass door. He unfortunately hadn't secured the curtain completely and water had leaked out onto the floor. Mom had come in afterwards and had to mop it up.

I had told Dad several times that he wasn't to eat or drink anything after midnight. Mom had also made several signs to remind him of this. One was taped to the fridge, one was taped to the bathroom mirror and one was placed on the kitchen counter. We were hoping that this effort would be sufficient.

When I arrived at my parents' home this morning, Dad was very agitated. My parents were arguing about whether Dad had eaten anything during the night. I interrupted the argument, but not before he told her to shut up. I had noticed that when Dad had raised his voice, Barron had timidly hidden under the coffee table in the family room.

While Dad was getting his jacket from the coat closet in the foyer, Mom started whispering to me. "When I came down this morning, I noticed that two donuts were missing from the package," she said. "I had just bought them yesterday. They hadn't been opened yet." She carefully peaked around the hallway to make sure Dad wasn't coming. "I asked him about it and he said that it must have been the dog. Vanessa, there is no way the dog could have opened the donut container. Your dad has been upset ever since."

My dad was honest to a fault, teaching me from an early age that lying was wrong. If he said that he didn't eat any donuts, then he truly didn't. At least, he didn't think that he had. I knew there was always the possibility that he may have eaten them, but just didn't remember.

Mom put Barron in the hall bath with some food and water. We had to coax him out from beneath the table as he was really scared. She then shut the door so he couldn't get out. They had only had Barron for a few months and Mom still didn't feel comfortable giving him the run of the house when no one was at home.

It was still dark when we slowly pulled out of the driveway. As we needed to be at the hospital by 7:15 a.m., I hoped to not hit too much traffic. We would inevitably be cutting it close.

After checking in, one of the staff members politely handed me a pager. We patiently sat in the waiting room and tried to get comfortable. Dad saw me drinking a plastic mug of coffee that I had brought from home. "Why didn't I get any coffee?" he asked.

"Dad, you're not supposed to have anything to drink before the surgery," I said. "Do you remember?" He acted like he did, but I would have to explain it one more time before they called him back.

He soon started to get a little antsy. "What are we doing here?" he asked.

"You're getting your hernia operated on," I replied. "Do you remember seeing Dr. Parker last week?" He slowly shook his head yes. "You decided that you wanted to get this taken care of once and for all. That's why we're here." Dad had repeatedly complained about the pain for weeks. Now, that we were finally doing something about it, he was acting like he didn't want to be here. It was frustrating. I knew that as sure as we cancelled the procedure, he would invariably ask when we could get it taken care of.

Before long, Dad was called back. After they got him prepped, we'd be able to visit with him one last time before the surgery. I had Dad carefully remove his dentures and put them in a small case that I kept in my bag. As I watched him slowly walk away with the nurse, I couldn't help but feel a little nervous.

About twenty minutes later, the pager suddenly went off. A nurse led Mom and I through several halls until we eventually reached Dad's room. He was lying down and smiled at the sight of us, seeming completely calm.

While we were there, the doctor came in and asked Dad a few standard questions to make sure he was lucid. Then, he took a special pen and drew a black mark directly on the right side of Dad's stomach. This was his precautionary method of reminding him and everyone else involved which side was going to be operated on.

When it became time to start administering the drugs, the nurse had us say our goodbyes. I gently kissed Dad on the cheek. "You're going to be fine, Dad," I said. "The next time I see you, your hernia is going to be fixed." We smiled at each other as I lovingly squeezed his hand. Mom said her private goodbyes as I stepped out into the hall. We were then led back out to the waiting room.

The procedure was scheduled to begin promptly at 8:45. I hoped to hear something in a couple of hours. As I made myself comfortable, I said a silent prayer that Dad would successfully make it through one more surgery.

A little while later, a nurse came out and said that everything was fine. The operation had been a success, but Dad was still sedated. Once he started to come to, we would be immediately notified.

About an hour later, we were led back to Dad's room. The nurse had a very concerned look on her face. "It sounds like he is saying 'No'," she said. "He has been repeating that ever since he woke up."

I stood next to Dad and warily looked at him, his pupils like pinpoints. He looked back at me, but showed absolutely no recognition, his mind appearing somewhere far off. "Daddy, it's Vanessa," I said. "Do you know where you are?"

"No, no, no," he cried. It was breaking my heart. He sounded terrified, like he was in a very dark place. I had absolutely no idea what was going on in his head. I couldn't even begin to imagine what he was experiencing right then.

I tenderly held his hand. "Dad, can you hear me?" I asked. No matter what I did, I couldn't seem to reach him.

He kept frantically looking around the room as he continued "No, no." I stayed by his side hoping my presence would eventually bring him back. I didn't know what else to do.

The moaning continued for about ten more minutes. I didn't want him to get any more upset, but I didn't feel like I was making a positive difference. Mom and I sat down in the plastic chairs next to his bed, but continued to keep our eyes firmly on Dad. He was not in a good place.

Within a couple of minutes, Dad started looking at me. I stood up and quickly returned to his side, wanting so much to believe that he knew who I was. "Dad, do you need something?" I asked. I couldn't seem to get anything out of him as he just stared at me.

The nurse was busy handling post operation matters. She had brought me a portable DVD player and asked that I watch a segment involving administering a daily shot to my dad once we got him home. I tried to watch the DVD, but it was so hard to concentrate. I needed to tend to Dad.

I had hoped that the more time that passed, the more Dad would return to his normal self. Unfortunately, he soon got belligerent and his tone completely changed. I dreaded what I suspected was coming. I quietly sat down and decided to once again leave him alone.

As the drugs continued to wear off, Dad actually began to talk more. He also became more combative as his words turned ugly. When they would get to be too much, I would reluctantly sit down and distract myself with the DVD. Then, Dad would invariably look at me and ask something. Thinking that things were going to be different this time, I would get up and return to his side. No matter what I said, he would end up saying something argumentative. It was a pattern that I had seen several times before. My stomach was in knots and I really didn't want to go through this again. I had known beforehand that the anesthesia would do this to him, but I couldn't do anything to change it. I felt so unbelievably worn down.

As Dad became more aware of his unfamiliar surroundings, he became more restless. "What are you two doing to me?" he asked.

"We're trying to get you better, Dad," I responded. "You had your hernia operated on. Once you recover from the procedure, you should feel much better."

"Why are you two doing this to me?" he repeated. I felt like he hadn't heard a word I said. No matter what my response was, he had something contentious to say in return. I knew that getting defensive was not the right thing to do. I had to dig so deep inside of myself to prevent that from happening.

The drugs were clearly doing this to him. This was absolutely not my father. My concern now was whether he would completely recover once the drugs were out of his system. Would this procedure end up stealing a little bit more of my dad just like the others had?

We tried several different positions, but it didn't seem to matter. Dad just couldn't seem to get comfortable. He was still hooked up to several monitors which wasn't helping any. I tried to adjust the bed so that he was sitting more upright, seeming to help for a little bit.

Before long, he wanted to get out of the bed to use the bathroom. The nurse had to help Dad as he couldn't walk by himself yet. Fortunately, the restroom was right across the hall. Until Dad could actually walk on his own, they wouldn't release him to go home.

After the nurse slowly led him back to the room, we got Dad situated in his bed. Within a minute, he was asking when he could leave. "Daddy, they won't let you leave until you can walk on your own," I said. "There are still drugs in your system. It may take awhile. You need to be patient." That was clearly not what he wanted to hear.

He was very agitated. As he continued to move around restlessly in the bed, the small monitor that was clipped over his thumb came off, ultimately causing the alarm to sound. I quickly reattached it, but not before the nurse came back in. "Dad, tell me what we can do to make you more comfortable," I said. He continued looking at me, seemingly unable to put into words what he wanted.

It left me trying different things on my own in hopes that one of them might actually work. At this point, it was a guessing game. Finally, I decided to sit him upright with the help of his nurse which seemed to calm him down for a little while.

I then had Dad drink some grape juice. He was very thirsty and that also seemed to help. "When can we go home?" he questioned. Dad had constantly asked this for over an hour now. I wasn't surprised as he always got like this in the hospital. He couldn't wait to get there, but then not long after he would arrive, he couldn't wait to leave. It never failed as he always seemed to get anxious in this environment. I knew that all of the noise and beeps and interruptions really bothered him. It was definitely not a peaceful setting.

A lot of outstanding issues still needed to be taken care of before we left. Since I would primarily be caring for Dad, I needed to make sure that I completely understood everything. The nurse gave me all of the instructions for Dad's care which included two new prescriptions, one a pain medication and the other Lovenox. As soon as she left the room, I searched my purse for an ibuprofen. My head was killing me.

After several hours, we were finally given permission to get Dad dressed. He was still a little shaky on his feet, so I had to help him with his clothing. Not long after that, the nurse had Dad carefully walk in the hallway. He still wasn't completely back to normal, but they agreed to discharge him anyway. I called Randy to see if he could pick Chris up from school. We were running late and I didn't want to have to take Dad through the car rider lane. It might unexpectedly set him off and I didn't want a scene at the elementary school.

I quickly drove the car around while the nurse brought Dad out in the wheelchair. On the familiar drive to Buford, he seemed much better. The thought of going home had calmed him down considerably.

After we arrived, I slowly walked Dad inside and got him comfortably situated in his recliner. Barron immediately jumped up on his lap. Dad seemed a little tired, apparently still under the effects of the anesthesia. I had a feeling that he'd be fast asleep when I returned.

I set off for Walmart to get Dad's prescriptions filled. I would start his Lovenox shots tomorrow morning. The pain killer would be hidden and only used in an emergency. The last thing I wanted was to introduce any more drugs into his system.

That night, Bob had driven over after work to check on them. He found Dad sitting in his usual recliner where he remained very quiet all evening. Most of the conversation was between Bob and Mom, with Dad just listening.

It really hadn't surprised me as Dad had looked that exact same way when I left him this afternoon. It was an extremely long day for him. He had gotten up very early and had gone through a lot during the course of the day. I assumed that as soon as his head hit the pillow, he'd be out and sleep through the night. At least, I was hoping so.

Thursday, February 17, 2011

It was eerily quiet as I slowly opened the front door. Normally it wouldn't have concerned me, but today I felt a little apprehensive. No sooner had I shut the door than he quickly came running down the stairs. "Hey Buddy," I said as I scratched his little head. He was all wiggles as I let him out back.

While Barron was outside, I carefully got my parents' daily medications ready. I was sitting at the breakfast area table when my dad suddenly walked into the room. "Hi Dad," I said.

"Hi Pootie," he replied, sitting down next to me and smiling. He seemed to be doing much better. I routinely checked his blood sugar before giving him his meds and orange juice. Everything looked good. "Are you in any pain, Dad?" I asked.

"Not really," he replied. I was so happy to hear this. I really hoped to refrain from having to give him any pain medication.

"Are you hungry?" I asked. "How about your usual breakfast?"

"That sounds good," he responded happily. With that, I made him a bowl of cereal and fruit, with a small piece of sweet roll on the side.

While he was busily eating, I went upstairs to check on Mom who was still lying in bed. "Mom, are you alright?" I asked. She was still very groggy. "Did you sleep okay?"

"I don't remember," she said. "I guess that means I did." We both smiled at that.

"Do you want to come downstairs for some breakfast?" I asked.

"Give me about five minutes and then I'll be down," she replied.

After breakfast, I had Dad sit on the loveseat as it was time for his first shot. It needed to be administered by 9:00 each morning. I had watched the DVD and read the directions three times, but still, I was nervous. I had never actually given anybody a shot before.

I rolled Dad's shirt up and rolled the waistband of his pants down to expose his midsection. Then, I took an alcohol swab and gently wiped the area thoroughly. Dad just sat there as calm as ever. The look on his face said that he had complete confidence in me even if I didn't. That alone gave me the strength to proceed.

I squeezed the skin together on the left side of his belly button. I then carefully positioned the syringe needle at a 90 degree angle to the pinched area of skin. I firmly pushed the needle through his skin until it was completely in. Then, I pushed the plunger slowly until all of the liquid was gone. As I pulled the syringe back out, Dad smiled at me. "I did it!" I squealed. It was just a simple shot, but it had felt like a major accomplishment to me.

While Dad's stomach was bare, I gently removed the bandage over the incision site. The staple was still intact and the area looked good. "Dad, tonight you can take a shower," I said. "Just don't take this bandage off. We can remove it tomorrow." He seemed fine with this. I knew a hot shower would undoubtedly make him feel brand new.

As I left later that day, I gave Dad strict instructions that he wasn't to lift anything. "You need to lie around and watch television or take a nap," I said. "Please do not go into the basement," I said in my scary voice. He then laughed.

As I walked out, I told Mom to keep a close eye on him and to call if they needed anything. It was so nice to have Dad feel comfortable again and not be in such pain. The surgery was officially behind us. I didn't know if there would be any repercussions from it or not. All we could do was move forward and pray that the anesthesia hadn't done any lasting damage.

Sunday, February 20, 2011

The smell of garlic toast had permeated every room in the house. Spaghetti sauce had now simmered on the stove for a couple of hours. It was the most relaxing and delicious dinner that we'd had in awhile. As I finished the dishes, I began to think about my dad, recovering so nicely from the hernia surgery. I had routinely given him his fourth shot of Lovenox this morning. It was old hat to me now. The bandage had been removed and it was healing fine. I'd take him to see Dr. Parker later this week to get the staple removed.

Later this evening, the phone suddenly rang. I immediately became alarmed when I saw that it was Mom. A phone call this late was never good news. "Vanessa, your father fell," she said. "He had gotten up to go to the bathroom. I was reading and heard a loud thud. When I went to check on him, I found him on the floor. The clothes hamper was on its side. He must have grabbed it as he was falling down."

"Mom, is he okay?" I frantically asked. "Did he hit his head on anything?" I began to panic.

"He seems okay right now," she replied. "I called 911 and the paramedics are here with him. They're getting ready to put Dad on the stretcher and take him to Parkland General Hospital. I'll follow them in my car."

"Will you stop by my house and pick me up?" I asked. My house was right off of Buford Drive and I knew that was the fastest method of getting to the hospital. I would probably see the ambulance drive by while I waited for Mom.

"Sure, I'll be there shortly," she responded. I then called Bob, who agreed to go over to their house later to get Barron. At this point, we didn't know how long they'd be gone.

Not long after I hung up the phone, I saw Mom's headlights in the driveway. I kissed Randy and Shawn goodbye and promised to call as soon as I knew anything. Chris was already sound asleep in his bed.

On the way to the hospital, Mom filled me in on the details of Dad's fall. "When the paramedic checked his blood sugar, it was in the low 40's," she said.

I couldn't believe it. In all of the time that I had checked Dad's blood sugar, it was never below 100, much less in the 40's. "Had he taken his evening meds tonight?" I curiously asked. One of his evening medications was for his diabetes. He took 10 mg. of Glipizide every night.

"Yes," Mom replied. "It was a normal evening. Nothing out of the ordinary had happened."

"I'm just thankful that you heard him fall and were there to help him," I said, knowing that it could have been disastrous if she hadn't.

Not long after we arrived at the emergency room, we were taken back to Dad's room. He was comfortably lying in the bed and was completely calm. "Dad, do you remember what happened?" I asked.

"Not too much, Pootie," he answered. "I had gone to the bathroom and was walking back to my bed. That's the last thing I remember. The next thing I know there are several guys standing around me."

"Are you hurting anywhere?" I asked.

"No," he replied.

"What part of your head did you hit?" I questioned. He pointed to the area above his right eye. I carefully looked at his head, but didn't see any visible marks. Even though the skin wasn't punctured in any way, I knew that there still could be an internal injury that we just couldn't see.

A nurse soon came in to check all of Dad's vitals and gather information from me. "Mr. Lee, we need to do a CT scan on you," she said. "Would that be okay?" Dad nodded his head yes.

Before long, an orderly came into the room to get Dad, wheeling him away in his current bed. "We'll be waiting for you right here, Dad," I said, gently touching his arm as he rolled by. He turned towards me and smiled lovingly.

Mom and I tried to relax while Dad was gone. Emergency rooms weren't known for their comfort. Unfortunately, it was probably going to be a long night.

A little while later, the orderly brought Dad back into the room, followed by the doctor who informed us that Dad's diabetes medication needed to be lowered. He had lost so much weight that his current dosage was now too high. The doctor would return once she had the results of the scan.

We all tried to get as comfortable as possible. Dad was a little chilly, so I went out into the hall and found him a couple of warm blankets. I tucked them snugly around him and he seemed content. The lights in the room were very bright. I tried to dim them, but unfortunately my choices were either on or off. I managed to find a small light above the sink that I turned on instead of the overhead light which made a big difference.

Mom and I had to sleep sitting upright in the standard plastic chairs. It was miserable, but Dad would never hear that from us. Every time he woke up and looked at me with his loving eyes, I could tell how bad he felt. He was truly sorry that we were so uncomfortable, but it didn't really matter how we felt. We were there for him and wouldn't leave his side. He soon closed his eyes and fell asleep.

Monday, February 21, 2011

As I glanced over at my parents, I realized that it was only a dream, my heart racing as I thought back about the terrifying incident. I was stranded late at night and my car wouldn't start. I had locked myself safely inside, or so I thought. The image of his face suddenly appearing against my window had awoken me. As I repeatedly blinked my eyes, I found myself safe and sound in the emergency room. Dad was still asleep, but Mom looked like she hadn't slept at all. She soon opened her eyes and glanced over at me. I smiled at her.

As it neared 6:00 a.m., I informed Mom that I needed to go home and help get Chris ready for school. I saw no problem with this as Dad had remained completely calm the entire night. My mom generously gave me the keys to her car. By now, Dad was awake as well. I gently kissed both of my parents goodbye and promised to be back by 8:15.

I hadn't even got Chris to school before my eerie ringtone sounded. We were actually in the driveway loading up. Mom sounded frantic. "Vanessa, are you coming back soon?" she asked. I could hear Dad's angry voice in the background, sounding extremely upset.

"I'm on my way to the elementary school, Mom," I replied. "I'll be back to the hospital in about thirty minutes. What's wrong?" When I had left them less than two hours ago, everything was fine. How could things have digressed so quickly?

"They moved your father to a regular hospital room," she said. "He thinks he is in a motel. He's very confused and very agitated. Please hurry, Vanessa."

My heart started racing once again. The whole time as I drove Chris to school, all I could think of was the chaos that was currently erupting in my Dad's hospital room. I prayed that God would get me back there in time.

When I later entered Dad's room, he looked completely disheveled. Why did this always seem to happen after I would leave? Before I could say a word, Dad looked at me and asked "Why am I in this motel?"

"Daddy, this is the hospital," I replied. "It's just a regular room that you've been moved into." I had to admit as I looked around that it was very nice. The room that we were in was in a newly renovated wing of the hospital. The walls had dark wood paneling on them and there was a nice sitting area by the window for guests, leaving me very impressed.

I pulled the recliner next to his bed and sat down. "I know it looks fancy, but you're still in the hospital," I said. "You had a bad fall and they want to keep you for another day." I actually had not talked to anyone yet, so I wasn't sure how much longer they wanted to keep Dad. "They couldn't keep you where you were. It was part of the emergency room. Besides, it wasn't comfortable. This room will be much better." My words seemed to slowly calm him down.

When the nurse came in, I asked her if Dad could have a bowl of cereal with a banana and some juice. He hadn't wanted the hot meal that was brought in earlier. "That's no problem," she responded. "I'll let them know." She smiled and quickly left the room.

By the time Dad finished his breakfast, he was in a much better mood. I then found the remote control and turned the television on. The more I could get this room to resemble his family room at home, the more comfortable he would probably feel. I knew it would go a long way in keeping him calm.

I noticed that Mom was sitting in another chair across the room from Dad, wiping her eyes with a tissue. She had clearly been crying. I didn't know what words were said before I had returned, but I imagined that she had received the brunt of Dad's anxiety attack. I didn't often see her in tears.

"What is wrong, Shirley?" Dad asked.

"I'm tired, Chester," she answered. "I'm tired of going through this. Nothing ever changes. You blow up at me. You say really mean things to me. Then, you apologize. Sometimes, you don't even do that. You expect me to just go on each time we go through this like nothing ever happened. I just can't do this anymore." Her voice was quivering.

Dad tried to make good of the situation, but nothing he said could fix this. It was quite possible that he didn't even remember everything that was said. My heart was breaking for my mother because I couldn't imagine what she had been living with for so long. It was breaking for my father as well. It certainly wasn't his fault that he had been inflicted with this terrible disease. Nothing about this heart wrenching situation was fair.

As time went on, we slowly got accustomed to the new room. Dad ate a good portion of his hot lunch. With more than enough for two people, he generously made sure that Mom ate some, too.

The nurse had come in earlier and led me to believe that they wanted to keep Dad for another day, but we were still waiting for the doctor to come in. Dad soon began to get restless. "When am I going to go home?" he asked.

"Dad, I think they want to keep you until tomorrow," I replied. "Once the doctor comes in, we can ask him." That seemed to pacify him for the moment.

Ten minutes later, Dad again let me know that he wanted to go home. "Why am I still here when everyone else has already gone?" he asked.

"Daddy, nobody has left," I said. "They are all still in their own rooms."

I could sense the combativeness starting to come out. "Pootie, if you walk around the hall, you're going to see that I'm the only one who hasn't gone home," he stated.

For the next hour, Dad continued to voice his belief that the other patients had already been discharged. Regardless of what I said, it hadn't changed his mind. At one point, I exhaustively left the room. He probably thought I was checking for myself. The truth was I needed a break.

As soon as I returned, he looked at me and said "Well?"

"Dad, I told you," I replied, feeling exasperated. "All of the other patients are still in their own rooms. Nobody has left." He just stared irately at me. I knew what he wanted me to do, but that was where I drew the line.

"Dad, I am not going room to room looking for patients that are still here just to prove a point," I said. "You need to trust me on this one." My patience was running exceedingly thin. I hadn't slept in over thirty-two hours and I felt completely run-down. Most of all, I was tired of this hospital game. It was always the same.

Dad started to say something, but then gave me that look that said it wasn't worth it. He was apparently mad at me. I then moved to the cushion in front of the window. Mom was already seated there reading the newspaper. She looked at me and could obviously tell that I was at the end of my rope. Nobody said a word after that.

Before long, the doctor came in to examine Dad, seemingly happy with his progress. I mentioned to the doctor that Dad wanted to go home today. "You don't want to stay here another day, Mr. Lee?" he asked.

"I'd rather go home if I can," he replied, appearing very calm with the doctor.

"Well, I don't see a problem with that," the doctor said. "If you're really sure you want to leave us?" He amiably smiled at Dad. Then, he turned to the nurse and told her to go ahead and prepare Dad's discharge papers.

The doctor then looked at me. "We are going to lower his Glipizide to

5 mg.," he said. "He'll still get it two times a day, in the morning and at night. Just keep checking his blood sugar. If it drops again, you need to call us."

As the time neared 2:15, they still weren't quite ready. "I need to go pick Chris up," I said, looking at my mom. "I should be back by 3:15. Just call me on my cell phone when Dad is discharged. If I get back before then, we'll come up here to the room. Otherwise, we'll wait in the pickup lane downstairs."

As I returned to the hospital an hour later, I got a phone call from Mom. "Hi Mom," I said. "Have they discharged Dad yet?"

"Yes," she replied. "We're trying to get him dressed right now." Her voice undeniably indicated something was terribly wrong. "How far away are you?"

"I should be there in about five minutes," I said. We agreed that Chris and I would wait for them in front of the lobby doors.

As I pulled up in front of the hospital, Mom and Dad were nowhere to be seen. I had Chris move to the backseat. My phone then rang again. "Vanessa, your father says he won't ride with you," Mom said. I could hear Dad in the background trying to argue with Mom while she was on the phone with me.

"I told her, Chester," Mom said. "She is already downstairs. Why don't we just ride home with her?"

"I already told you once, Shirley!" he exclaimed. "I'm not riding with her! I swear you can be so stupid sometimes." Mom said nothing at this, clearly trying not to upset him anymore than he already was. "Have her call Bob!" he demanded. "I'll ride with him."

"Chester, Bob is at work," Mom replied.

"Shut up, Shirley!" Dad yelled.

"You shouldn't talk to your wife like that, Mr. Lee," said one of the nurses.

"I'll talk to her any way I want!" he said angrily. I could hear two different people trying to calm Dad down, as he sounded out of control. It was happening again. As I listened to what was currently unfolding in his room, I began to feel nauseous.

"Vanessa, can you call Bob?" Mom asked. "He will not get in the car with you."

"I heard," I said. "I'll call you back as soon as I talk to him."

I realized that calling Bob was the best solution at this point. Chris was in the backseat and I didn't want him to witness Dad in his current state, knowing it would upset him. I was also afraid to drive with Dad in the car. I didn't want him to get upset with me and unexpectedly jump out of the car on the way to their home.

I called Bob and explained the situation. It was not the ideal time for him to be leaving work. Unfortunately, we had no other choice.

Before Bob got there, I looked up to see a nurse pushing Dad in the wheelchair. It was just a formality because as soon as they passed through the glass doors, he immediately got up and started walking towards the car. He had his blue pants on, with the hospital gown hanging loosely over them. Apparently, they weren't able to get him completely dressed. He walked up to the passenger door and I rolled the window down.

"Why are you doing this to me?" he asked.

"I haven't done anything to you, Dad," I replied.

Mom then walked up beside the car. "Vanessa has been here all night with you," she said. "She is trying to take care of you, Chester."

"Shut up, Shirley!" he again yelled.

"Mr. Lee, please don't talk to your wife like that," the nurse again said. He then stormed off, looking determined to take control of the situation.

By now, people were beginning to stare as Dad's voice grew louder, looking like a mad man.

As soon as Bob pulled up beside me, Dad got into his truck and quickly shut the door. He then told Bob to step on it. He desperately wanted out of there and he clearly didn't want anyone to stop him.

I was in shock at what had just played out. I was a total wreck. I looked over at Mom as she got into the car, looking completely run-down. As I slowly looked back at Chris, I prayed that he was okay, his precious blue eyes just staring at me. He didn't say a word. I knew I would have to talk to him later about what he had just witnessed.

My heart was still racing. I couldn't even sort through everything that had just happened. The one thing that I did know was that I absolutely despised this fucking disease. I wanted to scream at the top of my lungs. I hated it! I hated it! I hated it! It was destroying our lives. Every single day, it reared its ugly head and took a little more from us. Three months ago, I knew nothing about Alzheimer's or Sundowner's. Now, I knew more than I ever wanted to.

I drove the three of us to my home in Mom's car. Chris and I got out as Mom moved behind the wheel. "Mom, I am scared to death of you going home and being alone with Dad," I said. "Do you need to stay here?"

"No, that might make it worse," she replied. "I'll watch myself."

"Please be careful, Mom," I pleaded. "Don't say anything to Dad that might upset him. Call me any time. Okay?" She nodded and then kissed me goodbye.

An hour later, Bob called me on his way back to work. After they had arrived at the house, Dad was very restless. He got the mail and after looking through it, he secretly hid it under one of the seat cushions at the breakfast area table.

As soon as Mom had walked in the door, Dad immediately wanted to talk to her. She had told him that she was hungry and that they needed to eat dinner first. The truth was she just wasn't up to it at the moment. They could talk later.

I tensely called Mom later that night to find out that Dad was doing okay at the time. No further incidents had occurred, but she was walking on eggshells. I reiterated for her to please be careful. I was a nervous wreck.

Late that night after everybody had gone to bed, I thought about what had happened earlier, feeling that I might have made a big mistake. I knew that something was wrong with my dad. I knew that he needed to be tested. I actually had him in a hospital room which was the perfect opportunity. I could have gone into the hall and found the doctor and spoke to him without my dad hearing. I could have told him that there was a good chance that my dad had Alzheimer's, that I was worried and that he needed to be evaluated. They would surely have seen the signs. They could have kept him and done the necessary testing.

For some reason, I didn't. I had just wanted to keep him calm and I knew that prolonging his stay would have only upset him more. Maybe I should have taken advantage of the situation. In the long run, it might have been for the better. But, I hadn't said anything to the doctor. I had held back and now, I wondered if I would come to regret it. I was worried sick. It was going to be another sleepless night.

Tuesday, February 22, 2011

The sweet sound of Chris gently calling my name had startled me. As I slowly opened my eyes, I saw his precious face, obviously not feeling well. I pulled back the covers and he eagerly crawled in next to me. I then held him close. At a time in my life that was so full of despair, this simple act of cuddling with my youngest son was such a blessing. I truly hoped that this incredible warmth inside of me would remain. I had a bad feeling about today.

As I later drove to my parents' home, I was very nervous, having absolutely no idea how Dad was going to respond to me. The last time that I had seen him had not gone well. In fact, he was very upset with me. I hoped that a good night's sleep in his own bed had somehow made a difference.

When I pulled into the driveway, I noticed that the garage door was open, Dad sitting in a plastic chair just inside the door. I wasn't sure why he was out there. Maybe he was waiting on me.

"Hi Dad," I said, as I walked up to him. He said nothing, nor did he smile. He just stared coldly at me. It was impossible to mistake his look, obviously still mad at me. I sadly continued past him into the house.

When I walked inside, I found Mom in the kitchen. "Hi," I said, as I gently kissed her cheek. "How is Dad doing? I just walked past him and he didn't even acknowledge me. I can tell he's still upset."

"Actually, he seems okay this morning," she replied. "He's been very calm. I've made sure that I haven't said anything that would upset him."

"Well, that's good," I said. "I guess it's just me." I then carefully packaged my parents' medications. A minute later, Dad came inside and sat at the breakfast area table. I placed his pills in front of him with a glass of orange juice. He still wouldn't talk to me. I knew it was best to leave well enough alone, so I quietly went into the family room and sat down. I had decided that the last thing I wanted was to upset him anymore. I also felt terrible as Chris and I were both coming down with colds. I didn't have the energy for a confrontation today. I was determined to stay out of Dad's way and give him the time and space that he needed.

He soon followed me into the room. "I need to give you your Lovenox shot, Dad," I said. "We missed a day while you were in the hospital." He still said nothing, but sat calmly in the loveseat while I got the shot ready. I carefully administered it without any problems. "Do you want a Glucerna?" He shook his head yes. I hoped that he was slowly coming around.

After I gave Dad his shake, I went back into the breakfast area to get their evening meds ready. Before long, Dad went upstairs to take a nap. He still hadn't said anything to me. "Mom, I think I'm going to go on home," I said. "I need to take a nap and I really don't want either of you to get my cold." I looked lovingly at my mother, both of us still so drained. "It's probably best that I leave. Call me if you need me." I then hugged her goodbye.

Later that night, Mom did call me. "I talked to your father," she said.

"What happened?" I asked.

"I told him that he needed to apologize to you," she replied. "All you do every single day is take care of him. Even when you're sick like today, you still come over."

"You didn't need to do that, Mom," I said.

"Yes, I did," she responded. "He was being stubborn. Now, I want you to try and get some rest tonight. Don't worry about us."

"I'll try, Mom" I said. "I promise." With that, I hung up the phone.

Tonight, Shawn was inducted into the National Honor Society. I was so unbelievably proud of him. Unfortunately, Chris and I were feeling much worse. I knew that the best thing for us was to get in bed early. Randy had generously offered to take Shawn to the ceremony instead. I hated that I couldn't go as it would be one of the few times that I had ever missed one of the boy's activities. I truly hoped that it would be the last.

Wednesday, February 23, 2011

As I silently opened the front door, Barron ran up to me and smiled with that adorable under bite. I would never tire of seeing it or those liquid brown eyes, so full of love. Whatever unhappy feelings I had when I walked in this morning had quickly melted away. I continued my way into the family room where I saw Dad peacefully sitting in his recliner. I routinely checked his blood sugar and then gave him his morning meds. Physically, he looked very good. He had an unusually serious look on his face though. "Pootie, I want to apologize to you," he said. I attentively looked at my dad and waited for him to continue. He was completely calm. "I shouldn't have treated you the way that I did. It was uncalled for."

"Thank you, Dad," I replied. "I appreciate you saying that." I smiled at him lovingly as I knew how hard that was for him to say.

"Mom said that you and Chris are both sick," he continued.

I shook my head yes. "We both caught colds," I said.

"Are you feeling any better?" he asked.

"I feel really tired," I responded. "It'll probably just take a few days to get it out of my system."

"What about Chris?" Dad asked, absolutely hating when one of his grandchildren was sick.

"He's doing okay," I replied. "He managed to go to school today."

"Well, you need to take care of yourself," he said. "You don't have to stay here all day. Go home and get some rest."

At that point, I surprisingly noticed that Dad's right eye was black and blue. It wasn't until he had turned his head towards the light that I had seen it. "Dad, have you seen your eye?" I asked. It really looked bad. "Your right eye is all black and blue underneath. Is it hurting?"

"No," he replied. "I guess I haven't looked in the mirror today. I hadn't noticed it."

"It's probably from the fall that you had the other night," I said. "You must have hit your head on the counter when you fell." This really alarmed me as the bathroom counter top was marble and very hard. If he had accidentally hit the corner of it right next to where the hamper had fallen, he may have done some serious internal damage. The hospital hadn't mentioned anything about a concussion. I had an uneasy feeling that his fall was a lot worse than we had realized.

After breakfast, I gave Dad his daily Lovenox shot and then carefully checked the incision. It was healing nicely and the staple was still secure.

Today was the first day since Dad's fall that things had felt like normal. I had hated not speaking to him. It just wasn't natural. It felt so remarkably good to have everything cleared up between us. As I continued to look at Dad, I realized that even with his black eye, he was still the most handsome man I had ever known.

I remembered a day a couple of years back when I had conveniently stopped in the Kroger near my home. I was walking down the main aisle near the registers, on my way to the pharmacy. I suddenly looked up and immediately was taken aback by the handsomeness of this older gentleman. For a split second, there had been absolutely no recognition of who this man was. It was that first moment when you see someone, the incredible point before your brain realizes who it is and you truly have a "first impression" moment. It was those times that the most genuine thoughts within us came out.

In the blink of an eye, the moment then passed and I found myself looking at my dad. All I could think at that moment was "What an incredibly handsome man he is!" He still hadn't seen me at this point. He was dressed casually in a pair of nice pants with a button down shirt and looked so trim, his hair perfectly combed. I felt unbelievably proud that he was my father.

He soon looked up and saw me, both of us smiling. As we soon came together, we kissed each other and said our hellos. We then chatted for about ten minutes before we both went our own ways.

As I watched him leave the store, I remembered thinking how lucky I felt to be able to live in the same town and possibly run into my dad at any moment. I was so thankful that my parents had made the decision to move here, unquestionably changing my life for the better. I was even more thankful that he was my dad. I was truly blessed.

Thursday, February 24, 2011

He had an unusual look about him today that I couldn't put my finger on. I smiled, but got little response. Something was definitely different. It had started out like any other normal day. I had routinely checked Dad's blood sugar. He had taken his morning meds and had received his daily shot. Nothing at all seemed out of the ordinary.

For some reason though, Dad was not himself. He soon began complaining about his teeth as one of his dentures was evidently hurting him, this being the first time I had heard about this issue. Mom then got on the phone and called her dentist. Fortunately, they'd be able to see Dad in the morning at 10 a.m. which seemed to momentarily satisfy him.

He soon went upstairs to take a nap. In no time, he came back down, his teeth still bothering him. He was getting very restless. I gave him some ibuprofen to help with the pain after which he went back upstairs to try to get some sleep.

Later that day, I got an unexpected call from Mom. "Vanessa, your father wants to talk to you," she said, her voice clearly indicating that something was wrong.

"Pootie, your mother says she is not going to the dentist with us tomorrow," Dad said, sounding agitated.

"She's going with us, Dad," I replied.

"She decided that she was not going," he repeated slowly.

"I promise you that she is going, Dad," I responded. "I have never been to her dentist. She has to come with us so I know how to get there. Don't worry. Okay?"

"You're telling me she is going with us?" he asked again.

"Yes, Daddy," I replied, trying my hardest to reassure him over the phone. He sounded like he was on the verge of getting really upset. "Dad, why don't you go upstairs and take a nap? It might make you feel better." I then heard him hand the phone back to Mom, but I could still hear him faintly talking in the background. I had a terrible feeling that something bad was going to happen.

Mom then put the phone back up to her ear. "Mom, did Dad go back upstairs?" I asked.

"Yes," she whispered, "but he is moving very slowly."

"What happened?" I then asked.

"After you left, he came back downstairs," she replied. "It was probably no more than fifteen minutes later. He was not making any sense. Somehow, he got it in his head that I wasn't going to the dentist tomorrow. No matter what I said, he argued. Then, he got ugly and insisted that I would go to the appointment tomorrow."

"I think the best thing for him right now is to take a nap," I remarked.

"I agree," Mom said. "I'll call you and let you know how he is doing. Please don't call here. I'm afraid the phone will wake him up. It's right next to his bed."

"Okay, I won't," I said. "But please call me and let me know what is happening."

That afternoon, I got another startling phone call from Mom. "Your father will not stay in bed," she whispered. "He is up every five minutes. No matter what I am doing, he finds me. He is making me very nervous, Vanessa."

"Mom, I don't like the sound of this," I said. "You need to have a plan in case things get out of control."

"I do, Vanessa," she replied. "I have my keys in my pocket. I left my purse in the car. The deadbolt on the kitchen door is unlocked. If something happens, I'll make a run for it into the garage. I can lock the deadbolt from the outside so your father can't get out. By the time he finds any keys, I will already be in the car and have backed out of the driveway."

I tried to catch my breath as I listened to her, feeling sick to my stomach. This wasn't some stranger that she was talking about. It was my father. I felt so incredibly guilty talking about him behind his back. Even though I knew it was the disease and not really him, I felt like I was betraying Dad. I had to keep reminding myself that he was sick and not in control of his actions. My heart was breaking. As I reluctantly hung up the phone, the tears began to fall.

I called Bob at work to let him know what was happening. He didn't feel good about the situation either.

Not much later, Mom called again, this time from the bonus room. I could clearly hear that Dad had come into the room.

"Who are you talking to?" he asked sternly.

"I'm talking to Vanessa," she replied. He then told her to hang up the phone. "I need to go, Vanessa." She carefully set the phone down, but never hung it up.

I could hear Dad talking in a very controlling tone. It was undeniably the same tone that I had heard once before. "Shirley, you better not sell this house," he said.

"Chester, why would I ever sell this house?" she questioned. "I love this house."

"Well, this is my house and you better not sell it even if I'm not here," he said firmly. My skin began to crawl. This disturbing conversation and what was potentially about to happen was the last thing I wanted to witness. For both of my parents' safety, I unfortunately had no choice. Dad then slowly walked out of the room and Mom got back on the phone. I was scared to death. The voice that I had heard didn't sound like my dad, even though I knew it was him. I was now terrified for my mom's safety.

"Mom, do you understand how 911 works?" I asked.

"I don't think so," she replied.

"If, God forbid, something happens and you are ever in any danger, just pick up the phone and press the keys for 911," I said. "You don't have to say anything. Just set the phone down. They'll trace the call and get your address. Okay?" I was getting more nauseous by the second. I prayed that it would never come to this, but I also prayed that if it did, she would remember what to do.

In tears, I called the National Alzheimer's Hotline, the operator quickly transferring me to the Georgia Chapter of the Alzheimer's Association. After I explained the dire situation, the counselor put me on hold while she quickly phoned one of her peers. Not long after that, a conference call was set up with two counselors where they explained the necessary process should it get violent. If 911 were called, the paramedics would take Dad to the emergency room where he would be evaluated. If he were suspected of mental illness, they'd transfer him to the nearest psychiatric hospital for a complete mental evaluation.

I tried with all my might to be strong, but I couldn't stop crying. They looked up the nearest psychiatric facility which was called Woodland Hospital. They then instructed me to call them back if I needed anything else as they were only a phone call away. Someone would call tomorrow to check on us.

I then called Woodland Hospital and explained the current situation. The man on the phone checked and they actually did have a bed open. "The best thing would be if your dad came in voluntarily to be tested," he said. "Do you think that he would do that?"

"I honestly don't know how he would feel about that," I responded. Inside, I seriously doubted that Dad would commit himself to a facility to be tested. I didn't think he would have any problem doing it on an outpatient basis, but he wouldn't want to be away from home overnight. I wasn't feeling too confident.

After I got off the phone, I made a decision. After we took Dad to the dentist tomorrow morning, I would carefully bring up the subject of getting him tested. We had already discussed it awhile back and he had been amenable to it. If everything went well, we could drive over to Woodland Hospital afterwards, at which point I would try to talk my dad into committing himself into the hospital. It would all depend on his state of mind after the dental appointment. I knew that I needed for him to be on board with the decision. Otherwise, he would feel betrayed and probably never trust me again. I hated being in this difficult position, feeling like I was having to choose between my parents. It just wasn't fair. Nothing about this situation was fair.

As I busied myself making phone calls, I felt like I was preparing for the inevitable. I prayed that whatever happened, it would be non-violent. I was petrified over what might occur in the next 24 hours. The thought of the police being called on my dad scared me. He was not a criminal and shouldn't be around people that were. What if the police didn't believe he was sick and put him in jail? The terrifying thought of that happening made me ill. I didn't want that for my dad. He didn't deserve it. There had to be a better way to handle this.

I worried incessantly all afternoon. I couldn't call my mom because it might wake my dad up and I didn't want to make the situation any worse than it already was.

At 5:00 p.m., the phone suddenly rang, the caller id indicating that it was my mom. Dad had already taken his evening meds and he'd gone to bed for the night. Mom felt confident that everything was okay at that point. I was so unbelievably happy and felt such relief. I couldn't have asked for better news. I slowly began to breathe easier.

That evening about 7:00 p.m., Bob called me after having just talked to Mom. She had answered the phone and sounded okay. Her answers were a little short, but she said nothing to indicate that anything further had happened. I truly hoped that the phone ringing next to Dad's bed hadn't awoken him.

At about 7:30, I got another unexpected phone call from my mom. This time though, she was crying. "Vanessa, the paramedic needs to know if Dad is taking any kind of blood thinner," she said.

At that instant, my world and everything in it stopped. All I could think was that it had happened. Something terrible had happened. I knew without a doubt that nothing would ever be the same again.

Mom then passed the phone to the EMT. I carefully answered his questions and then asked one of my own. "What happened?"

"Can you come over here?" he asked in return. That was all he needed to say. Mom had actually called 911. I knew that something awful must have happened. I was in total shock. All day, I had felt like I was being pulled in a certain direction. Now that I was in the moment, I couldn't believe that something had actually occurred.

I solemnly looked at Randy. "It's happened," I said, as he hugged me tightly. No other words were necessary. For months, I had prayed that things would return to normal. I think inside though we both knew that one day it would come to this. Tonight, our lives were forever changed. There would be no more going back.

I then called Bob. He absolutely couldn't believe it since he had just talked to Mom. It must have happened right after he called. He was leaving home right then. I would follow him over.

As soon as we pulled into the subdivision, I saw flashing lights everywhere. Two fire trucks and three police cars were parked in the street, the entire road blocked. I swiftly drove up on the grass and cut through the yard to reach the driveway. All I wanted was to quickly get inside and see my parents. Bob then did the same.

The front door was wide open. As soon as I walked inside, I saw about six different uniformed men standing around. Mom was silently sitting on the stairs, appearing to be very shaken up. Dad was sitting in one of the dining room chairs putting on his brown loafers. His arms were covered in blood, but he was completely calm.

Dad looked at me and smiled. He said "There's my nurse. She takes good care of me." Dad seemed so genuinely happy to see me. "Anything you need to know about me, she's the one to ask." I wondered in disbelief how he could be in such a good mood after what had just transpired. I wondered if he even remembered anything that had happened.

One of the paramedics was currently trying to clean Dad's arms up. I assumed that Mom had scratched him in self-defense. Not only was his skin paper thin, he also took an aspirin every day which acted as a blood thinner. Both of these caused him to bleed so easily. Another paramedic simultaneously asked me questions about Dad's medications.

After they were done, they carefully walked Dad outside. I despondently watched as they helped him get into the back of the vehicle, never once complaining. He probably thought they were taking him to the hospital to get his wounds checked. I'm sure they would do that while he was there, but I knew the more crucial reason for him to be going.

One of the paramedics then approached me as he could tell I was upset. "What is going to happen to him?" I asked.

"He'll be taken to Parkland General Hospital," he replied. "They'll clean him up and then evaluate him."

"Will he be sent to Woodland Hospital?" I questioned.

"I doubt it," he responded. "Your dad doesn't belong there. Believe me. It's for people far worse off than him."

"Do you think he has Alzheimer's?" I asked.

"No, I don't," he replied. With that, he slowly walked away.

Everything that had been happening for months had culminated to this single point in time. I wanted so much to believe that the right thing would inevitably happen. Now, I wasn't so sure. I loved my daddy so much, but I knew that he desperately needed help. The worst thing would be for them to simply turn him away at the hospital without any further testing. I knew that the next time might not end the same way.

As soon as the fire trucks left, we had Mom pack a small bag with her personal things. The three of us then left for the emergency room. Barron would stay at Bob's house.

On the way over, I talked to Mom about the incident. "Mom, what happened tonight?" I asked. "Bob said he talked to you and everything seemed okay. Then, thirty minutes later, I get a phone call."

"When Bob called, your father was already up," she replied. "I was in my bed reading. I could hear him in his closet looking for something to wear to the dentist appointment. He kept coming into my room wanting me to help him pick out some clothes. I kept telling him no. The last time, I made the mistake of telling him that we could do this in the morning and that he needed to go back to bed. That set him off."

"What did he do?" I then asked.

"He came back into my room and got on top of me," she said. "He ended up straddling me in the bed. Then he started swinging at me with his fists. I put my arms up to block him. I told him to stop, but he wouldn't." Mom paused to catch her breath, still shaken up by the incident.

A part of me couldn't bear to hear the rest. This person she was describing was not my father. He could have never done that. Still, I needed for her to continue. I needed to know all of the horrid details. "What happened next, Mom?" I asked.

"I started scratching his arms in self-defense," she continued. "It was the only thing I could do. He was too strong for me. When his arms started to bleed, he finally stopped hitting me. Then, he ordered me to go to his room and get in his bed. He was blocking the side of the bed near the door, so I got out on the other side. I needed to do that anyway because that's where the phone was. He asked me why I was going the long way around the room and I told him he was in the way. He seemed to buy that. While his back was to me, I picked up the phone and pushed 911. Then, I set it down. I remembered what you had told me earlier. Your father never saw me use the phone."

"Then, I slowly got out of the bed," she said. "I wasn't sure how long it would take the police to arrive. I was hoping that if I moved slowly enough, they'd get there before I made it to his bedroom. I had no idea what he was going to do when I got there. He was yelling at me to hurry up. When we had made it to the top of the stairwell, I heard the doorbell ring. It was the police. They had gotten there in a matter of minutes." When Mom had secretly placed the phone down, it had allowed the 911

188

operator to overhear a portion of the attack. It was enough for the call to be considered an extreme emergency.

According to Mom, Dad had gone down the stairs and answered the front door. The police routinely questioned both of my parents as to what had happened. Mom told them her version. Dad unfortunately couldn't remember everything that had happened. The police had diligently checked every room in the house to verify their explanations and to make sure that no other rooms were in disarray. It probably looked a little suspicious that Mom was attacked, yet Dad was the one covered in blood. Once they were satisfied, the EMTs came into the house and checked both of my parents out. Not long after that, Bob and I had arrived.

As we walked into the emergency room, it was currently packed. Fortunately, we managed to find three seats together. It would have been so easy to ask the clerk if I could go back, but I honestly wasn't ready to see Dad. I was still so angry at him for attacking Mom. I just couldn't face him yet.

I soon went up to the desk and asked the receptionist on duty to give a message to the emergency room doctor. After he evaluated Dad, I urgently needed to talk to him. I needed to know the results. This predicament had gone on for too long. I wanted to make sure they were invariably going to do the right thing for my dad and finally get him the help that he needed.

About an hour later, the receptionist led us to a private room adjacent to the waiting area to meet with the doctor. "How is he?" I asked.

"He's very confused," the doctor replied. "He doesn't remember a lot of what happened. He actually thinks that your mother attacked him. He also keeps talking about going to the dentist tomorrow."

"What do you think is wrong with him?" I asked.

"There's a good chance he has Alzheimer's," he said. "He needs to be fully tested."

"Will he be sent to Woodland Hospital?" I inquired.

"Yes," he responded. "We're checking to see if they have an open bed right now." I already knew the answer to that.

The doctor had signed the 1013 form. Tomorrow, Dad would be involuntarily committed to the psychiatric hospital. He would finally get the mental evaluation that he desperately needed. It was certainly not the way I had wanted it to happen, but maybe it was for the best. Sometimes things happened in ways that were simply beyond our control.

As I left the emergency room, I felt heartbroken that I was also leaving my dad. An overwhelming emptiness inside my heart just wouldn't go away. I felt so guilty even though I knew we had no choice. I doubted if things would ever be the same again.

I took Mom home with me and once again put her to bed in Chris' room. I then went into my bedroom to change clothes. Afterwards, I distraughtly sat on the bed and began to pray. What started out in a calm voice eventually turned into a heated diatribe. "I don't know what you want me to do anymore," I said angrily. "No matter what I do, things continue to get worse. I need your guidance. Tell me what to do! Tell me what you want me to do!" It was at that point that I exhaustively collapsed onto the bed in tears.

Friday, February 25, 2011

I watched as Chris softly kissed her cheek, a certain tenderness about the moment making me smile. He had no idea why his Grandma Lee had slept in his bed last night or where his Papa Lee currently was. He knew nothing about the tragic event that had occurred last night. I wanted so deeply to shield this precious boy from all the ugliness of this horrid disease.

I soon left them alone while I called the emergency room, worrying about Dad all night long. The nurse said that he was doing fine and had just finished eating his breakfast. She then asked me if I wanted to talk to him, but I didn't think that was a good idea just yet. I knew that he would want to know when he was coming home and I couldn't lie to him. I thought it best to let things happen without my involvement, at least not directly. The right plans were already in motion and I needed to let them play out.

Mom had decided that she wanted to return home, seemingly doing much better. I knew that she would feel more comfortable in her own environment. After lunch, I drove her to Buford.

Late that afternoon, I again called the hospital. I had persistently called several times today and every report was exactly the same. Dad was calm and doing fine. They had expected him to be transported to Woodland Hospital very soon. Before I hung up the phone, I asked the nurse if she would tell my dad that I had called and that I loved him, truly hoping that the message would ease any anxiety he was feeling. I desperately needed him to know that I hadn't abandoned him.

That evening, Dad was eventually transferred to the psychiatric hospital, where he was admitted into their geriatric unit. The typical stay was 7 - 10 days, but it potentially could last for several weeks. It would ultimately depend on how well the testing went and how cooperative Dad was.

The standard procedure was to strip all of the current medications away from the patient. Each one would in turn be examined and reintroduced as necessary. That would allow the doctor to see if the combination of current meds was actually part of the problem. They would perform a complete mental evaluation on Dad. I felt confident that if a problem existed, it would be found at this hospital. I knew that the results of this testing could very well decide Dad's future.

Saturday, February 26, 2011

I calmly stood at the kitchen sink and looked out the window while drinking my morning coffee. Most of the trees were completely bare, except for the occasional pines scattered throughout the neighborhood. The tranquil scene before me still had such a soothing effect which I was grateful for. As I thought about the day's planned events, I was more than a little nervous.

I had called Woodland Hospital first thing this morning, but they wouldn't release any information to me until Dad formally gave his permission. The gentleman that I spoke with kindly walked over to Dad's wing and got him to sign the necessary form, which he did so willingly. The man then called me back and gave me Dad's patient number. We would need that in order to visit Dad and to get any future information about him. He also politely informed me that Dad's physician would be Dr. Franklin.

As soon as I got off the phone, I pulled up the website for Woodland Hospital, clicking on the tab for the current medical team. I couldn't believe it. The doctor that was assigned to my dad was Dr. Kenneth D. Franklin, the exact same doctor that Dad had been referred to awhile back. It was the actual doctor that we were on a waiting list to see. Dad ended up getting the very doctor that we had actively sought out so many weeks ago. What were the odds of that happening? I was thrilled at this news.

At noon, Bob, Mom and I drove to the hospital for the 12:30 – 1:30 visitation, only one of two times allowed each week to see patients. We needed to make sure we saw Dad every chance that we could. I had thought that for the first visit, it was probably best that Mom not come as we had no idea the state Dad would be in. Mom had vehemently disagreed. She was adamant that she see Dad at every single visit.

I had a hard copy of all of Dad's current medications. I wasn't sure whether the emergency room had sent them over when Dad was admitted or not, but I wasn't going to take any chances. I handed the paper to the girl at the desk and she promised to get it to Dad's doctor.

The environment at this hospital was very secure. We were routinely instructed that no personal belongings would be allowed in during visitation, including purses and cell phones. At 12:30, we were directed to go with an orderly. Normally, only two visitors were allowed back at a time. Somehow, all three of us made it through during today's visit.

The muscular orderly led us down several halls and through multiple locked doors. We were not allowed to go into the area where the patients stayed, but I managed to get a glimpse as we conveniently passed by on our way to a conference room. All of the rooms had two standard beds in them and they lined both sides of the floor. In the middle was a nurses' station, a dining area and a sitting area with a television and several couches. The patients had access to a hallway for walking that stretched around the entire area.

All of the visitors were securely taken to the meeting room. The patients had not yet been brought in. Within a couple of minutes, they slowly entered the room. I then saw my dad walk in with his pillow in his hand. He still had his black eye. As he lovingly smiled, I knew he was pleased to see us.

After we all hugged and kissed Dad, we sat down, with one of us on each side of him. We all repeatedly asked him questions about the facility. The food was so-so. His roommate was giving him problems. Everything was negative. After about five minutes, he said that he was ready to leave with us. We tried to explain that he needed to stay there for some testing. He got very upset and let us know that he didn't want to be there. No matter what we said, he argued. I tried to change the subject several times, but to no avail. He would give me a short answer then immediately change the subject back to leaving. The only thing he wanted to hear was that we were taking him out of this place. I had unfortunately seen this agitated side of him on many occasions.

After awhile, I grimly walked out of the room. Only ten minutes remained in our hour, but I knew it was futile to continue the current conversation. As I leaned against the wall by the nurses' station, a very attractive woman came up to me. She happened to be the director of the facility. "He is so agitated," I said. I could feel my eyes slowly filling with tears.

"Believe me," she responded. "It is normal. He's only been in here for one day. He'll adjust. We see this all the time." She was so kind and compassionate. "I promise you. We'll take good care of him."

As we were talking, Dad suddenly walked up to us. "Hi Mr. Lee," the director said. "How are you doing today?" Dad was actually very polite with her. I hoped that once we left, that demeanor would continue.

I then watched Dad walk towards a sitting area in the geriatric wing. Several patients were comfortably sitting on the couches. Dad soon began talking to them. I didn't know if one of them was his roommate or not. One of the gentlemen had a knitted cap on his head. Dad walked up to him and pulled the cap off. "Mr. Lee, we don't do that here," stated one of the nurses. Dad then tossed the cap back to the man, looking sheepishly. He would definitely need to be watched carefully.

Later that day, I took Shawn to his track meet, the Big Orange Relays at Parkview High School in Lilburn. His race actually wasn't until 4:40. He would be running an 800 in the 3rd leg of the Distance Medley Relay. It felt so good to spend some time with him. I had definitely needed to get away for awhile and the fresh air felt exhilarating. The earlier visit hadn't gone well at all. I truly hoped that my dad would be better during the next visit on Tuesday night. Unfortunately, it would be occurring at the time when Sundowner's usually began. I currently wasn't feeling too confident.

Sunday, February 27, 2011

In some ways, it felt like my father was a million miles away. The psychiatric facility was only about fifteen minutes from my home, but the restrictions and security to get to him made him feel almost unreachable. His agitated behavior at yesterday's visit had only reinforced that feeling. I had experienced such a difficult time connecting with him. I knew he'd have to be more cooperative if the testing were to be successful.

I nervously called Woodland Hospital and asked to speak to someone in the geriatric wing, after which the woman transferred me to one of the nurses. I gave her Dad's patient number and she quickly pulled up his chart. "He's already had his morning medications and eaten breakfast," the nurse said. "He is actually sitting at one of the tables and seems to be doing fine. He hasn't been seen by the doctor today. That will happen later in the afternoon." She hesitated for a moment as she continued reading his chart. "It looks like the doctor started him on Aricept yesterday." I completely froze.

"He can't be given Aricept," I said. "He had a terrible reaction to it awhile back. He doesn't do well with that drug. You have to have the doctor call me as soon as possible. The longer he takes that drug, the worse he'll get." I knew that it was critical that Dad stop taking it today.

Within a couple of hours, Dr. Franklin personally called me. "I understand that you have some concerns over your Dad taking Aricept?" he asked.

"Yes, I do" I replied. "I had Dad take Aricept a few weeks ago. He did not do well on this drug at all. It turned him into a completely different person. He became very agitated while he was on it. He argued about everything. When we visited him yesterday, he acted exactly the same way as he did when I had given him the Aricept before."

"I've actually heard about some patients reacting like this," he said. Dr. Franklin didn't seem too surprised and agreed to take Dad off of the Aricept immediately.

After I hung up the phone, I was so thankful that I had called, actually making a positive difference. The doctor had seriously listened to me. What happened today was proof that I needed to be an advocate for my dad. I needed to be his voice.

Dr. Franklin had impressed me immensely. He could have easily pushed me off to an assistant or a nurse, but he didn't. He called me directly. I couldn't remember many doctors that had ever done this. Even more impressive was his respectful manner, not the least bit condescending. On the contrary, he was so kind and seemed to really care about Dad. I felt grateful that he was the doctor assigned to my dad as I really liked him. It was becoming quite evident why he was in such high demand.

Later that day, I brought Dad some clothes and miscellaneous toiletries. When I had talked to the nurse earlier, she had mentioned that he needed some things. Unfortunately, I wasn't allowed to hand deliver the items to Dad, but instead, I had to leave them at the desk. I had never been inside an environment like this where security was of the utmost concern. It did make me feel comfortable knowing that Dad wouldn't be able to wander off.

Tuesday, March 1, 2011

The large number of elderly homes that existed around me that I'd never even noticed before surprised me, obviously travelling past them repeatedly over the years. At the time, they were simply overlooked as I had no need for them. Now, things were much different. As I began carefully researching different facilities, I felt an overwhelming sadness deep within me. I absolutely hated having to do this. It was so hard to get past the fact that Dad already had a home where he currently lived with his wife. Unfortunately, I knew that I had to be prepared for the worst. I still didn't know the outcome of the testing, but I did know the incident that caused him to be there.

When I talked to Mom earlier, she told me about some close friends of hers from high school. She had been in close contact with the wife for years. The husband was recently diagnosed with dementia. They had made the inevitable decision to sell their house and move into a smaller place together where she would be his primary caregiver. His main issue was forgetting how to do basic things that he had done his whole life. He didn't suffer from Sundowner's and wasn't violent in any way, so their immediate plan seemed viable.

I then thought about my parents' situation, wishing so much that they could do the same thing. Unfortunately, my dad's violent episodes made that impossible. This would be one more thing that I would discuss with Dr. Franklin. Was there a chance that these outbursts could be controlled with medication or possibly diet? Everything would be dependent on that answer.

I had recently checked several books out from the library on Alzheimer's. I started reading a section on caregiving. It said that the caregivers themselves were often at risk of serious illness and in the extreme, even death. It was because of the high levels of stress that this type of caregiving entailed. It was unquestionably a 24/7 job. Then, I ran across a statement that really hit home. It surprisingly said that an individual that was caring for another with Alzheimer's had a 63% higher chance of dying than someone not placed in that role. The caregiver could possibly end up dying before the person they were taking care of.

I then remembered the disturbing condition of my mother months ago when she was taking care of my dad by herself. Her health was terrible. In fact, she had actually reached a point where she appeared to be worse off than my father. I knew the decision wasn't as simple as whether my mother could take care of my father at home. It was also whether she would survive it. The decision would have to be the one that was best for both of my parents.

Tonight's visitation was from 6:00 – 7:00 p.m. I unfortunately had a prior commitment with Shawn and his track team. Bob and Mom would have to see Dad tonight without me. Remembering how agitated he had been at the last visit left me feeling very nervous about this one. Three days had now passed since he had last taken the Aricept. I really hoped that it would make a difference in his demeanor.

Later that evening, Chris and I were sitting in the outside stadium at Collins Hill High School. As we were getting ready to watch Shawn run, my cell phone suddenly rang. I saw that it was Bob and my heart immediately started racing. I wasn't sure I was ready for the news.

"Hey, we had a great visit tonight," Bob said. "Dad was completely different."

I felt such an amazing relief at that very moment. "Really?" I asked, feeling elated. It was absolutely the best news that I could have received.

"Yeah," he continued. "He was really calm. We stayed for the entire hour. Everything was very pleasant." It sounded like removing the Aricept had made all the difference in the world. Fortunately, Dad had probably only had a couple of doses introduced into his system.

What made the visit even more significant was that it had occurred in the evening when Dad normally suffered from Sundowner's. I truly hoped that his calm composure meant that the doctor had successfully found the right combination of medications for Dad. This was a very good sign.

Friday, March 4, 2011

The sign for Arbor Forest seemed to suddenly appear out of nowhere. As we slowly pulled into the parking lot, I immediately noticed the uniform row of rocking chairs out front. A couple of elderly women were sitting in two of them and amiably smiled as we walked towards them. The air of serenity surrounding this place was undeniable. It not only had an assisted living section, but also a memory care unit designed specifically for Alzheimer's patients. The secure environment would prevent Dad from inadvertently wandering off and possibly hurting himself. I thought the place was absolutely wonderful and I had yet to even walk through its front doors.

The memory care unit was a separate wing that was completely self-contained. It had sixteen individual bedrooms with their own full bath and thermostat. It also had a common sitting area with a television adjacent to a dining hall. Three entrance doors, all of which had code entry, provided secured access to the unit. In addition, at least two people were always on duty in the unit, including early morning hours.

The promising facility was only a few minutes from my parents' home in Buford and they currently had one opening. One of the directors gave us a tour of the unit and the vacant room which was very spacious and had a nice, wooded view. Beautiful gardens and walking paths were located in the back. We'd actually be able to visit Dad anytime and would also be able to take him out of the facility if we wanted.

Everyone that we met was incredibly kind and loving. At one point in telling them about my father, I had to stop and catch my breath as my eyes began to fill with tears. One of the female directors knelt down beside me and tenderly hugged me. "I know it's hard," she said, "but it is the best thing for your father. It really is. He will do great here."

I then asked about the logistics for transporting my dad to this location. They were very familiar with Woodland Hospital. One of the directors at Arbor Forest who served as the liaison between the patient and their doctors would go to the psychiatric hospital to meet and talk with my dad. She would also speak to his doctor and get a current status. Once my dad was ready to be discharged, they would drive their van over to get him. They had everything worked out to a tee.

As I drove home, I felt very good about this place, seeming like it would be a wonderful fit for my father. If he had to live away from home, this was the perfect choice. Such an incredible warmth radiated from within its walls. I felt optimistic that we could successfully make it a second home for Dad.

The only negative was that there wouldn't be a nurse or doctor physically on the premises. One physician actually did come to the facility every couple of weeks, but that was more for convenience. In an emergency, they would have to do the same as we did at home, they'd call 911.

They were generously holding the room for us until Monday morning at which point we would need to give them an answer. I needed to share all of this new information with my family. There would be a lot to think about this weekend. As much as I loved this place, it wouldn't be me who was living here. The ultimate question still remained. Would Dad want this to be his new home? I honestly didn't know the answer.

Saturday, March 5, 2011

I quickly grabbed my purse as Mom pulled up in the driveway. We had to hurry to make it to the hospital in time for Dad's visitation at 12:30. On the ride over, I glanced furtively at my mom, thankful that she was doing so well under the circumstances. I had learned so much about a person's inner strength from watching her. It wasn't measured by the level of a voice. It wasn't based on physical prowess. Sometimes it was as silent as the wind, never to be noticed. As I continued to stare at her, I saw an incredible strength in her that was deafening.

As Dad slowly walked into the large meeting room, he was apparently in good spirits. A small trace of his black eye still existed, but it was healing nicely. The three of us sat together in a corner, enjoying our privacy. Dad seemed so much better today, almost like his old self. Whatever they were doing here was definitely agreeing with him.

As we were busy talking, another patient soon walked up to Dad. His name was Rodney and evidently, he was Dad's new friend. The man was short, almost completely bald and had a smile glued to his face. He began to tell Dad how he planned to ultimately escape from the facility. "When all of these people walk out, I'm going to get right in the middle of them," he said. "Before you know it, I'm gonna be out the door."

"What are you going to do when you get out?" asked Dad. "Is your car here?" Dad mischievously smiled at the man as if he knew the answer already, clearly playing with him.

"No, I'll call someone to come and get me," he answered. "I've got money. So, do you think I can get away with it?" As I scrutinized Rodney, he obviously looked up to my dad. He was such an entertaining character.

"Well, I don't know," Dad replied. I continued to watch the amusing interaction between these two men. Dad just smiled at him. He didn't say much, but he apparently was in complete control of the situation.

After awhile, Rodney slowly walked off. The three of us just looked at each other and quietly laughed. In less than five minutes, he was back. "I think the nurses may be on to me," he said. "I may have to rethink this plan." I felt like I was watching a scene right out of a comedy movie. Rodney was genuinely hilarious. He even had Dad laughing. I was so glad that he was making the best of this tough situation.

Not all of the patients were quite as entertaining. Directly across from us was an elderly gentleman lying back in a recliner. His eyes were slightly open, but he wasn't moving much. Sitting with him was his faithful wife. I secretly watched her as she gently caressed his arms, never once leaving his side. I had overheard a nurse saying that a stroke had unfortunately left him this way. It was heartbreaking to see. As I carefully watched them, I imagined a long life spent together with several children and even more grandchildren. How incredibly sad the way that life turned out for some.

A friendly woman soon came up to us. "Is this your family, William?" she asked. Dad introduced us and we shook her hand. "Your dad is such a gentleman."

"Yes, he is," I agreed, smiling at her. "Thank you for saying so." Dad had always been the epitome of a true gentleman. It didn't surprise me in the least that even in this stressful environment, that side of him had shone through.

"He makes things so much better in here," the woman said. She then amiably looked at Dad. "I'll let you get back to your family." With that, she quickly walked off.

"It sounds like you are doing so much better, Daddy," I remarked. "I'm really happy about that." I had no sooner gotten the words out of my mouth when Rodney suddenly came back into the room.

As he approached us, we all started snickering again. It just couldn't be helped. "I think what I need to do is walk out with your family," he said as he looked seriously at Dad. "What do you think?" We all just shook our heads in amusement.

Towards the end of the visit, Dad curiously asked me what was next for him. I had always been completely honest with him and I wouldn't lie to him now. "There is a place called Arbor Forest that is wonderful," I said. "You would have your own private bedroom and bath. We could come see you anytime. The grandchildren could come, too. It would be so much different than this place. I think you'll love it, Daddy."

He smiled and actually seemed thrilled about this news. "That sounds good, Pootie," he replied. "I don't like being in this place." I knew that despite today's visit, he didn't want to remain at Woodland Hospital. The thing that did surprise me, though, was that he didn't mention going home.

Tuesday, March 8, 2011

As I casually walked into the room, the red, flashing light caught my eye. A new message had apparently been left while I dropped Chris off at school. I quickly pressed the play button only to hear the case worker from Woodland Hospital's voice. She left no details other than to return her call. My heart started racing, thinking the worst.

I immediately called her back, relieved to find out that everything was actually fine. She had simply needed to discuss some of the details regarding Dad's upcoming discharge. They had tested him for tuberculosis earlier today and he was peacefully sitting on one of the couches at the moment. "Has Dr. Franklin made any type of diagnosis for my dad?" I asked.

"No, he's still not done with all of the testing," she responded. "Right now, he is recommending that your dad not return home. He feels that he needs to be in a facility where someone can monitor him more closely."

"When can we meet with the doctor?" I asked. "We have several things that we'd like to discuss with him."

"Normally, the families do not meet directly with the doctor," she replied. "Instead, they meet with the case worker assigned to their family member. Everything is handled through them." I was a little shocked to hear this. How could anyone have a family member in a psychiatric hospital and not want to speak directly to the doctor potentially deciding their future? "If you would like, I can ask if the doctor would be willing to meet with you."

"Please do," I said. "It's really important to us."

The case worker called me back a couple of hours later. Dr. Franklin actually had no problem getting together with us. We then set the specific meeting up for this Saturday after our normal visitation with Dad.

At 4:00 p.m., Chris and I took Shawn to his track meet. He would be running the 800m at 6:30. Unfortunately, I would miss seeing Dad tonight.

Later that evening, I got a disturbing phone call from Bob. He and Mom had gone to the hospital to see Dad and unfortunately, the visit had not gone well. Dad was very anxious, his behavior very similar to our first visit with him. I was so disheartened to find this out. I truly thought that he was doing much better.

When I saw Dad the previous Saturday, he was in such a great mood, not seeming the least bit anxious. I did, however, tell him about Arbor Forest at the end of the visit. Had he thought about that ever since our talk? Sometimes, telling Dad future news too early only created problems. He would eventually become obsessed with it, wondering constantly if today was the day. Maybe I should have held off telling him so soon, but I wanted to be completely honest with him. This disease made everything so complicated. Or was it as simple as the Sundowner's showing its ugly self once again?

Thursday, March 10, 2011

I felt so terrible in the position I was currently in, having to ultimately decide the future of another person. The question wasn't whether Arbor Forest was the right facility or not, but whether we had reached the point of finally giving up on Dad returning home. We had prudently thought about the decision before us for days, finding it so difficult to reach that inevitable point. On Monday, I had informed Kevin, who was one of the directors at Arbor Forest, that we definitely wanted the room for Dad. After the previous visitation, we were convinced it was for the best.

It was undoubtedly the hardest decision that I ever made, a part of me feeling like I had betrayed my father. Even though I knew I wasn't the one that gave him this terrible disease, it was still unbearably difficult. All he ever wanted was to come home. That clearly wasn't the best decision for my dad or my mom, but I still felt incredibly guilty. How could I commit him to a facility and prevent him from returning to the life he had before? As the tears rolled down my face, I felt like a terrible daughter. I prayed that he would one day be able to understand and forgive me.

This morning, I drove Mom to Arbor Forest to sign the necessary papers and leave a deposit. The room was now officially Dad's, the decision bittersweet. As I watched so many of the residents come and go, I was pleasantly surprised at their outlooks. They seemed genuinely happy and content. I wondered if Dad would come to look this way in time.

Later that night, I found myself thinking about my father and how his life had changed so much. I began to think back on the night that Mom had called 911. I remembered seeing Dad walk away from their house that night as he got into the fire truck, the image still as vivid as the night it happened. My poor father had no idea at the time that he would probably never step foot in his home again. He had no clue as to the direction that his life was about to turn. None of this was fair. He didn't deserve any of it. It absolutely ripped my heart out.

I was so angry with him that night. I never once stopped to think about my daddy being all alone in the hospital or what he was going through. He probably had no idea why he was really there. He couldn't even remember everything that had happened. I should have been there for him that night. I should have at least held his hand and told him that I loved him. Was he scared? Had he felt abandoned? My only concession was that he wasn't thinking clearly and might not remember any of that night. I would forever live with that guilt.

Saturday, March 12, 2011

As soon as I opened my eyes this morning, the knowledge that all of my children were safe and sound under the same roof filled me with incredible warmth. It was such a comforting feeling to have them all home, one that I dearly missed. Preston had come in last night for an entire week. It was Spring Break at UGA and he was lovingly spending it with his family. Today, I felt complete.

Not long after getting up, I dropped Shawn off to take the SAT which would take several hours to complete. Randy would pick him up later and take him directly to the Jerry Arnold Challenge track meet. It would be a very long day for him.

At 12:30, Mom, Bob and I visited with Dad who acted completely different than he did on Tuesday night, appearing very calm. Some confusion was still evident, but he wasn't the least bit argumentative. He asked if he was still going to Arbor Forest and we assured him that he was. He surprisingly never once mentioned going home.

After the visitation, the three of us eagerly met with Dr. Franklin. He gave us the long-awaited news and confirmed what we all had suspected. Dad indeed was in the early stages of Alzheimer's. His diagnosis was actually mixed dementia which was a combination of Alzheimer's and vascular dementia. The vascular dementia was undoubtedly a result of his heart problems. His arteries had been almost completely blocked prior to the heart surgery, which probably prevented oxygen from reaching Dad's brain. The doctor felt that Dad had likely already suffered multiple minor strokes.

One of the tests had shown that his brain was smaller than it should have been which was highly indicative of Alzheimer's. It had also positively confirmed that Dad received a concussion the last time he fell. We had always suspected that he had hit his head on the bathroom counter. Now, we knew for sure.

"William has some days where there is not too much confusion," he said. "There are other days where there is a lot. It will eventually get to the point where it becomes a daily thing. I still have one more test that I want to perform on him, but I don't anticipate that changing anything drastically." The three of us continued to hang on his every word.

"I have been testing some medicine on him for his anxiety," he continued. "Right now, he is on Namenda to help improve his memory and Risperdal to keep him calm."

"I wanted to talk to you about the Risperdal," I said. "He had been put on that when he had his heart surgery. I had read where Risperdal was not approved by the FDA for people with dementia. Do you think it is safe for my dad to take?"

"There are risks with the Risperdal," the doctor replied. "That's true, but it does help with the agitation. The critical question is whether it is more dangerous for him not to take it."

I didn't have an answer to that, but he was absolutely right. I had never looked at it that way. It may not have been the perfect drug to give him, but we had already witnessed the danger to Dad and those around him when he wasn't given the Risperdal at all.

"Do you think that Dad could return home?" I asked.

"Who would you have taking care of him?" he asked in return. We all just stared at him. "If you want to hire someone to take care of him around the clock, then I think it's possible for him to go home. It can't be your mother though. I don't think she can take care of him." He then looked at Mom who didn't say a word. I knew he was absolutely correct in his assumption that Mom couldn't take care of Dad. She had already proven that. The additional stress of the past four months had definitely had a negative impact on her. Her health was starting to suffer and she was becoming more forgetful.

"We've looked into the cost of having someone there 24 hours a day," I replied. "It's outrageous. They could probably manage for someone to come in for part of the day, but I know that wouldn't be enough."

"In my opinion, it would be too dangerous for your dad to go home and live alone with your mother," he said. "I had a patient about a year ago that was in the exact same situation as your parents. The children brought him home. One night, he went into a rage and ended up strangling his wife. To this day, he still has absolutely no recollection of doing it."

He then cautiously looked at Bob and me. "You could end up losing both parents and in a terrible way," he remarked. He paused to give us a chance to reply, but we were completely speechless. "I think the best thing would be to put your dad in a home where he would get the care that he needs."

"Do you think that he will ever be able to come back home?" Mom questioned. "Is there a chance that with medication, he will get better?" Even after everything that had happened, Mom still wanted Dad to come home.

"There is no cure for what your husband has," the doctor replied. "We will try to prolong it, but we can't stop it from happening. It's only going to get worse. I know that's not good news." The doctor was completely honest with us and I appreciated it.

"We actually found Dad a room in a facility called Arbor Forest," I said. "The room is part of a memory care unit."

"I think that will be best for William," he stated. Then, he turned directly to me. "I want to give you my pager number. If you ever need to reach me, use it. I'll return your call as soon as I can." I was shocked as I had never had a doctor give me his personal pager number before. It was usually off limits. I graciously took the slip of paper hoping I would never need to use it.

He then handed me the complete list of medications that Dad was currently taking. I noticed that Namenda 5 mg. and Risperdal .25 mg. were at the bottom, both to be given twice a day.

"I am planning on discharging William on Monday," he said. "It will probably be sometime in the afternoon. I want to see him again in two weeks for a follow-up visit."

We all then stood and amiably shook Dr. Franklin's hand. "Thank you for everything," I said genuinely. The doctor had such a compassionate spirit about him, definitely unique. I had nothing but the highest respect for this man.

Later that day, I began looking over the list of medications that I had received from the doctor, soon noticing an error. A drug called Furosemide which was a water pill was on the list. Dad didn't take any water pills. One of the drugs that he did take was Finasteride and it was missing from the list. I felt concerned whether they had simply written it up incorrectly or whether Dad was taking the wrong drug all along.

I managed to eventually get in touch with the nurse that had written up the list. I felt relieved to find out that the error had simply been in the documentation. I immediately let her know that I had to have an updated copy or Arbor Forest would not accept the changes.

An hour later, I drove back to Woodland Hospital to pick up the revised list of medications. Before leaving, I verified that the list was indeed correct. I didn't want to have to come back again.

All of Dad's medications for Arbor Forest had to be specially bubble packed. They would unfortunately not accept them any other way. The nearest pharmacy that did this was Collier Village Pharmacy which was located in downtown Buford. I went over the entire list with them, including the two new prescriptions. I reluctantly turned over all of Dad's current pill bottles to also be packaged. His medicine would hopefully be ready for pickup in a couple of hours.

Later that day, everyone met at Mom and Dad's home in Buford. Both Bob and I, Randy and all of our children were there. With two trucks, we were hoping the move would be fast. Dad's bed, a dresser, nightstands, lamps, an extra table, two recliners and several boxes were all loaded up. His new room was conveniently only about five miles away.

As we unloaded the furniture, we were instructed to use the side entrance. However, we weren't allowed to leave the doors open while we were in the process of moving. Some of the curious residents had wandered down the hall to watch us. They obviously couldn't take the chance that one of them might get out. So, I dutifully stood at the door and every time someone was ready with a piece of furniture, I entered the code to let them in. I didn't mind the inconvenience. On the contrary, it was comforting to know how serious they took the security in this unit.

Before long, everything in Dad's new room was neatly in place. Mom was busy setting up the bathroom with the shower curtain and matching rug. The boys helped put sheets on the queen-sized bed. Pictures of the family were placed all about the room. By the time we were finished, it looked completely different. I truly hoped that Dad would feel at home in it, as much as that was possible.

On the way home, we stopped at Borders, which was currently going out of business. We were all in different sections of the store when my cell phone suddenly rang. I immediately looked at the caller id and my heart froze. It said Woodland Hospital. "Hello," I said.

"Pootie, I'm so glad I caught you," Dad said.

"Hi Dad, is everything alright?" I asked.

"I wanted to talk to you about my doctor," he replied. "I just saw him. You weren't able to meet with him today, were you?"

"Yes, we did," I reassured him. "We met with him right after we saw you this afternoon."

"You did?" Dad asked.

"Yes, Daddy," I replied. "Everything is in order. He is going to discharge you on Monday. We just got your new room set up. I think you are really going to like it."

"Oh, Pootie," he said, "that is so good to hear. I was worried that you didn't get to see him."

"No, everything is taken care of, Dad," I said. "You don't need to worry about anything." I truly hoped that my words had put him at ease. I desperately wanted the next two days to run smoothly.

"I love you, Dad," I said.

"I love you, too, Pootie," he replied back. With that, I hung up the phone. Dad believed in me and even more, he relied on me. I didn't want to ever let him down.

Monday, March 14, 2011

I could hear the cheerful chirping of the parakeet as we neared the common area. It had been years since my pet birds had filled our lives with such music. As I slowly walked by his cage, he seemed right at home. Several residents innocently looked up at us from their seats on the couches, a few remaining asleep. I smiled at these strangers as we passed them. They would soon be my Dad's new neighbors.

Mom and I had gone to Arbor Forest early this morning. We had some last minute things to do to Dad's room before he arrived. Mom had brought some more pictures and another lamp, while I had made a collage for Dad comprised of family photos and some classic barber pictures mixed in. It would hang right outside of Dad's door directly under his name tag. It was meant to represent Dad and what he loved most in life. All of the residents in the memory care unit had one. Hopefully, it would help to remind him which room was his.

Later that afternoon, Mom and I casually sat on a couch in the lobby. I had several phone calls to make and it was much more private there. It also gave us a prime view of the white van that they would eventually use to pick up Dad. Before long, Kevin cheerfully walked up to us and smiled.

"We're going to get him in about five minutes," he said. As he turned and walked away, I felt both happy and nervous.

A couple of hours later, I again made my way towards the lobby, expecting my dad to be arriving any minute. As soon as I opened the door, the image of Dad walking towards me left me pleasantly surprised. Following immediately behind him were Kevin and Anthony. Dad had a McDonald's shake in his hand and was smiling, the shake almost completely gone. They probably asked Dad on the way over if he wanted something to drink. I doubted they fully understood how important that simple gesture had been to Dad.

Mom and I eagerly hugged and kissed him, actually looking better than he had in weeks. Then, we gave him a quick tour of his wing. The unit was basically a long hall with eight individual bedrooms on one end and another eight on the other end. Between the two sections were a common area and a dining hall. We excitedly showed Dad his new room, where he soon decided to rest in his familiar blue recliner. The move had gone very smoothly, but Dad seemed a little tired.

Before long, the medical technician in the memory care unit came to Dad's room. She needed to get all of his medications processed into the system. I didn't want there to be any lapse of time after he moved in as missing even one dose of a medication could be serious. She politely introduced herself and then sat on the bed next to me. Dad and Mom watched silently as we went over every single medication that he was taking. She filled out all of the necessary forms and I reluctantly turned over all of the newly bubble packed medicine, having such mixed emotions. I had solely taken care of Dad's medicine for months now. It was hard to entrust it to someone else, even though I knew I had no choice.

Mom and I stayed with Dad in his new room the entire day. One of Dad's caregivers soon came to his door to formally meet him. Her name was Alexandra. She was an extremely kind person and had the bubbliest personality. It seemed like every other word out of her mouth was "Sugar". "How ya doin, Sugar?" "We'll be eating soon, Sugar." She talked to Dad with such respect, his reaction clearly indicating that he responded well to her.

Later that day, I eventually decided to go home. Randy had taken the week off to be with Preston and I very much wanted to spend some time with them today. I lovingly kissed Dad goodbye. He had done great all day.

On the way out, I saw Alexandra in the hall. She mentioned that they ate dinner about 5:00 p.m. "Don't you worry, Sugar," she said. "I'll go get him when it's time to eat." I couldn't help but smile every time I spoke with her. She was an absolute doll.

As I drove home, I thought about Dad's first day at Arbor Forest. He definitely seemed to be in the most appropriate environment for his condition. My dad had endured so much over the past four months as the disease had progressed a lot. I hoped that now that he was under the care of a good doctor and taking medication, the progression would slow down. I even hoped beyond the odds that he would miraculously start improving. I knew that the move was a lot for Dad to process and would probably take considerable time for him to adjust to everything. I truly prayed that his first night in his new home would go well.

Tuesday, March 15, 2011

He immediately barked as I walked in the door, his demeanor quickly changing once he realized it was me. His little body began wiggling from side to side as I knelt down and rubbed his tiny, black head. Barron had been so good for my parents. Not only had he provided them with such unconditional love, but he was a good watch dog as well. I felt a lot more comfortable with him in the house.

Mom and I soon left him for our drive to Arbor Forest. We found Dad calmly sitting in the recliner, smiling as we walked into his room. He had already eaten his breakfast by the time we arrived and was relaxing, dressed nice with his hair combed neatly. "Hi Daddy," I said. "How did your first night go? Did you sleep well?"

"Yeah, I actually did," he replied. "This bed is a lot more comfortable than what I had been sleeping in."

As I slowly looked around the room, I saw that most of the pictures were surprisingly missing. "Dad, what happened to your pictures?" I asked.

"I don't know, Pootie," he responded. As I began to warily look through his furniture, I soon found them, misplaced inside several different drawers. I also noticed that some bathroom items had suspiciously been moved into the drawers as well. I wasn't sure what had happened, but I wasn't going to pursue it anymore. I decided to just put everything neatly back in its place.

Not long after that, another one of Dad's caregivers knocked on the door. Her name was Susan. She wore the standard dress of khaki pants and a white polo shirt with her hair pulled back in a pony tail, her demeanor very soft spoken and gentle. She was so compassionate and kind that we hit it off immediately. She looked tenderly at Dad. "If you need anything, just ask me," she said. "Okay?" He shook his head slowly and smiled. I felt so relieved knowing that people like Alexandra and Susan were lovingly watching over my dad.

After about an hour, Mom, Dad and I all walked out to the common area. My parents sat down and Alexandra courteously handed them some water. A small table rested against one wall with a container of lemon water and cups on top of it. "We like to keep the residents very hydrated," she said. Alexandra then walked up to me. "How are you doing, Sugar?" she asked.

"I'm good," I replied. "Can I ask you something?" Mom and Dad were busy looking at the parakeet chirping in the corner.

"Anything," she replied.

"I'm wondering if Dad is in the right place," I said. "He seems so different than most of the other residents back here." She just looked at me, such warmth and understanding in those brown eyes of hers.

"Why don't we talk a walk to the other side," she said. "C'mon William and Shirley, let's show you some more of our facility." That was all it had taken. The three of us then followed Alexandra out of the memory care unit. We leisurely walked down the halls of the assisted living part of the facility. Some of the residents kept their doors shut for privacy, while others left them wide open. On the back hall, special 2-bedroom apartments existed for married couples.

Alexandra also showed us the walking path out back, the game room and a different dining hall in the front of the building. We met so many people on our stroll as Alexandra inherently seemed to know everyone. One impressive man was in his 90's and looked incredible, apparently walking everywhere. I remembered seeing him outside strolling down the street one day when Mom and I had come to the home.

The residents in the assisted living section were of various physical states. Some easily walked around with no assistance, some used canes and walkers, while others exclusively used wheelchairs. One patient had a registered nurse that stayed in his room during the day to help him. The one thing that they all invariably had in common was that their minds were still intact, for the most part. Some of them actually had some early signs of dementia, but none of them were a flight risk. That was the main difference.

When we got back to the memory care unit, Mom and Dad sat on one of the couches while I remained standing next to Alexandra. "Do you think that Dad would be better suited to the assisted living side?" I asked.

"He might be," she replied. "Let me ask you this. Would he ever get confused and wander off?"

"Unfortunately, I could see that happening," I replied. "If he wanted to go home bad enough, I wouldn't put it past him to just walk out on his own. He is a very determined man. Is there anything in place to prevent that from happening? Are the doors ever locked?"

"There is nothing to stop him from leaving," she responded. "The doors are locked at night on the outside, but not on the inside. All of the residents in the assisted living side are free to come and go as they please. The only thing they have to do is sign out so that we know where they are at all times."

"I'm not sure what to do," I said. "He just seems so out of place in here. Is he going to have anyone to talk to?"

"He will," she replied. "There are several people that are in their rooms right now. They're not all like this. We have activities every day and more of them come out during those. We also have services in the main lobby that they go to. Once he meets some of the other residents, he'll make some friends."

I was seriously having second thoughts about the memory care unit. It was so hard to know if we were doing the right thing. Most of the people that I had seen in this unit seemed to be in far worse shape than Dad. On the other hand, I knew he was at high risk for wandering off and getting lost. I felt like we had no choice. I knew he was extremely confused and probably felt abandoned as I could see it in his sad eyes when I would leave him.

When it was time for lunch, Alexandra decided to take Dad to the other dining area near the lobby. All three of us sat together at the table. Everyone that we met was very talkative and friendly. The head chef, Carl, soon came out to meet us. He just happened to be Alexandra's husband. The two of them were quite a pair. Before she walked away, she reminded me that we would have to walk Dad back to the memory care unit when we were done. Otherwise, he might inadvertently try to follow us out when we left.

Late that afternoon, Preston and I went to Shawn's track meet. The coach had actually scheduled him to run in two different races. He did so awesome, actually setting a personal record for himself in one of the races. I was so proud of him. It felt wonderful to spend some quality time with my older boys.

That evening, I got an alarming phone call from Mom. After I had left Arbor Forest today, she had decided to stay with Dad for awhile. Not long after that, he unfortunately had an episode. It was like a light switch flipping on. It had happened that fast.

Dad had started expressing that he wanted Mom to spend the night. He was very confused about the current living arrangements. When she told him that wasn't a good idea just yet, he got very agitated with her and eventually told her to leave.

Mom was clearly upset by the incident. "He's confused, Mom," I said. "He's lived with you for 54 years. He doesn't understand why you're not living together now. It's only been two days since he moved into Arbor Forest. He just needs some time to adjust."

"I hope you're right," she said, sounding so depressed. I knew the incident had taken an emotional toll on her. They always did.

Wednesday, March 16, 2011

As I carefully started the engine, that familiar rumbling sound came to life. Looking around the inside of the truck, so many things reminded me of Dad, the miniature Alf doll that he'd had for years, the Tom T. Hall CDs, even his sunglasses. When I closed my eyes, I could still smell the faint scent of Dad's cologne. He was here with me, as were so many memories locked away in this cab. I had decided to drive Dad's truck to Arbor Forest this morning as Preston had a dentist appointment and needed my car.

Every time my Honda had acted up, Dad would generously let me borrow his truck. It didn't matter what type of inconvenience it created for him, he had always put my needs first.

When Randy and I were first married, we drove a red, Volkswagen van that we had bought from his parents. A few months into the marriage, Randy was leisurely on his way to work one morning. While he was driving, the engine accidentally caught on fire. He managed to get out of the vehicle safely, but not before the entire van had burnt up, the fire department having to be called out. Unfortunately, it was a total loss and we only had liability insurance on it.

My dad had graciously given us his 1973 Chevy truck to use. We had agreed to pay him $100 a month for a year for a total of $1,200.00. A few months later, Randy and I were driving back from his parents' home in Molino one Sunday night. We were on Highway 29 when an elderly man in the oncoming turn lane broadsided us in the driver's side right behind the cab, never even slowing down. It sent us swiftly spinning. After three rotations, we finally stopped about fifty yards away, landing right in front of the Race Trac gas station. Neither one of us were wearing our seatbelts. It was a miracle that we weren't seriously hurt. The truck, however, was totaled.

Again, my dad lovingly came to our rescue, this time giving us his 1973 Thunderbird. We agreed to the same payment plan of $100 a month, even though half of the time, he wouldn't accept the money. Dad had always been there for us. I knew that he would do absolutely anything for me. I was trying to be there for him every day.

When I walked into the memory care unit, I found Dad sitting at a table in the dining area peacefully drinking a cup of coffee. When he eventually finished, we went back to his room. As soon as we walked in, I immediately saw that several things had been moved. As I started opening each of the dresser drawers, followed by the nightstand, I noticed that every single drawer had items that didn't belong. Amidst his clothing were various bathroom items and family pictures. I even found shoes in some of the drawers. From the outside, everything looked fine. On the inside however, everything was a complete mess. "Dad, did you move things around in your drawers?" I asked.

"It wasn't me," he responded. "It's that woman. I caught her coming in here and moving things around." Dad was convinced that someone had come into his room. I honestly wasn't sure what was going on.

Later that morning, Susan pulled me aside. "Are your parents getting a divorce?" she asked.

"No," I replied, looking surprised. "What made you think that?"

"After your mom left yesterday, your dad came down to the common area and sat down," she said. "We started talking a little and he told me they were getting a divorce." I knew that Dad had been upset, but I had no idea why he would have said something like that. Divorce was never discussed during their marriage. It would have never been an option.

At noon, Alexandra came by and told us lunch would be served in a couple of minutes. Dad and I soon walked down to the dining area. We were seated next to Janet and Margaret who were both really sweet women. Dad ate his entire lunch without saying a single word. I tried to engage him in conversation, but he just didn't seem comfortable. Every now and then, Margaret would say something, but for the most part, it was Janet and I. She was very talkative. At one point, she looked at me and said "You have the most beautiful blue eyes," in her strong Southern drawl.

"Aw, thank you, Janet," I said. "So do you."

"I got them from my daddy," she said, rubbing my arm. I had clearly made a new friend.

Dad and I spent the entire afternoon together. I took him out back for a little bit where a gazebo and a wrought iron table with chairs was set up. We casually sat in the cushioned seats for awhile, enjoying the sunshine. It was a beautiful day and the fresh air did him a lot of good.

When it neared dinnertime, I informed Dad that I needed to be going. He never said so, but I could see it in his sad eyes. He didn't want me to go. "I'll be back in the morning," I said. "I promise." I then gently kissed him goodbye, leaving him sitting on one of the couches in the common area. It absolutely broke my heart.

As I slowly walked away, I thought about a similar time when Preston was two years old. I had dropped him off at day care one morning before work. He was in a new room and hadn't quite adjusted yet. I had truly hoped that once I left, he would be fine. Both of his teachers were currently in the room along with several other children. As I reached my car to leave, I glanced back at the building and noticed Preston's sad face in the window looking out at me, tears streaming down his cheeks. It ripped my heart in two. I absolutely couldn't leave him like that.

I quickly turned and went back inside and he immediately ran to me. I picked him up and we just hugged each other tightly with no other concerns in the world. I eventually left that morning, but I made sure that Preston was in a good place before I did.

Today, unfortunately, felt very similar. I was leaving one of my loved ones in the care of someone else that I had placed great trust in. The only difference was the age.

Later that evening, I found myself reflecting heavily on Dad's situation, praying about it every day for months. So many times, I had felt like I was hanging on by a mere thread. I had heard repeatedly that I couldn't make decisions based on my emotions. I was unquestionably too close to the situation. Instead, I needed to use my head and make informed choices, but sometimes it wasn't so easy.

Yesterday, I had started second guessing myself and thinking that maybe the assisted living part of the facility would be better suited for my dad. A lot of the people in the memory care unit were in a much more advanced stage and I thought Dad would be able to relate better to the people in the other section. After the unfortunate episode yesterday afternoon, I felt like God was telling me that my dad was right where he needed to be. He may not have had his freedom, but he was ultimately safe.

Thursday, March 17, 2011

I soon began to feel very at home within the walls of Arbor Forest, never before having any idea that the world inside existed. Several directors had called me by name today as I casually made my way through the lobby. Once inside the memory care unit, the caregivers had done the same. So many of the residents had smiled at me as I walked past them, one even gently caressing my arm. I felt a part of a much bigger family, a very special family.

When I arrived at Dad's room, I noticed that his door was closed, immediately causing me alarm. As I cautiously opened the door, I saw no sign of him. I noticed that his bed was neatly made with his throw pillows dispersed on top. Then, as I rounded the corner, I could clearly hear the shower water running. I slowly began to breathe again.

"Daddy, I'm out here," I yelled through the door.

"Okay, Pootie," he replied. "I'll be out in a minute."

While I patiently waited, I checked his room, his drawers again in disarray. Items that had previously hung in his closet were now in his dresser. I began the tedious process of straightening them up once again. This seemed to undoubtedly be my new daily routine.

Dad soon came out of the bathroom. "Dad, has anyone been coming in your room?" I asked, curious if his story would remain the same.

"That woman is still coming in my room," he said. "Last night, I found her lying in my bed. I think she is the one that is moving my things around."

"Well, what happened after you found her?" I asked.

"I told her to get out of my bed," he replied. "She wasn't allowed to stay in here." Dad seemed so sure of himself. I honestly didn't know whether he was completely imagining this other woman or if someone had actually come into his room. I had a hard time believing that if someone was in Dad's bed that none of the caregivers would have mentioned it to me. Dad's mental condition had never caused him to have delusions before. As soon as I got a chance, I'd walk down to the common area and ask some questions.

Dad's closet was located right off of the bathroom. When I walked back to it, I noticed that it was completely empty of clothes. All that remained were some metal hangers. I had already found some of his shirts in the drawers, but several pieces of clothing were still mysteriously missing. I soon found the items in the dirty clothes hamper. I took the next fifteen minutes to get Dad's closet back in order.

Dad was very calm all day. At one point, we were quietly relaxing in the chairs in his room. He looked over at me and apparently wanted to say something. I had still not talked to Dad about his diagnosis, just waiting for the right time. "How long am I going to be here?" he asked.

"I don't know, Daddy," I replied. "Do you remember the doctor at Woodland Hospital?" He nodded his head yes. "Well, he gave you a complete mental evaluation while you were there. Did he ever talk to you about the results?"

"No, I don't think so," he answered.

I slowly took a deep breath. This definitely wasn't the type of conversation that I ever thought I would need to have with one of my parents. "You have Alzheimer's, Daddy," I reluctantly said. "The doctor's actual diagnosis is mixed dementia. Alzheimer's is a part of that. Do you remember having the heart surgery back in December?" He again shook his head yes. "Your arteries had a lot of blockage. As a result, the doctor thinks that you may have had some minor strokes. They were small enough that you probably never realized that you were even having them. Unfortunately, they caused some damage." I knew that this was a lot for my dad to take in at one time.

"A lot of the things that you have been dealing with are caused by the Alzheimer's," I continued. "All of the forgetting that you have been doing for so long is because of the disease. You also have a condition called Sundowner's. Sometimes during the day, usually at night, it causes you to get very anxious. During some of those times, the anxiety turns into agitation and you lose your temper. You usually don't even remember some of the things that happen during those episodes."

"Dr. Franklin doesn't feel it is safe for you to go back home," I carefully explained. "He feels that you need someone to keep an eye on you 24 hours a day. Mom just isn't able to do that. We thought this place would be a good fit for you, at least for now."

"What will your mother do?" he asked.

"Well, for the time being, it's probably best that Mom stay at home," I replied. I had never talked to Dad about the dreadful incident that had occurred during his last night at home. I wasn't sure if he was really ready for that. "We don't know what will happen in the future, Daddy. The doctor has you taking some medications to help heal your brain. Hopefully in time, things will improve. We just have to take it one day at a time."

I had tried to be completely honest with my words, without revealing more information than was necessary. Dad remained very quiet and showed absolutely no emotion. I truly hoped that he understood the situation and the critical decisions that were made.

Before long, he nodded off. I took that opportunity to walk down to the common area and talk to Susan. I mentioned Dad's claims that someone was coming into his room and that it had even escalated to the point of that person getting in his bed. She was unaware of anyone going in his room and certainly not in his bed. She would have definitely heard about that if it had happened.

She did let me know that Dad sometimes got confused when he was walking back to his room. The rooms were all arranged into groups of four, with two on each side of the hall. Dad's room was the first room on the right in the second grouping of rooms. Susan had furtively watched him walk back and accidentally go into the first room on the right in the first grouping of rooms, which was Janet's room. Her bed was coincidentally in the exact same location in her room as Dad's was in his room.

Susan also mentioned that Dad was beginning to pace at night which didn't surprise me at all as that was usually when the Sundowner's kicked in. One of the nice things about this facility was that someone was always awake in the common area for Dad to talk to when he got up in the middle of the night.

Today at lunch, Alexandra had Dad sit in his new spot which was a table located in the back of the dining area directly in front of the window. Donald, Joseph and Frank soon joined him. It was appropriately going to be the "Guy Table". Dad conveniently sat in the seat nearest the window. From his vantage point, he had a clear view of the entire dining area. It really was the best seat in the house. "This is going to be your new place, William, for every meal," Alexandra said with a smile. "What do you think, Sugar?"

"This looks great," Dad replied, seemingly pleased with the new setup. I gained more respect for Alexandra every day. This was clearly more than a job for her. She was doing whatever it took to help Dad adjust positively.

Later that afternoon, Preston and I took Shawn to his track meet at Parkview High School. He was slated to run the 1600m at 5:10. He victoriously walked away with first place in his heat, with no one even coming close. I was so unbelievably proud of him.

As I quietly lied in bed tonight, I thought about how different things were now. A few months ago, I probably would have been hard-pressed to even spell Alzheimer's correctly. Now, I relentlessly studied this horrid disease daily. Every time my dad started to exhibit a new symptom, I thoroughly researched it to find out if it meant that he was progressing into a different stage. The more I knew, the better I was able to deal with it. Unfortunately, the downside to doing this was that as I sometimes read ahead, I got a glimpse into the agonizing future that awaited my daddy. It was heartbreaking.

Friday, March 18, 2011

I lovingly held his hand as we set off down the road, the area changing so much over the years. It surprisingly had been considered country at one time. There had definitely been a small town charm about it which was part of the appeal for me. I didn't mind working in the big city, but I preferred the solitude and peacefulness that this area offered for my home. As we slowly drove by the busy Mall of Georgia, that country feel was evidently gone forever.

Before long, Randy and I arrived at Arbor Forest. It was actually the first time that Randy had seen Dad in his new home. Dad was in a great mood as we took him out front and leisurely sat in the rocking chairs. Anthony soon saw us and generously brought everyone a glass of iced tea. The immense level of respect that the directors showed the residents was moving. "Thank you, partner," said Dad. It was a common term that my dad sometimes used to address people. I had heard it many times over the years. It meant that he had high esteem for this person. It meant that he considered him a friend.

At lunchtime, we took Dad back inside. The normal routine in his unit was to have snacks a couple of times a day and three square meals. Several caregivers had mentioned that Dad was hands down their best eater. He really loved the food as was evidenced by him completely cleaning his plate at every meal. He was still so thin, but I hoped in time that he would put on some additional weight.

Today, some extra desserts were sitting on the tray. Alexandra came up to Dad and secretly whispered something in his ear. A minute later, she placed another dessert in front of Dad. He and Alexandra seemed to speak the same language and were fast becoming good friends.

After lunch, Mom drove to Arbor Forest to spend the afternoon with Dad. They sat in the common area for awhile and then spent some time in his room. Later that day, she took him out back to get some fresh air. Dad soon began to get agitated and tried forcefully to get out of the gate. Fortunately, a padlock stopped him. He got very argumentative with Mom and no matter what they did, he didn't seem happy. Eventually, he told her that he didn't know why she came because she didn't care about him. She ended up leaving.

At 9:00 that night, I got a startling call from one of Dad's caregivers saying that he had been very agitated. Earlier that evening, he was totally out of control. Dad was loudly banging on the front door of the memory care unit wanting someone to let him out so he could speak to whoever was in charge. The caregivers had eventually settled him down and he had gone back to his room. They just wanted to keep us apprised of the situation.

About twenty minutes later, I got another unexpected phone call asking me to come to the facility. They desperately needed me to calm Dad down as he had become agitated once again. Since their doctor hadn't yet seen Dad, they didn't have any emergency medication to give him. He was yelling, going into the other patient's rooms and slamming their doors. At one point when going back to his room, he had gotten confused and gone into Janet's room instead where she was asleep in her bed. Dad confusingly started going through her dresser drawers thinking that she was in his room and he began yelling at her. They eventually had to lock all of the other patient's rooms. The last straw was when he pushed one of the caregivers. She informed us that if we couldn't calm him down, they would have to call 911.

Randy and I quickly drove to Arbor Forest. By the time we got there, Dad was sitting in the dining area and seemed calm. His eyes had that intent, serious look to them, his pupils extremely small. He looked so confused. "Daddy, why don't we go back to your room?" I suggested. He slowly stood up to walk with us. As we came up on Janet's room, I noticed Dad stopping. "Dad, your room is up there," I said as I pointed up ahead. He then started walking again and we continued on to his room.

Every room had a gold name plate and a picture on the wall right outside their door. Unfortunately, Dad's name tag was still on order. The picture was meant to be symbolic of the patient. I had made a collage for Dad that contained pictures of his children and grandchildren with a picture of my parents in the center. "Daddy, have you seen this picture?" I asked, pointing at the frame. He looked at it and slowly nodded yes. "It will always be hanging right outside of your room. So, if you don't see this, then it isn't your room."

With that, we moved inside and sat down, Dad and I in the chairs and Randy on the bed. I asked Dad what had happened tonight and he again said that a woman had come into his room. I tried to explain to him that he had gotten confused and gone into the wrong room. He got angry and accused me of believing the caregiver over him. He then told me that the mysterious woman had changed his room number. I thought it best to leave this issue alone.

"Daddy, do you know why they called us tonight?" I asked. He slowly nodded his head no. "One of the caregivers said that you shoved her."

"It wasn't like that," he said. "She was trying to block me from going into a room and I just tried to move her."

"You can't do that, Dad," I stated. "You can't put your hands on them. The next time, they said they'll have to call 911." He just blankly stared at me and I couldn't tell if I was reaching him or not. "If they call 911, there's a chance that they'll take you back to the hospital. You don't want to go through that again. Do you remember the last time this happened?

You had gone into Mom's bedroom and she ended up dialing 911." My dad and I had still to this day never discussed this incident as I was never quite sure how to bring it up. I had decided to wait until the opportunity presented itself, now seemed like that time.

"I never put my hands on your mother," Dad replied.

"You did, Dad," I said. "That's why she made the call. You hit her and she called 911. Then, they took you to the hospital."

"I never hit your mother," he argued, his voice slowly rising.

"You did, Dad," I said. "That's why she called the police."

"I have never in my life hit your mother!" Dad yelled.

The room went completely quiet. You could hear a pin drop. And then, it suddenly hit me. It wasn't that he was in denial. Dad had absolutely no recollection of attacking Mom. I had thought about the events of that night so many times. Never once did I even imagine that the disease had completely blocked the confrontation from his memory.

I knew immediately that I had messed up, not handling the situation well at all. I looked over at Randy and he was shaking his head at me. I was at a complete loss for what to do.

Dad then looked at Randy. "Ran, I'm sorry you had to be a part of this," Dad said.

"It's okay, Chester," Randy replied. "I'm just sorry about everything that you've gone through tonight."

Before long, Dad got up and slowly walked out of the room. "Vanessa, you can't argue with your Dad like that," Randy said. "When he's going through one of those episodes, he's not himself. He doesn't know what he's saying. You can't have a serious conversation when he's like that. Plus, you brought something up that he may not even remember." I knew he was obviously right, but it was still hard. I had always been completely honest with my dad. This horrible disease was changing everything. I was slowly learning that some things were best left unsaid.

"You're right," I said. "I got caught up in the moment. I had no idea he didn't remember the incident that night." I could feel the beginning of a headache coming on as I firmly rubbed my temples trying to stave off the inevitable. "I'm just too emotionally involved with everything. You're not here every day like I am, Randy. It's hard. It's so hard to always do the right thing."

Randy and I then walked down the hall to the common area where we found Dad sitting on one of the couches. A couple of other residents and a caregiver were currently watching television. I nervously sat next to Dad as he stared back at me, his blue eyes piercing. He didn't say a word, but his eyes spoke volumes as if to say I had betrayed him. The look on his face said he couldn't believe I thought him capable of hitting Mom. I had never seen Dad look at me with such disappointment. I truly hoped I was wrong.

After about thirty minutes, Dad appeared completely calm, so Randy and I decided to go home. I felt terrible about what had transpired, but I was also worried about making it any worse. I thought the best thing would be to wait until tomorrow to talk about it. I didn't want to upset my dad any further. I slowly stood and said "Goodbye, Dad." He intentionally said nothing, but continued to watch me until I rounded the corner at the end of the hall.

On the way home, Randy tenderly held my hand. "Are you okay?" he asked.

"No, I'm not," I replied. "When this all started with my dad, we were thrown into it. Everything just happened so fast. We've never had a chance to catch our breath." I took a second to gather my thoughts. "It's been nonstop ever since. I'm doing the best I can, but this is all so new to me. Sometimes, I feel like I'm failing at it. He has enough to deal with without me making it worse. No matter how hard I try, I continue to make mistakes. I'm just so tired." He raised my hand to his lips and gently kissed it. I leaned back on the headrest and closed my eyes. The rest of the drive would be in silence.

Saturday, March 19, 2011

I worriedly sat down in the living room and, once again, thought about the disturbing events of last night. I then paged his doctor, needing to let him know about the incident at Arbor Forest. I knew that Dad needed time to adjust, the new environment clearly being a lot for him to take in at once. So much had already happened to him and unfortunately, it was still occurring. I then looked over at Randy who had apparently been talking to me. I was so deep in thought that I never even heard him. About that time, the phone rang as if on cue.

Dr. Franklin was very surprised since Dad had done so well at Woodland Hospital. He decided to double the amount of Risperdal that Dad was taking in the evening to .5 mg. The .25 mg. in the morning would remain the same. I explained that he would have to fax over a new order to Arbor Forest for the change to actually take place. They would not accept a verbal directive over the phone.

The doctor then told me to give the facility his pager number in case they ever needed to get in touch with him. My respect for this man had just increased again. I didn't know any other doctors that gave their personal pager numbers out as freely as he did.

I also mentioned to Dr. Franklin that Mom and I were going to see Dad every day. Contrary to what we had thought, this wasn't a good idea. He felt we should limit it to once a week to give Dad a chance to get used to the new facility. It would also allow the caregivers some time to get to know Dad and his behavior. Instead of us always being there taking care of him, we needed to let them do their job.

It was unfortunately a very sad situation. We wanted to be there for my dad to make things better, but we may have actually done him a disservice. I didn't know if staying away was the right thing to do or not. I also didn't think I could manage only seeing Dad once a week. I did know that a number of other people had suggested it as well. I'd try to compromise and reduce the visits to 2 - 3 days a week and see if that allowed him to adjust better. It hurt deeply to think of my dad alone, but I chose this place because of the caring people and I ultimately had to have faith that he was in good hands.

I also had another concern related to our visits. We were always taking Dad out of his unit either to the assisted living walking trail and gazebo, the front of the building with the rocking chairs or the front lobby whenever a special activity was planned. I think he got so used to it that he didn't realize he couldn't leave the unit without supervision. We probably should have allowed more time for Dad to get used to his normal routine before we started adding changes.

After briefly talking with the doctor, I made the decision not to go to

Arbor Forest today. I was already stretched very thin and desperately needed a break. Knowing that Bob would be going to see Dad later helped tremendously to ease the guilt I was feeling.

I struggled to make sense of what had happened last night between my dad and me. Dealing with Alzheimer's was hard enough, but the Sundowner's created another dimension that sometimes felt unmanageable. It seemed that the basic defense mechanisms that we used in dealing with people in our everyday lives were the exact opposite behavior that was necessary for a dementia patient. I had seen firsthand how difficult it was to reason with someone when they were in the throes of a Sundowner's episode. It wasn't about what was right or wrong, but about restoring that person to a calm state. Awhile back, I had read that the most important way to do this was to redirect the patient. Until last night, I never realized how true that statement was. This had been a definite learning experience for me.

Later that afternoon, Bob went to visit Dad. He seemed much calmer than the previous night, but he still appeared very confused. As they were casually sitting on a couch in the common area, Bob suggested that they go to his room. Dad's surprising response was that he didn't have one.

After awhile, Bob walked down to Dad's room by himself. As he walked through the door, he noticed that Dad's bed was not made. Then as he moved closer, he realized why. At some point, the sheets had been soiled. Fortunately, Bob found an extra set in the closet to make the bed. Nothing about the accident was mentioned to Dad. Bob and I both felt that he was probably embarrassed and intentionally didn't tell anyone. The worst part about this incident was that it indicated that Dad was possibly progressing into the next stage of Alzheimer's. The disease wasn't slowing down.

Sunday, March 20, 2011

I felt more than a little nervous at the thought of what awaited me, having no idea what state he would be in this morning. The more I learned about this disease, the more I realized that I never knew what to expect from day to day. That was Alzheimer's. Sometimes you just had to put your feelings and fears aside and plunge forward. I was determined to make things right with my dad.

As I entered the memory care unit at Arbor Forest, I carefully began looking for him. After checking the common area, I walked back to his room where I found him lying back in his blue recliner. He looked up at me and smiled. "Hi Pootie," he said.

"Hi Dad," I replied. "How are you doing?"

"I'm okay," he responded, sounding very calm. I thought about apologizing for the other night and wisely decided against it. I had no idea how much of it he remembered. I hoped none of it. The last thing I wanted to do was remind him about the incident. It seemed that oftentimes with Alzheimer's, the best choice was to move ahead and not dwell on the past.

Before long, Alexandra rhythmically knocked on the door. She cheerily came into the room and told us about the church service that would be starting at 11 a.m. "The preacher does such a good job," she said. "I think you both would really enjoy it."

I soon walked Dad down to the lobby on the other side of the facility. The room was so crowded that we couldn't find two seats together, so I gave Dad the closest one. I then took a seat at the table behind him.

I kept my eyes on Dad throughout the service. He really seemed to enjoy it. About twenty minutes into it, I noticed that Dad had nodded off. As I curiously looked around the room, I saw that he wasn't alone. I then saw Alexandra looking at me as she winked and then smiled. While sitting in the common area so many times this past week, I had noticed the other residents comfortably napping. At the time, it hadn't seemed like Dad had really fit in. Now as I watched him closely, I realized that this was our new norm.

After lunch, I took Dad out back to our special place. His fingernails hadn't been trimmed in awhile. Normally at home, he would do it himself every week. I had put a pair of clippers in my purse last week just in case. He now sat perfectly still for me in the wrought iron chair. Afterwards, we talked freely as we enjoyed the beautiful weather. He was so relaxed in his new sanctuary.

He soon got chilly and asked to go back inside. The back door used a code to get in that was different than the one to get out. Unfortunately, it wasn't working, so I knocked on the door several times. I soon heard one of the residents on the other side of the door, but I knew she definitely couldn't help me. Eventually, one of the caregivers approached. She told me the code to try, but it still didn't work. She ended up using the code to get out in order to open the door for us.

Not many of the residents in the memory care unit went out back. Apparently, the code had changed, but no one knew the new one. I would have to remember to find that out before our next outing.

Late that night, I got a troubling phone call from Arbor Forest. Dad had gotten confused about his room again and had mistakenly gone into Janet's room. When he found her in bed, he thought that she was in his bed. He vehemently told her to get out, but she didn't move. She was very scared and soon began to cry. Before anyone could stop him, Dad firmly picked her up out of the bed and set her on the floor, the whole time telling her that she needed to stop getting in his bed.

The caregivers quickly moved Janet to one of the couches in the common area. She was still shaken up, but had not been harmed beyond that. The caregivers then called their director and she made the decision to call 911.

They had to lock Janet's door in order to convince Dad that she wouldn't return which helped to calm him down. Janet's family was notified and completely understood the situation. They were agreeable to her sleeping on the couch this one night.

By the time the EMTs had arrived, things had settled down considerably. They thoroughly checked both my dad and Janet out. As they talked to Dad, he was still very confused, adamant that Janet had been in his room. Since no one was hurt, they decided against taking my dad to the hospital. He eventually made his way back to his own room where he would remain the rest of the night.

Monday, March 21, 2011

The feeling of uncertainty enveloped me as I thought about last night's incident. The confusion by itself was difficult enough, but when you added in the agitation, it became a different matter altogether. I had already decided on my first order of business for the day, actually my last thought as sleep finally fell upon me last night. I needed to make sure that Dad's anxiety medication had been changed.

When I arrived in the memory care unit, I went directly to the medicine cart to talk with the medical technician on duty. All of the patient's medications were locked up in the cart, along with a notebook that contained instructions for taking them. I had the girl look up Dad's section to verify whether or not his nighttime Risperdal had been changed. I was alarmed to find out that it hadn't. I didn't know whether they hadn't received the fax or if they just hadn't implemented the change yet. Nothing in the notebook reflected the doctor's latest order.

I brought up last night's incident and pressed upon her how critical it was that Dad's medication be changed. She assured me that she would talk to the director immediately. I also gave her the doctor's pager number again in case they needed to get in touch with him.

As I looked around, I noticed that Dad was not in the common area or the dining area, so I walked back towards his room. As I reached his door, I saw a huge piece of paper taped to the front of it, covering most of it. In big, bold letters, it said "William Chester Lee's Room". It had colorful flowers and balloons drawn on it. Some words were also written on it in black ink. I couldn't understand what they meant, but it was clearly Dad's handwriting. It appeared as though one of the caregivers had made the sign for Dad to help him identify his room. The person had even gone so far as to have Dad write something on it so that he would feel a part of it. I really hoped that it would work.

When I walked into the room, Dad was lying in his bed. "Daddy, are you okay?" I asked.

"My lower back is hurting," he replied.

"What happened?" I then asked. Dad didn't know that one of the caregivers had called me about the incident last night. I would let him bring it up first before I mentioned it.

"I found that woman in my bed again last night," he responded. "When she wouldn't leave, I picked her up myself. I think that's what hurt my back."

"Do you want something for the pain?" I asked.

"Yes, Pootie," he replied. "That would help."

"Let me go down and talk to the med tech," I said. "I'll be right back."

I found the technician still at the medicine cart in the common area. "Hey, is it possible to give my dad some ibuprofen?" I asked. "His back is really hurting him."

"Unfortunately, we aren't allowed to give him anything unless we have a PRN for the medicine already set up in his chart," she replied.

"What is a PRN?" I inquired.

"It's an order from a doctor for a specific medicine on an as needed basis," she replied. "It's not something that is scheduled. It's there for the patient if they ever need it. Most of the residents here have a PRN for some type of pain medication."

"Okay," I said. "Am I allowed to set that up for my dad?" She slowly shook her head no. "Even if it's just an over-the-counter pain medicine?"

"No, it has to come from one of his doctors," she replied. "It not only needs to say which medicine, but also the dosage. You can either bring the unopened medication to me or we can request it from Collier Village Pharmacy." I suddenly felt very frustrated.

"That's going to take awhile to get in place," I said. "He needs something now. Can I just give it to him myself?"

"Sure," she replied. "Just know that you can't leave it in his room. You either have to bring it to us and we'll store it in the cart for you or you can take it with you. The residents are not allowed to have any type of medication in their room."

As I walked back to Dad's room, I felt very disturbed thinking about the medicine policy. I clearly understood the importance of having a doctor's order for all prescription meds, but it just seemed that forcing the same rules with over-the-counter drugs was a bit much. Something that should have been relatively easy to implement was made very convoluted.

I then called Mom on my cell phone and asked her if she would bring some ibuprofen with her when she came up later. I'd have to remember to contact one of Dad's doctors to get an order so this wouldn't happen again.

As I looked around Dad's room, I noticed that everything was in shambles. Shoes were piled in the corner. One of the nightstand drawers was missing, which I soon found lodged underneath the bed. I struggled to get it out as it was really a tight fit. I didn't know how Dad had managed to get it under there in the first place. One of the dresser drawers was also missing, which I later discovered behind the recliner. I looked through the remaining drawers and they all contained an assortment of items. A tube of toothpaste and a shoe was inside the top nightstand drawer with the other drawers looking very much the same.

I didn't ask Dad what had happened, but quietly put the items back where they belonged. I began to see a correlation between the condition of Dad's room and the previous night's stress level. The worse the anxiety, the messier the room was.

The closet was again empty of any hanging clothes and the dirty clothes hamper was full. A bag was sitting by the front door with hangers and clothes in it. I made a decision to fold all of the items normally kept on hangers and put them in his dresser. If this was Dad's way of telling me that he didn't want things in his closet, then I would respectfully listen to him. I didn't want to do anything to create extra anxiety in him. After all, this was his room and I needed to give him some control.

Before long, Dad decided to walk down to the common area to watch television with the other residents. I took this as a good sign as he was starting to feel more comfortable around them. After we sat down, Dad lovingly placed his arm around me. I looked at him and he smiled. Then, he scrunched his nose at me in that affectionate manner that he always did. We were good again.

"Tomorrow, some students from a local Christian school are coming to sing in the front lobby," I said. "Would you be interested in listening to them?"

"That sounds great," Dad replied. "I think I'd enjoy that."

"Okay, I'll get here early so we can go together," I said.

When I got ready to leave, Dad insisted on walking me to the front door. I made sure that he didn't see the code when I entered it. At the door, I gently kissed him goodbye. Even after I had walked a few feet past the door, Dad still stood watching me with the door open. I stopped and turned around to face him. "Daddy, you need to shut the door," I said. I didn't know whether he didn't want me to leave or whether he wanted to get out. He smiled and slowly let it close. As I walked down the hall towards the front entrance, I imagined my dad walking down his hall back to his new life. I longed for the day when it got easier to leave him.

Friday, March 25, 2011

I smiled at her loving face, as it was becoming more familiar to me every day. Regardless of what she was doing, she always made it a point to say hello and ask how I was doing. Her happiness and spirit had permeated the halls in the memory care unit, making a special environment of one normally filled with so much grief. "Let me get that for you, Sugar," Alexandra said as she amiably opened the door for me. My hands were completely full with Dad's clean laundry. She followed me in as we made our way down the hall.

As I walked into Dad's room, I noticed that his bed was stripped of all sheets, with even the bedspread missing. I checked the dirty clothes hamper and all of the bedding was stuffed tightly inside, making it completely full. I had been doing laundry for Dad for over a week now. The memory care unit had their own washer and dryer in a little closet off of the dining area. His laundry was supposed to get done twice a week, on average. In an emergency, it would be handled more often.

Every day, I typically found clothes in the hamper and separate bags by the door. I didn't want him to be without clothing or sheets, so I routinely took some of his laundry home with me to wash. Mom had done the same. The amount of clothes that I found was more than what he should have been wearing. I didn't know if he was having accidents or whether they were getting placed there in the nighttime when he was anxious.

After making Dad's bed for him, I filled one of the trash bags that I had found in a bathroom drawer with the dirty clothes and bedding. As soon as I got home, I would once again do his laundry and bring it back to him in the morning.

While Dad was busy eating lunch, I took the opportunity to talk with Susan. I was curious how he was doing when we weren't there. According to her, he was starting to do better, although he did get a little more agitated as the day progressed and it neared sundown. For most people, that was the time of day when they began to relax and enjoy the evening. For someone with Sundowner's, like my dad, it was the beginning of his daily nightmare.

While researching this condition, I had found that the term was originally associated with behavior after sundown which, for the most part, was true. Unfortunately, as I had seen many times, they now believed that the behavior could occur at any point during the day. I had seen my dad agitated during all hours. The norm, though, was that it started anywhere from 3 – 5 p.m. From that point until the next morning, he usually had several bouts of restlessness where he couldn't sleep and would do a lot of pacing.

I mentioned to Susan that the doctor had recommended us limiting our visits to once a week. As soon as I said it, she smiled. "I have to agree with the doctor," she said. "I think it would be better if your dad had some time to get used to all of us. It's probably harder for you than it is for him. Just give him some time to adjust."

That afternoon, Dad had several more visitors, including one of his neighbors. They had casually visited in the common area for awhile. Not long after that, Mom brought their dog, Barron, up to see him. It was the first time in a month that Dad had seen his pet. As soon as Barron saw him, he excitedly ran and jumped up on his lap, both so happy to see each other.

Today was a good day for Dad. Not only was he calm, but he seemed genuinely happy. He had only been at the facility for a week and a half, but seemed to be getting more used to it every day. Mom and I had both cut back on our daily visits. It was so unbelievably hard on the days that I didn't visit Dad. As I would busily go about my normal routine, I would constantly wonder what he was doing and whether he was alright. Even though I felt it was for the best, it was still very difficult as I felt guilty every day that I wasn't with him. Susan was absolutely right. It was probably much harder on me than it was on Dad.

Saturday, March 26, 2011

I stared out the window as the trepidation slowly started to take hold. Bob would be picking me up soon. As if on cue, I felt the arms of my husband from behind firmly wrap around my waist. He could always tell when I was worried as I wore my emotions on my sleeve. Today would be Dad's first appointment with his psychiatrist since his stay at Woodland Hospital. I intentionally didn't mention it to him yesterday so that he'd be as calm as possible. It wasn't until noon and I knew we'd have plenty of time to get him ready this morning.

When Bob and I arrived at Arbor Forest, we found Dad relaxing in his room. Fortunately, he was neatly dressed and had already eaten breakfast. I mentioned to him that Bob and I were going to be taking him out of the facility to see Dr. Franklin. He actually seemed fine with the news.

As I put all of Dad's clean laundry in the drawers, I curiously checked the dirty clothes hamper. It was about half full which was a good sign. I wouldn't need to take any laundry home with me today.

On the ride over, Dad sat in the front seat and casually looked out the window the entire time. We travelled down Buford Drive which was a direct route from Arbor Forest to Woodland Hospital. Dad had driven on this road so many times over the years, making several comments about places he clearly recognized.

As we later waited in the lobby at Woodland Hospital, Dad looked a little alarmed. I wasn't sure if he recognized this area of the facility or not. "Don't worry," I said. "We're just going to see the doctor for an appointment and then we'll leave." I smiled at him and added "You're coming back with us." That seemed to ease his mind.

The appointment actually went very smoothly. Dad was noticeably quiet as he sat across from Dr. Franklin, not talking unless the doctor specifically asked him something. Even then, his answers were short and to the point. I, in fact, did most of the talking. When I needed to say something to the doctor in private, I simply lowered my voice. I knew that Dad's hearing was getting bad and he wouldn't be able to hear me if I intentionally talked low. By discreetly handling it this way, Dad wouldn't feel like I was talking behind his back.

I told the doctor about all of the confusion that Dad had experienced with his new room. I also mentioned that his anxiety was setting in before sundown. Based on that, the doctor changed the time of his evening dose of Risperdal to 5 p.m. instead of the previous time of 9 p.m. with the dosage amounts remaining the same.

I really liked Dr. Franklin. We agreed to come back in twelve weeks. "You have my pager number if you need to get in touch with me before then," he said. I truly hoped we wouldn't need to do that, but just knowing that he was only a phone call away was very comforting.

Since Dad had missed lunch at Arbor Forest, Bob decided to stop at McDonalds on the way back. Dad actually hadn't had a fast food burger in months. Bob ordered him a Quarter Pounder with Cheese and some fries. They both hungrily ate their food in the truck on the way back. Dad finished every single bite of his lunch.

When we eventually got back, Bob dropped Dad and me off at the front door while he parked his truck. We wanted to get Dad settled before we left. Today was the first time that we had taken Dad off of the premises since he had moved here. I had been a little nervous knowing that if he was in the middle of a Sundowner's episode, it could have been extremely dangerous. As it turned out, he remained very calm the entire time. My ultimate goal was to bring Dad to my house for a home-cooked meal, something that we had repeatedly done ever since he had moved to Georgia. I wanted to show him that some things were never going to change.

Sunday, March 27, 2011

The smile on his young face always warmed my heart, knowing the reason why made it all the more special today. As I watched Chris get ready to leave, there was no denying the excitement within him. After he had neatly dressed, he'd gone into the bathroom and carefully combed his hair, wanting everything to be just right. When he walked back into the living room, I embraced him tightly. He was going to see his Papa for the first time in over a month.

This was a good week for Dad as he seemed to be adjusting more and more every day. As soon as Randy and Chris walked into his room, he started smiling. "Hey Lil' Monkey!" Dad happily said. Chris eagerly ran up to him and sat on his lap. They hugged each other closely. Dad then looked up at Randy. "Hey Ran."

Randy extended his hand to Dad and they shook. "How are you doing, Chester?" Randy asked.

"I can't complain," he replied.

"I hear you need a shave," Randy said.

"It's been awhile since I had one," Dad commented.

Dad had actually not had a shave in weeks. He had asked me a couple of days ago if I thought Randy would do it. I knew it would make a world of difference in him. Mom had brought Dad's electric razor in earlier this week. Randy soon found it in one of the bathroom drawers. A stool with a stuffed dog resting on it sat in the corner of his bedroom, which Randy conveniently moved to the middle of the room for Dad to sit on.

As Randy gently began to shave Dad's face, Dad sat very still. Chris was casually sitting in the blue recliner directly in front of him. Dad continued to watch him and occasionally scrunched his nose in that affectionate way that he always did.

After about fifteen minutes, Randy had Dad look in the mirror, his smile saying everything. He was definitely pleased with the results. "Aw, Randy, that looks good," Dad said. He then took some aftershave that was sitting on the bathroom counter and put a little on his face. About that time, Chris walked up behind him looking curious. Dad put a dab of the aftershave on his cheeks as well. "Now you smell good, too."

Before long, they leisurely walked to the common area. Dad comfortably sat on one of the couches with Chris sitting on his lap, his pride overflowing. Several of the other residents began watching the two of them. "Is this your grandson?" asked Helen, one of the women living on the other end of the hall.

"Yes, indeed," replied Dad. "This is my Chris. I call him 'My Lil' Monkey'." He then affectionately kissed Chris on the cheek and Chris smiled. Dad loved showing his grandchildren off to the other residents. There was such a difference in my dad in just two weeks. He definitely seemed more comfortable in his new environment and was so much more social with everyone. Now, my pride was overflowing.

That evening, I thought about Chris' earlier visit with Dad. A memory suddenly popped into my head, seemingly out of nowhere. Sometimes the human brain amazed me, how it locked our memories away and brought them out at just the right time. Today, I had surprisingly remembered one of Chris' field trips when he was in Pre-K at Discovery Point. It had been Christmastime. All of the children had made special Christmas cards earlier in the week. The planned outing was to an assisted living facility in Buford.

The children had excitedly ridden over on the day care bus, while a couple of parents had followed behind. As we made our way inside the facility, we were greeted by several friendly faces. We were then led down a long hall to an area on the other side of the building. The door was secretly opened with a special code, after which we all walked down another long hall that opened up into an area where several elderly people had gathered. They were currently seated all about the room. Some rested in wheelchairs, while others sat on couches and chairs. All of their eyes were steadily glued to their young visitors.

The children soon made their way to the front of the room and started joyously singing their Christmas carols. Everyone looked on with smiles on their faces, probably reminiscing about memorable times in their past. After a few songs, the children each delivered their special Christmas card to someone in the room. By the time they were done, everyone had a priceless card in their possession. It was such a unique moment to watch these people suddenly come to life at the hands of these young children. You could see it in their eyes that it had meant the world to them.

It wasn't until this very moment that I suddenly realized that the assisted living facility that Chris had gone to was Arbor Forest. The area that the children had happily sung in was the memory care unit. Chris had been in the exact same area that my dad now called home. Never would we have imagined that just three short years from that remarkable day, Chris would again be coming back to the same unit, only this time to visit his Papa Lee. Life could be so unpredictable at times.

Thursday, March 31, 2011

As I stood looking around the room, I saw chaos everywhere, the image being that of a home ransacked by an intruder. Everything before me was strewn about. I wondered how long it had taken to get this way, possibly all night. I took a deep breath as I slowly contemplated where to start.

The first thing I did was get Dad's bed in order. He was out of clean sheets, but fortunately I had washed a set in the laundry that I brought back. I then bagged up the dirty laundry to go home with me.

As I looked through some of the drawers, I noticed that everything was out of place. Then, it suddenly struck me. It seemed that no matter how many times I had arranged the drawers back in an order that I preferred, I would still come in to find them in disarray. Was it possible that to Dad, they were already in order? If I left things in the drawers as they were, would he still move them around or would they remain in the same place?

I had always been a perfectionist, but maybe, just this once, I needed to see things as they looked through my dad's eyes. Instead of viewing things as they appeared from the outside in, I needed to look at things in the Alzheimer's world from the inside out. Today, as hard as it was for me, I would intentionally refrain from putting everything back in its place.

Before long, Alexandra came by and announced that it was time for lunch. As we arrived in the dining hall, Dad immediately made his way to his reserved spot in front of the window while I pulled up a chair next to him, an honorary member of the "Guy Table". I would occasionally tease Dad about the seating arrangements. The truth was he felt very comfortable with this setup. The other men at the table normally didn't talk too much and I think Dad preferred it that way.

I was usually the one that started the conversations. I would curiously ask Donald about his days in the Navy. I wasn't sure what profession Joseph had had during his life. He talked so low that I would have to bend my head down so that my ear was positioned right in front of his mouth. Even then, I didn't always hear him. I had to admit that sometimes, I shook my head without knowing exactly what I was agreeing with. Unfortunately, I was never able to engage Frank in any type of talk. Most of my words, however, were directed towards my dad.

Some of the residents had a difficult time feeding themselves at mealtime. The caregivers would have to take turns giving them a bite to eat. Dad's eating skills were still great. Not only could he feed himself independently, he was very neat in doing so. A lot of times, the staff would generously bring me a plate of my own. On the days when I didn't eat, Dad would usually load up his fork with food and hold it up to my mouth to lovingly share it with me. Lunchtime had become a very special time for us both.

After the meal, I took Dad out back and neatly trimmed his nails. I didn't have to persuade him in the least as he usually jumped at the chance to go outside. I had luckily found an extra pair of sunglasses in my car for him. At times, it could get very bright out back. He absolutely loved the serenity that the outdoors provided. This was part of our new routine that Dad inevitably looked forward to every time I came to see him. I felt very optimistic over how things had gone this week.

After I picked Chris up from school, we went to Mill Creek High School for the Gwinnett County Track and Field Championships. Shawn would be running the second leg of the 4x800m relay at 4:00. No matter what my schedule was like or how many things I had going on, I tried hard to never miss one of the boys' events. It was especially important to me to always be there for them.

I sadly thought about the fact that Dad had never gone to a cross country or track meet for Preston or Shawn. The reason was simply that I had never invited him to one. They were different than normal sporting events. The cross country meets were for one race only, a 5K. Typically, the spectators would follow the runners around different parts of the course. There wasn't a single location that allowed you to sit and see the entire race. Instead, you had to steadily follow the runners and I knew that all of the necessary walking would have been hard for my dad.

The track meets had the added advantage of having a stadium to sit in and comfortably watch the races. However, most runners only competed in one race. You could easily travel an hour to only watch a race lasting a couple of minutes. I had thought that these types of events would be too hard on Dad.

Sitting here now, I realized that Dad would probably never again get the chance to watch his grandsons' race. I wished so much that I had taken advantage of the opportunity when I had it. Sometimes, we took life for granted. I now felt painfully aware of how quickly it could change.

Friday, April 1, 2011

I was casually sitting on my bed early this morning putting on my sneakers when my cell phone suddenly rang. The Breaking Benjamin ringtone clearly indicated that it was Preston, sounding very upset. He was calling to let me know that an unfortunate incident had occurred in his dorm room last night. At about 1 a.m., his roommate had staggered into the room, heavily intoxicated. He carelessly knocked the television off of the stand. Then, he unexpectedly threw up in the trash can, after which he passed out on the futon. Knowing he had an important test first thing in the morning, Preston rolled over and tried to go back to sleep.

About two hours later, Preston was again awoken. As his roommate slowly got up from the futon, he suddenly lost his balance and grabbed Preston's bed. He then made his way to the other side of the room near Preston's closet. When Preston opened his eyes, he surprisingly saw his roommate standing in front of his white dresser, urinating on the front of it. By the time he had finished, he had also managed to pee on Preston's shoes and most importantly, all of his notebooks for his classes. His roommate then fell back on the futon and passed out once again. Preston was forced to leave the room due to the foul odor.

Before long, the RA at the end of the hall found out what had happened and called the building RA. Because of the seriousness of the situation, campus security was immediately called. They cautiously entered the dorm room, which smelled strongly of urine and vomit, and found the roommate still passed out on the futon. He was eventually awoken and taken away.

Preston unfortunately had to take a critical test at 8 a.m. after only getting two hours of sleep. It upset me so much. This boy had disrespected my son the entire year. Time and time again, he would agree to get his act together, but unfortunately he never did. Preston dealt with more than any student should've ever had to deal with. He had consistently honored the "code" the entire year. Regrettably, he had eventually been pushed to his limits.

Later that morning, I visited Dad, where we casually sat on one of the couches in the common area. He could easily tell that something was bothering me. I told him all about the incident in Preston's dorm as he listened so intently, the undeniable look of concern in his eyes showing how much it bothered him. He didn't like to hear when someone was treated so badly, especially when it was one of his family members. Dad deeply loved all of his grandchildren.

When Dad had moved to Atlanta, Preston was only nine years old. He had regularly played soccer since the age of four. For eight years, Dad had religiously watched all of Preston's games. At the beginning of every season, he would ask me for the game schedule so he could make sure he planned ahead. Unless he was seriously sick, he never missed one.

At the end of every game, Dad would patiently wait for Preston to come across the field. Then, he would say "You played good, Prez." Dad had called Preston this name for as long as I could remember, always warming my heart when I heard it.

Dad and I ended up calmly talking for over an hour. He seemed so lucid today, reminding me of so many other talks that we had had throughout our lives. No matter what was going on with my dad, I didn't ever want to give them up.

Before I left, I went to Dad's room. It was a nice surprise to find his bed actually made. As I curiously looked through the dresser drawers, I noticed that everything was still disorganized. Various items from the bathroom were still mixed in with the clothes. What struck me, though, was that the mess I was seeing was the same mess that I had seen yesterday. It actually didn't look much different at all. Was I trying to inflict my orderliness on my dad? Today was undoubtedly another step in my learning process.

Later that afternoon, I took some homemade cookies to Chris' second grade class for his birthday. Chris swiftly ran up and hugged me as soon as I entered the classroom. The children had loved the break from their schoolwork. Several of them also came up and lovingly put their arms around me. It was a definite reminder of how sweet and simple life could be at this age.

A couple of hours later, I made the trip to Athens to get Preston. I had promised to come pick him up after his last class. He very much wanted to come home for Chris' birthday and also needed to get away. Under the circumstances, I felt that a couple of days break would be good for him. The dust needed to settle and I needed my family together this weekend.

Saturday, April 2, 2011

He had a sincere love for the sport that had existed his entire life. Whether it was playing it himself when he was younger, watching it on television or sitting in the stands while one of his grandchildren played, baseball had always been a big part of him. As recently as last season, he had gone to almost all of Andrew's games. He truly loved watching him play.

It just so happened that Andrew had a baseball game this morning. Bob and Mom were planning on going to Arbor Forest beforehand to get Dad and drive him to the game. I felt somewhat apprehensive thinking about today's plans as it would be another important milestone for Dad. If everything went according to plan, it would be the second time that Dad was taken out of the facility.

As they walked by the common area, one of the caregivers suddenly stopped them. "I just wanted to give you a heads up," she said. "He's been packing his things up all morning. He thinks he is leaving for good. We couldn't even get him to come down and eat breakfast." Bob and Mom were immediately alarmed. This was not what they had expected.

When they soon arrived at Dad's room, all of his belongings were indeed packed and sitting by the door. Bags were everywhere. In addition, the hamper was filled to the brim. It was positioned alongside his two trash cans, which were also full. Dad was impatiently waiting in the recliner, looking frazzled.

"Hey Dad," Bob said. "Why are all your things packed up?"

"I'm ready to leave," he replied. "This is not my home."

"Dad, we were just taking you to watch Drew's game," he said. "Then, we were bringing you right back."

This was clearly not what Dad wanted to hear as he began to get more agitated. "I don't want to come back," he replied angrily. "I want to go to my home." He was adamant.

"You can't, Dad," Bob responded. No matter what Bob said, Dad invariably argued with him. He was very upset. I had made the mistake of telling Dad about the game earlier in the week, thinking it would make him happy and give him something to look forward to. I had no idea that it would lead to this.

Dad looked completely exhausted. He apparently hadn't slept much throughout the night as it would have taken him a considerable amount of time to pack everything up. They absolutely couldn't take Dad out of the memory care unit while he was in this state. It wouldn't be safe. There was also a good chance that he would put up a fight when it got time to bring him back.

"I'm sorry, Dad," said Bob. "We can't take you out when you're this upset. Maybe we'll try again for another game."

Bob and Mom had no choice but to leave without Dad. It was not a good exit. Dad remained in his recliner and crossly stared at them as they slowly walked away. He said nothing.

I thought about the mass confusion that Dad was undoubtedly experiencing. All he wanted was to live his life again as he had before the 911 incident. He simply wanted to be there for his grandson. I couldn't imagine the lack of control that he was feeling. It absolutely broke my heart.

I soon made a call to Arbor Forest and spoke to one of the caregivers. I was really worried about Dad. They assured me that not only would they check on him as soon as we hung up, but they'd keep a close eye on him the rest of the day. I had thought about bringing Chris to see him later, but now I was a little nervous. The last thing I wanted was for Chris to see his Papa in an agitated state. The rest of us were used to it, but it would be devastating for Chris. I truly hoped that Dad would calm down and be able to sort things out. Today would be one of those days when Dad was best left alone.

With everything that was going on, we decided to celebrate Chris' 8th birthday quietly with the family, taking him to his favorite restaurant,

Zaxby's. When we got back home, Chris opened up his presents, after which we had cake and ice cream. Mom, Bob and the boys came over to watch Chris blow out his candles. The empty spot at the table seemed to emanate sadness. Dad had never once missed celebrating Chris' birthday with him. Even when Chris was born, Dad had driven up to the hospital by himself to see him for the very first time.

Chris' birthday this year was a very low-key event, but he didn't seem to mind. I decided at that moment that I would take Chris and some of his cake to Arbor Forest tomorrow. We would celebrate with Dad one day late.

Later that evening, Preston got an unexpected text message from one of his roommate's friends, actually giving him a hard time. He even had the nerve to bring up the "code" and how you just didn't cross that line. Preston firmly stood his ground as the messages continued between them. I was really proud of the way he had handled this whole situation.

Preston had already contacted his RA and was trying to get moved to another dorm room. Only one month was left in this semester, but I felt uneasy about him returning to the same environment. I knew that this was going to be one of those times in my life where I ultimately had to step back and allow my son to handle the situation on his own, completely relying on my faith. Not only did I believe in Preston, but I also believed in God. That faith would carry me through this distressing ordeal.

Sunday, April 3, 2011

Chris carefully held the cake in his lap as we drove to Arbor Forest. The look on his face was clearly one of excitement, knowing that he'd soon celebrate his birthday with his Papa. I, on the other hand, had a very nervous feeling inside, a feeling that I now lived with every day. It never went away. As each new day began, I never knew what it would bring. I also never knew what I would find when I walked through the doors of the memory care unit.

Taking care of parents could be so hard at times, nothing really preparing us for it. Before we had children, we read books extensively on what to expect and how best to care for them. With parents, there didn't seem to be any advance notice. It just sort of happened one day and you found yourself in a situation where you were caring for them. As with all new life experiences, I sometimes made mistakes. I was slowly learning and adapting to my new role in the sandwich generation.

Chris and I had brought Dad a couple of slices of birthday cake. I wasn't sure what his demeanor would be today. My plan was that if he were still agitated, I would have Chris wait at the other end of the hall near the front door while I took care of Dad. This way he wouldn't be able to witness any agitation. I could usually tell within a few seconds what state Dad was in. If he were upset, then Chris and I would have to leave.

As it turned out, Dad was completely calm. As soon as he smiled and greeted us, I knew that everything was okay. Chris soon handed Dad the plastic container of cake and a fork. He then proceeded to tell him excitedly that it was his birthday yesterday and he was now eight years old.

Dad ate all of the birthday cake, even giving Chris a few bites. He thoroughly enjoyed it. I wasn't the least bit surprised since, like me, my dad had a sweet tooth.

While Dad and Chris visited, I busily unpacked all of his belongings which were still sitting by the door. I filled the drawers with his clothes, put his toiletries back in the bathroom and moved the hamper and trash cans back in place. He remained completely calm the entire time. We never talked about what had happened yesterday. I truly hoped that he wouldn't remember it as I knew the events that occurred during a Sundowner's episode were sometimes blocked from his memory. Hopefully, this was one of those times.

Dad's brothers and cousins would be travelling to Atlanta this coming weekend to see him. The timing seemed perfect as Dad could really use some special family time. I also wanted him to realize that this was yet another thing that wasn't going to change. I wisely decided not to mention the visit until later in the week. I definitely didn't want a repeat performance of yesterday.

This evening, Randy and Shawn drove Preston back to Athens. I was incredibly nervous, not knowing what he would find when he returned to his room. I honestly hoped that Preston would stay in one of his friends' rooms tonight. Randy made sure he was safe before he left to return home.

Late that night, I got a text message from Preston saying that his roommate never showed up. Preston had boldly decided to sleep in his own room tonight. I completely trusted his judgment and prayed that he would be okay.

Monday, April 4, 2011

I constantly tossed and turned throughout the night, waking up several times thinking about Preston. I finally decided after the last time that sleep was obviously not going to come. I soon made my way to the kitchen to put a pot of coffee on. Riley appeared in the doorway to keep me company as she was never too far from me. As she eagerly took her morning bone from my hand, my day had officially started.

When Preston got back from his 8:00 class, he was stunned to find most of his roommate's belongings gone. Later that day, his roommate and a friend unexpectedly came by the dorm room. He was surprisingly very apologetic to Preston and had even bought him a new pair of shower shoes. He then let Preston know that he was moving somewhere else. My son now officially had the room to himself.

I felt such a tremendous relief that everything had worked out for the best, neither Preston nor his roommate harboring any ill will feelings. It had definitely been a long year for him, but finally the aggravation was over. I truly believed in the power of prayer.

Shawn and Chris were happily on Spring Break this week. Randy had taken some vacation time to spend with them. Earlier this morning, Shawn had track practice. He'd specifically asked me to wait for him, very much wanting to visit Dad this afternoon.

When we arrived at Arbor Forest, we found Dad leisurely sitting in the common area. As soon as he saw us, a huge smile broke across his face. "Hi Pootie," he said. He then noticed Shawn standing behind me. "Hi Shawnee."

"Hi Grandpa," Shawn replied, as he took a seat next to Dad on the couch. I pulled a chair from the dining area over so that I was sitting next to them. The room was completely full. I was so glad to see Dad out here on his own visiting with the other residents. It was truly a good sign.

Shawn began to tell Dad about everything that was going on with him at school. I sat back quietly and watched them. It seemed like just yesterday that Shawn had come to his Papa asking him for his help with an extracurricular project. He had been in the Cub Scouts when he was in 2nd grade. When it came time for the derby races, he needed some assistance and Dad had generously offered to help him. They worked for hours on end in Dad's basement to make the car. Shawn had even found an old Lego driver complete with helmet that they carefully placed in the driver's seat.

A week after the car was finished, it was time to race. Dad had eagerly come over to go to the competition with the boys. Shawn ended up winning 3rd place in Show and was awarded a special trophy. It not only made Shawn's day, but Dad's as well. To this day, that car still proudly rests on one of Shawn's shelves.

While Dad and Shawn were busy talking, I decided to check his room. I had put everything up neatly yesterday and wondered if I would find it that way again today. As I carefully looked through the drawers, I again found some stray items. It certainly wasn't as bad as it was some mornings when I came in. I decided to leave everything as I originally found it. I was no longer going to try to control how and where Dad's things were placed. In Dad's world, everything was arranged the way he wanted. From now on, I was going to respect that.

When I came back out to the common area, I noticed that everyone's eyes were clearly on one of the residents named Helen. Helen was a petite woman with shoulder length, gray hair. She normally sat in a wheelchair, but today, the caregiver had placed her directly on one of the couches.

She was currently very agitated. Several of the residents suffered from Sundowner's. When they occasionally got upset, they sometimes displayed a foul mouth. It was not at all uncommon to hear one of them dropping the f-bomb. These were mainly the female residents.

The caregiver was trying to pick Helen up and place her in her wheelchair. She needed to go back to her room to be changed, but Helen didn't want any part of it. "Get your hands off of me!" she said angrily.

"Miss Helen, I'm not hurting you," the caregiver said. "We have to change your clothes."

"If you lay one more hand on me, I'm gonna call the police and have you arrested," Helen said. She was small, but very feisty. Normally, she was very sweet. I had had many conversations with her in the past. Today, she had just been pushed too far.

"Do that," the caregiver said. "I'll tell them how you treated me."

"I'll knock you on your ass," Helen said sternly. "I want to speak to my son right now."

"Miss Helen, your son is at work," she said, as she proceeded to pick Helen up. Helen then smacked her on the arm. The caregiver somehow managed to get her in the wheelchair. I could hear Helen loudly yelling at her the entire time they moved down the hall towards her room.

I looked at Dad and he shrugged his shoulders and smiled. Most of the caregivers in this unit were very good at dealing with Alzheimer's and Sundowner's. The girl today was clearly not that experienced. Even I with my limited knowledge could spot that. Instead of arguing with Helen, she should have redirected her. It could have possibly prevented her from getting more agitated.

I recently read that when someone with Alzheimer's gets agitated, it was crucial that they be calmed down quickly. If that agitation rose to a certain level and remained that way for an extended period of time, it could harm the brain even further. Even if you managed to calm the person down, the damage may have already occurred. I was beginning to understand why so many of these residents had medication to keep them calm. It wasn't just for the benefit of the caregiver. It was also to help keep the Alzheimer's from getting any worse.

Thursday, April 7, 2011

He usually didn't venture out of his room too much except for meals. As I made my way down the hall, Joseph surprised me as he walked towards me using his walker. He had a big grin on his face and apparently wanted to say something to me. I moved close to him and leaned my head near his mouth. Unfortunately, the only words I could make out were "room" and "food". I smiled at him and nodded my head before eventually continuing down the hall, having no idea what I had agreed to.

I found Dad sitting on the floor in his closet, trying diligently to put socks on his feet. He already had three on the left foot and five on the right. He was having a difficult time getting more socks on top of the ones that he was already wearing, looking so confused. "Let me help you, Daddy," I said.

I bent down and gently started stripping off the extra layers. I left him with one matching white sock on each foot. "What shoes do you want to wear?" I asked.

"The brown loafers," he replied. Unfortunately, his shoes weren't lined up in his closet anymore. I soon found the matching loafers that he wanted and helped him put them on. I then helped him get up off of the floor.

While we were in the bathroom, I showed Dad the bag of pull-ups that I had brought. I placed a stack in his top nightstand drawer with the rest placed inside the bathroom cabinet under the sink. He was having so many accidents lately that I felt this would help with the laundry. "From now on when you get dressed, I want you to use these instead of your briefs," I said. He nodded his head in agreement. I wasn't sure if he would remember or not, but I knew that the caregivers would as they were actually the ones to suggest them.

After lunch, Dad and I decided to take a walk on the trails outside of the assisted living section. This particular walking area was much larger and I thought it would be good exercise for Dad.

Dad did great as we walked for several laps. We eventually decided to rest for awhile in the gazebo in the back, the weather beautiful. While sitting together, we talked about several different things currently going on with Randy and the boys. Dad seemed very lucid today.

Then, he looked directly at me. "Why am I here, Pootie?" he asked calmly. "I don't understand why I'm not at home." It was completely out of the blue and I was not expecting it.

"Daddy, you have Alzheimer's," I replied. "You aren't able to take care of yourself like you used to." He continued to stare at me. "It causes you to forget things. Some of those things are very important. The disease also causes you to get anxious. When that happens, you usually get very agitated. Dr. Franklin feels that you need someone to watch over you. Mom isn't well enough to do that anymore." I took a deep breath.

"We had some very close calls at home during the past several months," I continued. "We spent a lot of time in the emergency room. We just can't take that chance anymore. I don't want anything bad to happen to you, Daddy."

At that moment, he slowly looked away. Then, I noticed why. He soon wiped away a tear that had fallen down his cheek. My daddy was crying.

I hated so much that he was hurting, wanting more than anything in the world to take away his pain. I knew I could do nothing to stop what was happening to him, feeling so unbelievably helpless. All I could do was watch this horrible disease take a little bit more of him every day. I despised it so much.

My dad had come to me because he wanted the truth, knowing that I couldn't lie to him. And I never would. My words had not given him the solace that he desperately wanted. They had probably even taken away some of his hope. The reality was that no matter how much I wanted to, I couldn't change the course my dad was on. All I could do was hold his hand and walk by his side.

We both remained seated in that gazebo, looking out at the beautiful trees. Nothing else was said. All that could be heard was the chirping of the nearby birds. I placed my dad's hand in mine and he gently squeezed it. Before long, my own tears began to fall. It was these times that were by far the hardest.

Spring of 1950

Dad had played baseball for years. He was a good all around player. He caught well; he fielded well; he even hit well. Unfortunately, he was not a long ball hitter.

One day, his father decided to do something about that. Dad had a game scheduled for later that day. Before the game started, Grandpa calmly called Dad aside. "I'll tell you what," he said. "If you hit a home run, I'll buy you a car."

Dad stared at Grandpa with wide eyes, completely shocked. "Really?" he asked. "You're telling me that if I get a homer, you'll buy me a car?"

Grandpa convincingly shook his head yes. "I will," he reiterated.

Dad slowly walked away. Every few steps, he turned and skeptically looked back at Grandpa. Grandpa just stood there and smiled at Dad.

By the 8th inning, Dad had yet to get a home run. He had successfully hit the ball several times, just not out of the park. Grandpa then walked up to the dugout and got Dad's attention.

Dad walked over to talk to his father privately. "I've been thinking about our deal," Grandpa said. "I've decided to change it. If you get a home run, I will buy you a brand new car."

Dad laughed incredulously. "You aren't serious?" he asked.

"Yes, I am," Grandpa replied. "If you hit a homer, I'll get you a new car."

Dad's smile stretched from ear to ear. He couldn't believe this latest proposal. He excitedly returned to the game, while Grandpa returned to his seat.

It soon became time for Dad to bat again. The crowd was silent. Grandpa watched with anticipation. As soon as the ball went over the plate, Dad immediately made contact. The ball went sailing up in the air. It kept going farther and farther. Dad stood in amazement and watched it. Then, it suddenly happened. The ball dropped down on the other side of the fence. Dad had actually hit it out of the park. The only problem was that it was about six inches to the left of the foul line. Dad had just missed it.

Dad then did what only a kid desperately wanting a car would do. He turned around and anxiously looked up into the stands at his father. The baseball game was still going on, but Dad's attention was somewhere else. He hoped beyond hope that his hit would satisfy the deal.

Grandpa's heart was racing, never anticipating this happening. He looked down at Dad. Then, he slowly shook his head no. Dad's heart suddenly dropped. He had come so close to getting that new car. He had actually never hit the ball over the fence before. Today, he had missed a new car by only six inches. What were the odds?

Friday, April 8, 2011

I saw him from across the room, immediately taken aback at how handsome he appeared. He had never looked as relaxed in this environment as he did at this very moment. I lovingly smiled at my dad as I made my way towards his dining table. He was currently drinking a cup of coffee with Joseph and looked so happy to see me. I amiably spoke to the other residents as I passed them. I was aware, based on the amount of time that I spent in the memory care unit, that a lot of these residents didn't get many visitors. I already knew all of their names and was beginning to develop a special relationship with them. I made it a point to take the time to talk with the other residents whenever I saw them. A simple hello and some kind words meant so much.

Before long, Dad let me know that he needed to go back to his room. While he was in his bathroom, I swiftly made his bed and straightened up his room. "Pootie, can you help me with this?" Dad called from the next room.

I walked into the bathroom and found Dad having trouble buttoning his pants. As I got closer, I noticed that the button he was having trouble with was for a second pair of pants currently underneath the outer garment. "Dad, you have two pairs of pants on," I said. He looked very confused. "Why don't we take this extra pair off?"

I had him carefully sit down on the bed while I took his shoes off. I then got the second pair of pants off of him. I hadn't noticed anything odd in his clothing when we had walked back to his room earlier. Unfortunately, he had lost so much weight that he could easily wear both pairs of pants without either one fitting too tight.

I then took Dad out back to trim his nails, knowing he would want to look and feel his best when he found out about his unexpected weekend visitors. The weather was currently perfect as it was warming up and the sun was out in full force. This simple weekly ritual had turned into our special time together.

"Dad, I have a surprise for you," I said. He looked at me like a wide-eyed little boy waiting in anticipation for some amazing news. "Your brothers and cousins are in town. They should be getting to the motel very soon. Once they get settled, they're going to come up here and see you." He happily began to smile.

"Are they going to take me home?" he asked.

"No, Daddy," I replied. "They're just coming to visit you. Uncle Shelby, Uncle Ronnie, Jeanneen and Johnny will all be here." I wasn't sure where he had gotten the idea that they'd be taking him home. I had hoped that that confusion had been totally resolved last weekend.

Not long after I left, I talked to my Uncle Shelby on the phone. I gave him the address and the code to get into the memory care unit. I also told him about the incident the previous weekend and the comment that Dad had made to me earlier in the day. The thought of them taking Dad out of the facility if he was still confused greatly concerned me. They would have to make that call when they saw him.

Later that day, my Dad's family arrived at Arbor Forest. They had apparently decided to stay inside the unit for today's visit. They met Alexandra for the first time and absolutely loved her. "William, you didn't tell me you had such handsome brothers," she said. "You're going to have all of the ladies on the other side breaking down the door to get in here, Sugar."

They all laughed. Dad hadn't seemed this happy in quite awhile. The unconditional love that existed between them was palpable. It proved that it didn't matter where they were just as long as they were together.

A peacefulness settled inside of me knowing that this weekend I could spend time with my husband and children and not worry about my dad. It wasn't something that I felt very often. I knew that he was in good hands. I also knew that this time with his brothers and cousins would be very special to him. Inside, I hoped that Dad would get a good night's sleep and that his belongings would remain unpacked in the morning.

Saturday, April 9, 2011

They had planned on spending the entire afternoon with him. Even though their last visit had only been three months ago, there was a lot of catching up to do, with so much happening recently. Not only had he been diagnosed with Alzheimer's, but the disease had progressed significantly. As my uncles and cousins slowly made their way down the hall inside of the memory care unit, they soon heard Dad's voice addressing one of the caregivers, his tone clearly indicating he was beginning to get agitated. They had arrived just in time.

As soon as Dad saw them, everything suddenly changed. He immediately smiled and stood to hug them. Whatever was bothering him before had quickly dissipated. Their arrival had managed to calm him down before the agitation had escalated any further.

After several minutes of standing, Shelby made a suggestion. "Do you feel like taking a walk, Chester?" he asked. "We can sit in the rocking chairs in the front of the building." Dad was more than willing to go with them. They knew the change of atmosphere would undoubtedly be good for him.

From the front of the facility, they could easily see the comings and goings of not only the employees and visitors, but also some of the other residents. There was always someone to watch. When they were all seated, Ronnie handed Dad a smoothie that they had brought just for him. "Is that what I think it is?" he asked as he perked up. He immediately took a long sip through the straw. "I do love these."

"They're good for you, too, Gump," Ronnie added.

Not long after they came outside, Alexandra stuck her head out to say hello, soon becoming part of the irrepressible laughter. She was getting a glimpse into the close relationship between my dad and his brothers. Before going back inside, Alexandra politely mentioned that dinner would be around 5.

The five of them leisurely remained outside for a couple of hours. It had turned out to be a gorgeous day. They told stories, laughed, ribbed each other and then laughed some more. It could have easily continued well into the night.

As it neared dinnertime, they decided to bring Dad back inside. He was in good spirits and had remained very calm all afternoon. He was, however, beginning to get hungry. It was actually no problem getting him to go back into the unit. He loved the food here and was beginning to adjust to his new schedule. The four of them promised to come by in the morning before they left town, their presence making Dad's weekend very special.

That evening, I rode to my parents' home in Buford to visit Mom. While casually sitting on the couch in the family room, I looked through a stack of magazines on the table. I interestingly came across a brochure for Canada. It was an old pamphlet from a trip that my parents had taken not long after they had moved here.

My mom had always wanted to travel, whereas Dad wasn't quite so eager. When she had initially proposed the idea of a trip through Western Canada via train, Dad had actually agreed. We had all been so surprised. It was the first trip that they had taken together in awhile.

They had flown to Calgary and then ridden a train through the Canadian mountains. Every day, the rail tour had taken them someplace new, Branff, Lake Louise, Jasper and Kamloops, to name some. Eventually, they had reached their last stop which was Vancouver. From there, they would ultimately fly back home, the entire journey lasting ten days. It had been quite an adventure and one that I knew they would always remember.

For several years after that trip, Dad had adamantly turned down all invitations to travel. His brother, Ronnie, had asked him to go to Paradise Island on the tip of Nassau on so many different occasions. Dad always declined as it was simply out of his comfort zone.

In 2007, Dad had agreed to take a train to New Orleans for their first grandson, Chad's wedding. He did not want to drive and he definitely didn't want to fly. The train seemed a reasonable alternative. It was to be a short trip and one that he would very much enjoy.

Mom and Dad had arranged for Randy to pick them up from the train station once they returned. He had arrived early and was in the station looking down below through a large window. From his location, he could easily see the passengers getting off of the train.

Before long, he saw Mom and Dad who happened to be the last passengers to exit the train. They began slowly walking towards the station, with Dad leading. It was dark outside and by now, all of the other passengers had already made it back to the station. At the point where they should have followed the signs and turned left, they didn't. Dad continued to walk forward which would eventually lead them underneath the station. Randy could do nothing but watch.

Dad then accidentally stepped off a small ledge and fell face forward into the dirt and rocks. Mom soon made it to his side and carefully helped him get up. He had unfortunately skinned the palms of both of his hands. Dirt was smeared on the front of his pants. Dad had gotten confused. He was in a place that he had never been before and he had gotten confused. He would not soon forget this troubling incident.

Years later, Dad's brothers generously planned a trip to Las Vegas just for the three of them. They knew Dad was getting older and this might possibly be their last chance. At first, Dad had seemed completely fine with it. As the date got closer however, he began to have doubts. He had told me on several occasions that he just didn't feel comfortable going. He had even asked Randy if he'd be interested in coming with him. He felt confident that Randy would take care of him and never leave his side. Unfortunately, Randy couldn't take the time off from work.

Within a few weeks of the planned trip, Dad regrettably had me email his brothers. He had decided, once and for all, not to go. By this time, all of the plans were already made and it was too late to cancel. Dad just didn't feel good about going. He had his comfort zone and Las Vegas wasn't in it.

As it turned out, the trip to Canada was the last major trip that Mom and Dad ever took. Now looking back, I wondered if Dad somehow knew that something was happening to him. We were all so shocked when he had agreed to go on this trip. I could think of so many other places that he would have probably preferred to travel to. Had he decided to go on this trip just to please my mom? Had he known all along that it would be his last vacation?

Sunday, April 10, 2011

As Chris and I alertly walked down the cereal aisle, I soon found the item I was searching for. I grabbed a box of Special K Vanilla Almond cereal from the top shelf as it was one of his favorites. Some of the caregivers and I had previously discussed Dad's pacing at night. Whenever he would anxiously wander down to the common area, the caregiver on duty would always ask him if he wanted a snack. Mom had even brought some peanut butter crackers and left them in his room for just this reason. Sometimes he would eat them, other times he wouldn't. Regardless, it didn't seem to stop him from wandering down the hall.

We had decided to try something new with Dad last week. My dad had always loved his cereal first thing in the morning. We agreed to keep a box of it in one of the cabinets in the dining area. It was a comfort food for Dad and we hoped that it would create a comfortable feeling inside of him in the middle of the night and help to keep him calm.

The new routine was that whenever Dad wandered down to the common area at night, the caregiver would ask him if he wanted some cereal. Some nights, she had generously fixed it for him and other nights, he had managed by himself. Between bowls in the cabinet, spoons in the drawer and milk in the fridge, Dad had all of the necessary supplies. After fixing his snack, he would calmly sit in his reserved spot in the dining area and eat. Once he was done, he would routinely take his dish and spoon to the sink and rinse them out. Then, he would either leisurely sit on the couch for a little bit or go back to his room. The food in his stomach definitely helped to make him tired. It had actually worked very well for over a week now. He was running out of cereal though and I needed to get him some more. The idea that something so simple had made such a difference left me pleasantly surprised.

Dad was in a good mood this morning when we arrived. He vividly told us all about his visits this weekend. Several times, he laughed out loud as he was relaying something that had happened. It was so good to see him this happy. It was reminiscent of so many other joyful times the five of them had spent together.

When Chris and I left later that afternoon, Dad was sitting in the common area, appearing very calm. The caregiver was thoughtfully playing a collection of older music on the CD player. The songs were evidently popular with a lot of the residents. As I looked around the room, they all seemed so relaxed. A couple of the women were even tapping their feet to the music, clearly enjoying this trip back in time.

Later that afternoon, Mom came to Arbor Forest to visit Dad, bringing Barron with her. At one point, they took him out back for awhile. When they came back inside, Mom immediately noticed that Joseph was standing in front of his room, which was conveniently located right next to Dad's room. Dad took the leash from Mom and walked Barron down the hall towards him. As Mom soon approached them, she heard Dad tell Joseph that he wasn't allowed to hold Barron. Joseph didn't say anything. He just stood there silently. This wasn't like Dad at all. He was beginning to get agitated.

He eventually walked back into his room, with Mom following closely behind. She tried to engage Dad in conversation, but he had no interest. He was very restless. Before long, he determinedly left the room.

About five minutes later, Dad surprisingly returned with one of the other residents. Her name was Margaret and she slowly entered the room using her walker. He vehemently told her to stay put in his room while he found out what was going on. He then left again.

Mom could tell that Margaret was very scared. Neither one of them knew exactly what was happening. What they did know was that Dad was trying to take charge of the situation, whatever it was.

In no time, Mom heard Dad yelling loudly in the hall, urgently wanting to speak to someone in charge. Nothing he said made any sense as he sounded so confused. Mom nervously stuck her head out in the hall to get Dad's attention, but he wouldn't come back in the room.

Mom eventually decided to leave since Dad was completely ignoring her. As she was walking down the hall, Dad began yelling at her to come back. She continued walking and he continued yelling at her. When she finally made it to the front door, she quickly entered the secret code. Once she stepped outside, she made sure that it shut behind her completely. In no time, she could hear Dad on the other side banging on the door and yelling for her.

Mom walked away very disturbed and quickly looked for someone in charge. She suddenly saw Alexandra in the lobby. "He's a wreck right now," Mom said. "He's so upset and he's trying to get out. Can someone go check on him? I'm really worried."

"I'll send someone right now, Shirley," Alexandra replied reassuringly. "Don't you worry about a thing. We'll take good care of him."

When I called the memory care unit later, I found out that Alexandra had asked Anthony to check on Dad. He had gone into the memory care unit and indeed found Dad very agitated. He calmly asked him if he wanted to take a walk with him. That was all it took.

Anthony amiably walked with Dad to one of the break rooms on the other side of the facility. The assisted living residents were currently having an ice cream social. The different atmosphere had done wonders to calm Dad down. Anthony generously dished up some ice cream for the both of them. He then took Dad out front to the rocking chairs where they ate together.

When they were finished, Anthony kindly drove my dad around the facility in the golf cart. Whatever had upset my dad earlier was long forgotten. Anthony had made Dad feel special at a time when he needed it the most.

When I heard this news, I was completely in awe. It took a very special and dedicated person to take someone in a highly agitated state and redirect them. Anthony had managed to turn the dangerous situation completely around into a positive, happy one.

Some of the people that I had met at Arbor Forest were so incredibly loving. They were also very skilled in dealing with Alzheimer's. The length that they would go to take care of their residents truly amazed me. The situation today could not have been handled any better. I was learning from some of the best.

Wednesday, April 13, 2011

He absolutely adored each and every one of them, always going to such great lengths to be involved in their lives. His grandchildren meant the world to him. Earlier in the week, I had proposed an idea to Bob. I thought it might make Dad feel good if he had some homemade pictures and notes from his grandchildren hanging in his room. Only one picture was currently on his wall, but hopefully soon that would change. I really wanted to make the room more comforting to Dad.

The plan was for the grandchildren to bring in something new each week. Dad would then decide where he wanted the homemade picture placed. I hoped that not only would it brighten the room, but it would also lift his spirits.

Yesterday afternoon, Chris had made his first picture for Dad. He chose one of his favorite photos of the two of them taken at one of his birthday parties at Chuck E. Cheese's. He was joyfully sitting in Dad's lap as they both looked out on the stage with smiles on their faces, reminiscent of a very happy time. Chris had carefully taped the picture onto a piece of red construction paper. Underneath the photo, he had written "I love you so much, Grandpa!!!! Love, Chris."

I had also made Dad a picture, taping the last photo that was taken of Dad with Bob and me on a large piece of construction paper. Next to it, I had placed one of my favorite pictures of Curtis. On the piece of paper, I had written the message "Any man can be a father, but it takes someone extremely special to be a Dad! We love you, Daddy!"

After picking Chris up from school, we stopped at McDonald's to get a vanilla milkshake, knowing how much Dad loved these drinks. We were planning on surprising him with it.

As we excitedly walked into the common area, we spotted Dad napping on the couch. Chris gently nudged him and said "Papa, wake up." Dad slowly opened his eyes, so happy to see Chris standing in front of him. They ended up sharing the whole shake and hugging each other the entire time. Dad was in Heaven.

Then, Chris lovingly showed Dad his special picture. Dad didn't say anything at first, but he was obviously deeply moved. After a few seconds, he looked at Chris and smiled. "My Lil' Monkey!" Then, he affectionately kissed him on the cheek.

"Let's go hang it in your room, Papa," Chris said. He then took Dad firmly by the hand and led him down the hall.

Dad showed us where he wanted the pictures and I let Chris tape them on the wall. Dad seemed genuinely pleased. I hoped that they would remain hanging on his walls. Even more so, I hoped that they'd be a constant reminder of how much we loved him even when we weren't there to tell him.

Friday, April 15, 2011

I found him sitting in his blue recliner with two different shoes on, appearing very calm. At one time, mismatched shoes would have bothered him, but those days were long since in the past. As I thought about Dad's upcoming appointment later this afternoon, I was glad I had intentionally refrained from telling him about it. It had made a big difference in his demeanor. Knowing that we would be leaving the building later, I suggested he change one of the shoes. This time, he chose the navy blue boat shoes. They were easy to get on once I found the missing one in his bottom nightstand drawer.

Dad remained peacefully seated while I made his bed. His sheets had already been taken off before I arrived. I then noticed that his hamper was missing. This was a pleasant surprise as I wouldn't need to do extra laundry today. I knew the caregivers were taking care of it.

While I put the clean sheets on the bed, Dad just stared at me. The loving look on his face as he watched me always touched my heart, expressing how secure and appreciative he felt that I was taking care of him. When I finished, I strategically placed his throw pillows on top. Among them was the red, heart-shaped pillow from his triple bypass surgery. "All done," I said.

"You do take good care of me, Pootie," he replied.

We casually sat in his room for awhile and talked. I soon informed him that he had a doctor's appointment. "We need to see Dr. Martinez," I said. "You haven't seen him since the hospital changed your diabetes medicine."

"When do we need to leave?" he asked.

"In about thirty minutes," I responded. "There's no hurry." I was a little nervous about taking my Dad to the appointment. It would be the first time I had taken him out of the facility completely by myself. I truly hoped that he would remain calm while we were gone.

Within the hour, Dad and I left Arbor Forest. I made sure to keep the conversation light and happy on the way there. He calmly stared out the window most of the time. Driving in a car wasn't something that he got to do much of these days. He was thoroughly enjoying it.

Fortunately, we didn't have much of a wait today. I knew that would not have gone over very well with Dad. Dr. Martinez soon made his way into the examining room. It had been months since Dad had seen him and a lot had happened since then.

The doctor curiously asked me about the change in Dad's diabetes medication and I told him the reason. "Dad got up in the middle of the night to use the bathroom," I said. "On the way back, he got dizzy and fell. When the paramedics came, they checked his blood sugar. It was in the low 40's. He was taken to the hospital and they adjusted his Glipizide to 5 mg. They felt that 10 mg. was too strong based on his weight."

Dr. Martinez quietly studied his notes. "I'd like to try him on another medication," he said. "It's a little more reliable and won't need to change based on his weight." Instead of the Glipizide, Dad would now be taking Januvia 100 mg. "This medication isn't covered completely by insurance. It runs a little higher. I'm going to give you some samples for the first month to make sure there are no complications."

"Okay," I said. "I need to have an order from you with the changes. Dad is now living in a facility that has a memory care unit." I carefully looked at Dad to make sure he was okay with the conversation, his eyes telling me to continue. "He was diagnosed with Alzheimer's in March. The facility has a strict policy. They won't administer any type of medication without a doctor's order."

He gave me the same distinct look that I had seen from some of Dad's other doctors. He was probably wondering why something so simple had been made so complicated. Unfortunately, that was our reality. "I can't just tell them," I stated. "It has to be a written order from you that states the old medication to stop and the new medication to start." I knew that if the order wasn't just so, Dad's meds wouldn't get changed. I also knew that it would be up to me to make sure everything happened exactly as it should.

By the time Dad and I got back to Arbor Forest, he was hungry for lunch. The appointment had gone very well and he had remained calm the entire time. While Dad was eating, I talked to the medical technician on duty about Dad's new prescription, also giving her the physician's order. I then had to take the prescription and Januvia samples to Collier Village Pharmacy to get them bubble-packed, after which I would need to bring them back to the med tech. It would undoubtedly be a long afternoon.

Later that day, Shawn, Chris and I made the trip to Athens to pick Preston up. Preston very much wanted to visit Dad this weekend. He had come to Arbor Forest on the day that we all moved Dad's furniture in, but had yet to personally see him in his new home. It had actually been months since they had seen each other. I knew it would mean a lot to Dad to have him visit as they had a lot of catching up to do. I also looked forward to having all of my children under the same roof.

Saturday, April 16, 2011

A slight chance of rain had existed earlier, but the skies now looked completely clear. Andrew's baseball game would go on as planned. It meant that another significant event could possibly happen today. Early this morning, Bob and Mom had gone to Arbor Forest to visit Dad. Bob was going to try once again to take him to the game. We intentionally hadn't said anything about it all week. Today's plan would be completely contingent on Dad's state when they arrived. If he was calm, then Bob would suggest going. Unfortunately, this was the way we had to do things now.

When they arrived, Dad was calmly sitting in the dining area just finishing up his breakfast. He was so happy to see them. "How would you like to go see Drew play some baseball today?" Bob asked.

"Really?" Dad replied. Bob shook his head yes. "I'd like that a lot."

They managed to get Dad to the park without any complications. He had been so excited! The game had gone very well and Dad thoroughly enjoyed himself. It had definitely been a good idea to take him out of the facility today. He had remained calm throughout the game with no accidents occurring. Afterwards, Andrew had run up to his Papa and hugged him tightly. It was a very special moment for both of them.

Later that afternoon, Preston and I went to Arbor Forest to visit Dad. As soon as we walked into the common area, we saw him on one of the couches. He immediately looked up and smiled. "Hi Prez," Dad said.

"Hi Papa," Preston replied. Dad stood up and they hugged each other. "How are you doing?"

"I can't complain," he said, as he rolled his eyes jokingly at me and smiled.

Dad sat back down on the couch with Preston sitting next to him. The only other vacant seat was across the room on another couch. I took that seat and began to talk to a couple of other residents. I wanted to give Dad and Preston some special time alone.

"Mom made you some pistachio salad," Preston said as he held up the plastic container in his hand. Dad's face suddenly lit up. It had always been one of his favorites.

"Why don't we go back to my room and have a little, Prez?" Dad suggested.

When we got to Dad's room, Preston handed him the pudding and a spoon. He sat down in his recliner and began eating right away. "Pootie, you've done it again," he said. Dad was in a very calm and happy mood, looking exceptionally well.

Preston and Dad continued their conversation, actually talking for over an hour. The mutual love and respect that existed between them was evident today. I had always loved watching my children and my father together. With everything that had happened, it was now all the more special to me.

Just like Shawn, Preston had come to his Papa in 5th grade needing some assistance with a school project. His class was currently studying World War I. The assignment entailed building a model plane similar to one that was used during that time period. Not only had Papa helped him build a plane from that war, he also built another one from World War II. Some of the decals had flaked off over time, but those planes still sat on a shelf in Preston's room. He would forever treasure them.

"So, when do you have to go back to college, Prez?" Dad asked.

"I have to go back tomorrow night," he replied. "I have a couple of more weeks of regular classes and then a week of finals. Then, I'll be home for the summer." He looked at me and smiled.

I thought about taking Preston back to college tomorrow, definitely having mixed emotions. I always felt incredibly sad when he would leave. Ever since the beginning of the semester in January, I now experienced an additional feeling when I said goodbye to him. A peaceful feeling would overcome me, almost a relief, knowing that he'd be safe and secure at college and that none of our ugly, devastating Alzheimer's world would be able to touch him. Even though I missed him terribly, I wanted to spare him the anguish and pain that had become a part of our daily lives.

Tuesday, April 19, 2011

I first saw her at the dining table, surprising me at first. I was the only female to date that had ever graced the seats of the "Guy Table". As I slowly approached them, I smiled at my dad who was already seated in his reserved spot. Immediately to his left sat a woman whose name was Dorothy, apparently new to the unit. I took the seat directly across from her.

We surprisingly ended up talking the entire time about anything and everything. She was actually very nice. The thing that struck me the most was how completely coherent she seemed. At no point during any of the conversation had she sounded the least bit confused.

"Your father has the prettiest blue eyes," she said, looking at my dad and smiling.

"Yes, he does," I agreed. I would later find out that Dorothy's room was right next door to my dad's room.

After lunch, Dad and I went back to his room for awhile. "How is your mother doing?" he asked.

"She's fine, Daddy," I replied. "Did you remember that Mom was going to have her thyroid procedure today?" He shook his head yes, but he still looked a little confused.

Mom had an overactive thyroid condition caused by Grave's disease. We had actually known about it for awhile, but were just waiting for the right time to schedule the procedure. She had finally decided to do something about it this week. This morning, she had taken a radioactive iodine capsule to treat it, with the premise that the thyroid would soak up the iodine and shrink. The hope was that it would eventually stop producing the excessive amount of hormones. If it shrunk too much, she might actually have to take a supplement.

"Mom has been having problems with her thyroid," I said. "She had the procedure done this morning. She isn't allowed to be around anyone for one week since she is considered radioactive." He seemed to understand this, but I knew it probably wasn't the best news for him. One week would undoubtedly feel a lot longer to Dad than it would to the rest of us.

"She can't come up to see you, but she is planning on calling you on the phone," I continued. I then retrieved an index card from my purse. "I made this card for you with all of our phone numbers on it. I'll give it to one of the caregivers and they can keep it on the cart. Anytime you want to talk to one of us, you tell them and they'll get you the number. Mom's is the first one in the list." I then appropriately pointed to Mom's name on the card. "How does that sound?"

"That sounds good," he responded. I hoped that this would be a good solution to us not visiting him every day. I wanted Dad to inherently feel like we would be there for him anytime. All he had to do was call.

Later that evening, Mom called me and said that she had talked to Dad on the phone earlier. She didn't have to wait long as he was actually already seated in the common area. They had casually talked for about five minutes. He had seemed very happy throughout the conversation. It had worked out very well.

I mentioned to Mom that I had met a new resident today named Dorothy. "She seems very alert and lucid, Mom," I said. "I think it will be good for Dad to have someone to talk to. She was really nice and she seemed genuinely interested in talking to Dad. She is actually in the room right next to him." There had been a slight pause in Mom's response, but I knew better than to read anything into it.

"I think you may be right," she replied. "That's the one thing that is lacking in his environment. Other than the staff, he doesn't have a lot of people to talk to, at least not at his level."

Friday, April 22, 2011

No sooner had I reached Dad's door than I heard the music. It was clearly coming from the room next to his, Dorothy's room. It was just loud enough to let me know that the room was now occupied. It might have been my imagination, but I distinctly thought I heard the faint sound of a woman singing. I then closed Dad's door as I walked into his room. He was calmly sitting in the blue recliner and smiled when he saw me. I soon let him know he had an appointment this morning with his cardiologist. I had specifically refrained from telling him about it until now which would give him an hour's notice from when we needed to leave.

Apparently, that was too much time. Within fifteen minutes, he began getting very anxious. "Dad, we have plenty of time," I said. "I promise I'll get you there before 11."

While we were waiting, I quickly changed his sheets. It seemed as though the accidents were happening a lot more frequently. I carefully bagged up the soiled items to come home with me.

"Shouldn't we be leaving?" he inquired, not more than five minutes later.

"No, not yet," I replied, deciding to change the subject. "Dad, how do you like Dorothy?"

"Well, sometimes she says things that I don't care for," he said.

"What do you mean?" I asked.

"I think she may think that something is going to happen with the two of us," he answered. "She says things that aren't really appropriate." Dad was completely serious. I was stunned.

"Really?" I asked. "I've talked to her several times and never noticed anything like that. She seems so nice and on the up and up." He rolled his eyes a little and shrugged his shoulders.

"Sometimes she makes me feel uncomfortable," he said. I definitely hadn't seen that side of her. I wasn't sure what to believe.

"Don't we need to be going?" Dad asked again.

"No, Daddy," I stated. "If we go too early, then we'll just have to sit in the doctor's office and wait. It's more comfortable here." As much as he wanted to go, I knew that he wouldn't like sitting in the lobby or the examination room any more than I would.

I realized today that not only couldn't I tell Dad about an appointment prior to the actual date, I also couldn't give him too much notice on the actual day of the appointment. From now on, I would tell him thirty minutes in advance. Otherwise, he just got too anxious.

The appointment today had gone very smoothly. Dad's blood pressure numbers looked good, the doctor very happy with Dad's progress. He was down to two blood pressure medications and those would invariably remain the same.

By the time we returned to Arbor Forest, it was lunchtime. While we were seated at the table, I overheard some of the caregivers talking about an incident that had occurred the night before. One of the female residents was apparently going through a Sundowner's episode and ended up hitting another woman. I then noticed that one of the women at the next table had a bandage over one of her eyes. The woman that had committed the assault was not in the room. I looked around and found only two empty seats. Based on that, it was easy to determine which woman was involved. I had a feeling they were intentionally trying to keep them apart today.

Sometimes when I would visit Dad, I'd ask him how the previous night had gone. At times, his answer would surprise me. Some of the incidents that he described were a little hard to believe, the situations sounding very chaotic. At the time, I thought he was just confused. Now, I wasn't so certain. With every day that passed, I found that a lot of what happened back here mimicked what happened in the outside world. It was still human beings living together in close quarters with their differences. One thing was for sure, I never found it boring back here in the memory care unit.

After lunch, Dad and I casually moved to one of the couches in the common area. Before long, Dorothy came and sat down next to me. She began by telling me that she wasn't supposed to be in this unit. The assisted living section had no current openings, so they moved her back here for the time being. I felt a little surprised at that. I knew that in order to be placed in this memory care unit, it required a doctor stating that the resident not only had Alzheimer's but was in danger of wandering. I couldn't detect any sign of either in her. She still seemed completely lucid, in addition to being very sure of herself. I honestly didn't know what was going on, but I would definitely keep my eyes on her, especially after my dad's last comment.

Sunday, April 24, 2011

I had looked forward to today for a long, long time. It was a day that I had secretly promised myself and my father would one day take place. Dad was coming to our home for dinner. I had butterflies in my stomach. It would be the first time since he had moved into Arbor Forest that he had come here. I felt both nervous and excited at the same time.

Randy and Shawn had promptly left at 2 p.m. to get Dad. When they arrived, they found him in his room, which was currently a mess. He was beginning to show signs of agitation as he couldn't find his upper denture anywhere. Randy thoroughly searched the room. He looked in every drawer, under the bed, in the bathroom, even under the mattress. It was absolutely nowhere to be found. They unfortunately had no choice but to bring Dad without it. Luckily, he still had his lower denture and a few random teeth on top. I hoped that he'd be able to manage until we could get it replaced.

The three of them rode quietly to our house in the truck. Dad was still a little anxious, but Randy had done a good job distracting him and calming him down. I hated that Shawn had to witness the anxiety. He had only seen Dad like this once before.

Dad had been coming over to eat ever since he had first moved to Georgia. His favorite meal was meatloaf, corn, green beans, mashed potatoes and gravy, rolls and pistachio salad. Unfortunately, he hadn't been served this meal in months. I had attentively cooked everything just the way he liked it. I wanted today to be very special for my dad.

As soon as they arrived, Randy carefully helped Dad up the stairs. Riley was at the top excitedly waiting for him as she always did. "Hey girl," Dad said. "How ya doing, Riley?" She wiggled and conveniently turned around so he would rub her backside. She had missed her Papa so much.

Dad had generously taken care of Riley for one week every summer ever since he had moved to Buford. The last thing I would always say to him before I left was "No scraps, Dad." When I would return from vacation, I would inevitably find out that Dad had shared all of his meals with Riley, even his breakfast donuts. It was hard to get upset over that. It was their special time together and she adored Dad.

Chris and I lovingly hugged Dad hello. He then made his way into the living room while I finished dinner. We had planned on eating early. I knew Dad was slated to take his evening dose of Risperdal at 5 and I wanted him to be back at Arbor Forest for that. He was comfortably settling into a routine and I knew it could create unnecessary tension if he wasn't back in time.

When dinner was ready, Dad sat in the same spot near the window that had always been reserved for him. In some ways, it was like old times. Only today, Mom wasn't sitting next to him. She unfortunately wasn't able to come because of the iodine treatment. She was still very much in the radioactive period, so I would take a plate over to her tomorrow.

As I watched him eat, I soon started to notice other differences. Even though Dad still managed to eat by himself, he ate much slower than he ever had. He also didn't talk much. In fact, the majority of the time, his head remained down looking at his food. He was concentrating so hard, looking very similar to the way he looked when he ate at Arbor Forest. My dad had aged so much since his heart surgery.

I remained seated next to Dad until he had finished eating. We were inevitably the last two to leave the table. His plate was almost completely empty, thoroughly enjoying the meal. I had devotedly made his favorite and he had truly loved it.

After dinner, we again moved to the living room where Dad finally began to loosen up. Riley remained by his side the entire time, leaning against his chair. Before long, Bob and Andrew came over. Dad was freely laughing with everyone and was in such a good mood. All of the earlier agitation was completely gone. All that remained was a man enjoying the company of his loved ones.

Dad soon began to ask what time it was. When I mentioned that he'd be getting his evening meds once he returned, he said he thought it was time to go. We clearly knew that was our sign. It was important to get

Dad back to his room at Arbor Forest while he remained calm. Bob had generously agreed to drive him back.

After they left, I warily thought about the visit, experiencing so many different emotions. I felt happy that the dinner had gone so well. I wanted Dad to invariably know that this was yet another thing that didn't have to change. I also felt a lot of sadness. Even though I tried to convince my dad that some things would always remain the same, I knew inside that wasn't entirely true. My dad was unfortunately changing every day. Sometimes, the changes seemed so miniscule that I hardly even noticed them. During other times like today, it was very obvious.

I had been told repeatedly that Alzheimer's could not be reversed. At best, we could only slow it down. I knew enough to expect that more changes would inevitably occur. As much as I researched this terrible disease and tried to brace myself for what would ultimately come next, it was still difficult. I knew that I needed to adapt to our new future, but sometimes, it was so hard to let go of the past.

Wednesday, April 27, 2011

Not long after the school bell rang, Chris quickly hopped into the car. "How would you like to go see Papa right now?" I asked.

"I'd love it," he replied. "Can we get him a milkshake?"

"Absolutely," I said. "What flavor should we get him today?"

"Hmm," he thought for a minute, "chocolate." I nodded my head in agreement and he lovingly smiled at me.

Along with the chocolate milkshake, Chris had brought Dad a new homemade picture. He had taken a large sheet of construction paper and carefully traced his hands in the middle. Then, he had colored them a peach shade. Around his hands, he had drawn hearts in various sizes and colored them bright pink. Above the hands, he had written "Do you know how much I love you?" On the bottom of the sheet were the words "I love you Grandpa!!!! Love, Chris". When Chris had traced his hands, he had spread them wide open to indicate how much he loved his Papa.

As soon as we walked into the room, Dad suddenly brightened up.

"Well, look at what we've got here," he said. Chris handed him his goodies and immediately sat on his lap. He was such good therapy for Dad.

While casually talking with him, I noticed that he still didn't have his upper denture in. "Mom found an extra set of teeth in your bathroom," I said. I then handed him the upper denture that was in my purse and he eagerly tried it on. It actually fit. When Mom had given it to me earlier, I had no idea how old it was. Dad opened his mouth and clicked his teeth together to show me. "They look good, Dad. Do they feel okay?" He nodded yes.

Later that afternoon, the three of us walked down to Dad's room. I needed to call his endocrinologist. I had been routinely monitoring his blood sugar and was concerned with the latest readings. Ever since Dad had started taking the Januvia, his blood sugar was surprisingly higher than usual. The levels during the day were consistently above 300, whereas normally they stayed close to 200.

I had also noticed that Dad was extremely forgetful lately. He had actually made some statements that sounded very bizarre. That, along with the fact that the Januvia was about seven times as expensive as his previous medication, bothered me.

I called Dr. Martinez's office and, as expected, I had to leave a message. In that recording, I not only mentioned my concerns but also voiced my recommendation. I had politely asked if it was possible to put my dad back on the Glipizide. He had endured so much lately and I saw no reason to unnecessarily change his medication. Sometimes, it seemed as though the doctors were more concerned with having their patients on the latest and greatest drugs than what was actually best for them.

Within thirty minutes, the doctor's assistant called me back. Unfortunately, the doctor didn't agree with me. Instead, he added another medication to work with the Januvia. The new prescription was for Actoplus Met 15 mg. Before I hung up, I made sure she understood what was involved in order to add a new medication for Dad.

While we were relaxing in Dad's room, I soon began to hear music next door in Dorothy's room. "How often does she play her music?" I asked.

"All the time," he replied. Then, we both laughed.

"Is she still making you feel uncomfortable?" I asked.

"Yes, that is why I want your mother to come," he said. "I'm hoping that once she meets Shirley, she'll stop with the comments." I still wasn't sure what was going on, but I did know that my dad didn't need any more drama in his life. He already had enough issues to deal with.

Later that evening, I talked to Preston on the phone. He only had one more week of regular classes and then finals. I absolutely couldn't wait. We would actually be moving most of his personal belongings home this weekend. It would be so nice to have all of the boys at home this summer. I felt like I had neglected them over the past six months and I really wanted to get my life balanced out better.

Monday, May 2, 2011

With every step closer, the loud pounding increased. As I soon arrived at the door to the memory care unit, I could distinctly hear someone on the other side intensely banging on it. I immediately became alarmed, concerned it might be my dad. I felt a little afraid to open the door. "Do you need some help?" I asked, loud enough to hear me through the door.

"I need for you to open this door right now!" she demanded. The loud voice was clearly Dorothy's and she was currently very irate. I then entered the code and opened the door, after which she rapidly brushed by me without so much as a word. I had never before seen her like this. I turned and watched her determinedly walk down the hall. After she turned left towards the lobby, I proceeded into the unit.

I found one of the familiar caregivers in the dining area diligently sweeping the floor. "I just wanted to let you know that Dorothy just left through the front door," I said. "She sounded very upset."

Another caregiver had overheard me and soon walked over. "Thanks for letting us know," she said. "I'll go get her." With that, she quickly walked down the hall and left the unit.

The remaining caregiver stopped sweeping and turned to me. "She's mad that she can't get out," the caregiver said. "We've had some problems with her lately. She doesn't understand that the residents back here are not allowed to just leave whenever they feel like it. She wants to be able to come and go as she pleases." The caregiver paused for a moment to catch her breath, clearly feeling exasperated. "We have found her on the side of the road picking flowers. One of the employees had to bring her back in. She was also giving the code out to some of the other residents back here. The other day, one of them managed to get out. We had no choice but to change it. If she asks you for the new code, don't tell her. She is going to have to abide by the same rules as everyone else back here."

I soon continued down the hall to my dad's room, where I found him casually relaxing in his recliner. We sat together and talked openly for awhile. Before long, we heard the familiar music begin next door, accompanied by the occasional slamming of drawers. Dorothy was back and she was obviously still rattled.

"I understand that she has been upset lately," I said. He nodded his head yes. "I think it might be best if you kept your distance from her." I had never said that about another resident, but I was slowly developing a bad feeling about Dorothy.

"I already try to do that," he replied. "I have nothing to say to her." I tenderly reached for his hand and smiled at him. He then lovingly scrunched his nose back at me.

"Pootie, I've been thinking," he said. "I don't have anything to do around here. I think I'd like to get a job."

He had totally caught me off guard as it was the last thing I ever expected to hear from Dad. "What kind of job?" I asked.

"I don't know," he replied. "I've always been good at fixing things. Maybe, I could help out that way."

"Well, that's a possibility," I remarked. "I can talk to Kevin or Anthony about it if you'd like. See what we can come up with."

"That sounds good," he said.

I would definitely have to give this some considerable thought. In talking with Dad, he was clearly very serious about this. He needed to feel needed. It was as simple as that.

When Kevin first gave us a tour of the facility, he had shown us the hair salon. It was a small room, but it had everything you could possibly need. I had mentioned that Dad was a barber and Kevin had offered up the idea of Dad possibly cutting some of the residents' hair. It had sounded good at the time, but now I wasn't so sure. Allowing one resident to cut another resident's hair posed too much of a liability. I didn't even know if Dad could stand on his feet for extended periods of time anymore, in addition to whether he still had the dexterity to cut hair. I truly hoped that barbering wouldn't be one of his suggestions.

On the way out of the facility that afternoon, I talked to the activity director, Lauren, when she had asked me how my dad was doing. The subject of Dorothy inevitably came up. "I think she is actually a bad influence on your father," she said. "She feels that she should be able to get out of the unit whenever she wants. I think she is trying to persuade your father to feel the same way."

I was totally shocked. That was one of the main reasons my dad was in the memory care unit, to prevent him from wandering off. What Dorothy was doing posed a huge safety risk for him. "I don't understand," I said. "According to her, she isn't supposed to be back there. She's just waiting for a room in assisted living to open up."

Lauren smiled at me and slowly shook her head. "She is right where she needs to be," she stated. "Believe me, Vanessa. We've talked to her son and he is in agreement. She's been leaving the facility. Several times, we've found her in bushes right off of this busy road picking flowers." I followed her gaze to the street out front. She was absolutely right about it being busy. The thought of my dad walking along this stretch of road deeply alarmed me.

As I drove home, I was very confused. Dorothy had appeared completely rational to me. If what Lauren said was true, then she was a lot smarter than I had given her credit for. Now, I would definitely have to keep an eye on her. I also wanted her to stay away from my dad.

Wednesday, May 4, 2011

It felt so good to be together as we casually drove down the road. Shawn was usually at practice after school, but now that track season was over, I looked forward to spending more time with him. Today, I had actually picked him up from his school before Chris. I lovingly smiled at the two of them as we made our way to Arbor Forest.

We soon found Dad in the common area along with several other residents. The caregiver that was on duty had put some dancing music on the CD player. Her name was Jackie and I had never seen her before today, usually working the night shift. Jackie lived in the apartment complex right down the road from the facility and would conveniently walk to work.

She affably came up to us while we were sitting and started telling me about an incident that had happened a few days ago. Dad was comfortably sitting on one of the couches in the common area and had his legs crossed. Jackie had noticed that his feet looked very swollen. "William, is there something wrong with your feet?" she asked. He looked down at them and shook his head no. After taking his loafers off, she then realized what the problem was. Dad had multiple pairs of socks on. "I peeled one sock off and held it up to him and said 'That's one'. Then, I took another sock off and said 'That's two'. What number did we get up to, William?"

"I don't remember," he replied sheepishly. Dad was laughing uncontrollably at this point, as were the rest of us. This woman was so entertaining. I felt like we were watching a stand-up act in a comedy show. Everything that came out of her mouth was funny. Dad was clearly enjoying her as much as the boys and I were.

"We got up to five," she said. "I told him that shoes aren't meant to fit comfortably over five pairs of socks." After she had helped him remove the extra socks, the loafers had then slid on easily.

I truly loved watching the way this caregiver interacted with Dad. Even more so, I loved the way that he responded to her. It made me feel good to know that she was attentively watching over him at night.

Before long, Jackie surprisingly got up in the middle of the room with one of the female residents. Jackie was a tall woman and towered above the other lady, but it didn't matter. The resident was having a good time. Soon, others had happily joined in. Chris boldly went up to a resident named Christine who was a tiny woman and not much bigger than he was. They both danced in the hall for the entire duration of the song.

As the next tune began, Jackie came over and somehow got Dad to stand up. He was very reluctant, but she wouldn't take no for an answer. They remained dancing in the middle of the room for a couple of minutes, long enough for me to capture the moment on my cell phone.

She then moved on to some other residents, her goal to eventually have everyone dance at least one song. At one point, I had noticed Dorothy quietly sitting on the other side of the room. When Jackie made her way over to Dorothy, she didn't hesitate a bit, immediately rising up to the occasion and dancing very well.

Jackie seemed to have a knack for dealing with the ins and outs of Alzheimer's and it showed. Everyone was having a great time. I honestly laughed more today than I had in a long time, as was also true for Dad.

While we were leisurely listening to the music, another caregiver in the dining area had motioned for me to come see her. "Look what we found in one of the cabinets," she said.

I couldn't believe I was actually looking at Dad's upper denture. I had assumed that he had taken it out and laid it on the table while he was eating and that it was long gone. "I can't believe you found it," I replied smiling. It was turning out to be a very good day.

I decided to secretly hide the denture in one of the drawers in Dad's bathroom. The one he was wearing seemed to fit fine. At least, we would have a backup. I then walked back to Dad's room alone, not wanting to disturb the good time he was having.

After hiding the extra teeth, I decided to hang Chris' latest picture to Dad. With all the excitement in the common area, we hadn't had a chance to show it to him. It would be a nice surprise at some later point when he invariably found it.

On the outside of the card, Chris had drawn a steering wheel, a tire and some other car parts. He had written "Honk!!!! Honk!!!!" in the middle of the page. On the inside, he had drawn a convertible car. The caption read "I've got you a convertible! Have a nice trip!!!! Love, Chris".

As I taped the latest picture on the wall, I slowly stood back in wonder and looked at the growing collection. They definitely added extra warmth to the room. My goal was to eventually have the walls covered with love letters to Dad.

Thursday, May 5, 2011

The feeling was one of sheer comfort as I walked inside. I had made the decision awhile back that if this was to be Dad's new home and these residents were to be his new neighbors, then I wanted to know them as well. In the past few months, I had done just that. I knew all of these precious people and they all knew me. Two of those women recently passed away. Even though they got to a point where it was somewhat expected, it was still heartbreaking when it actually happened. I found myself trying to remember how they had acted during their last few days here in the unit. I wanted to be able to recognize those signs and know when the end was near. I knew that one day I would unfortunately see them in my dad.

The residents in this unit were all at varying stages of Alzheimer's. I now watched all of them very closely as they displayed many similar characteristics. As they neared the end, they would inevitably get to a state where they weren't really there. Their appetites would slowly diminish and their bodies would become restless. Then it would just be a matter of time.

Another resident was doing very poorly right now. She lived in the room diagonally across from my dad. A couple of days ago, her bed was moved out of her room and replaced with a hospital bed that had railings on the side. She was getting very restless in her sleep and had actually fallen out of her bed a few times.

The other day, I was sitting next to her in the common area. She innocently looked at me with little girl eyes and started talking. I couldn't make out what she was saying, but it didn't seem to matter. She continued to talk to me and would occasionally laugh in her own little world. I dreaded the day when I would walk into the unit and she wouldn't be here. I knew the sad reality was that it could happen any day.

I watched my dad and secretly compared him to the other residents. He wasn't at the level that so many of them were, but I could definitely see a change in him as his memory was getting much worse. Some days, it was more evident than others.

Today, Dad and I were casually seated in the common area waiting for lunch to be served. Dorothy came down and said "Hello blue eyes" as she looked at my dad. He didn't respond other than to look at me and smile. We had become accustomed to her ways as she flirted with Dad every day. Even though the circumstances had separated my parents, Dad still considered himself married until death.

On a couple of recent occasions, Dorothy had asked me for the new code to the memory care unit. "I can't give it to you, Dorothy," I stated. "You need to take that up with someone in charge. If they say it's okay, then I'll let you out, but I can't give anyone back here the code." She clearly wasn't happy with my answer, but the director had specifically instructed me not to give her the code. I knew it could be dangerous for her as well as the other residents. I definitely wouldn't want her taking my dad out of the unit. She soon dejectedly walked away from us.

"Have you had a chance to talk to anyone about a job for me?" Dad asked.

"I actually have spoken to Kevin about it," I replied. "He said he would give it some thought." One of the caregivers at night had also mentioned that Dad had brought the subject up with her. "We're still working on it." He seemed satisfied for the moment.

The truth was I was having a hard time coming up with the right job for Dad. The few tasks that I had come up with probably weren't the type of work that Dad was looking for. Likewise, the jobs that he was interested in were probably things that Dad used to be able to do very well, but might not be possible anymore. It was a sensitive area and one that I tried to handle very delicately.

Later that afternoon, Mom called to tell me that she and Barron had visited Dad. It unfortunately had not gone well. Not long after she had arrived, Mom had suggested they go out front and sit in the rocking chairs. Dad had taken Barron by the leash and led him outside. As soon as Dad had sat down, Barron jumped up in his lap. Dad then began asking Mom about finding him a job. It was very much on his mind and he was beginning to get persistent about it. Not getting the answer he wanted, Dad started getting upset.

He then took Barron by the leash and started walking him towards the assisted living standalone apartments, which were located in the back, down a steep slope. Barron began swiftly leading him down the road and Dad's pace soon quickened, appearing as if he was going to lose his balance. Mom had run after him and managed to get him back to his rocking chair, but not before he had become very winded and very agitated.

"Mom, I don't think it's a good idea for you to take Dad out front anymore," I said. "He could have fallen or worse, he could have taken Barron out on the main road. It could have been very dangerous." Sometimes, Mom seemed oblivious to Dad's condition. I had to remind myself that she was also getting older.

Friday, May 6, 2011

The balloons slowly swayed back and forth as I walked past them, the area completely transformed and almost unrecognizable. Arbor Forest was graciously throwing a combination brunch and talent show for the family members of those living in the memory care unit. The entire common area was decorated with long tables moved into the center of the room, white table cloths draped over them and beautiful arrangements sitting on top. We were having a party!

Our reserved seats were at a table with three other residents. Mom and Dad sat across from me, both of them dressed so nicely. One of the residents sitting near us was accompanied by her daughter who was very witty. It seemed as though every other sentence out of her mouth left me laughing. The other two residents were a married couple that lived on the opposite hall from Dad. Unfortunately, they didn't have any additional family present.

This particular couple ordinarily sat at the table next to Dad's in the dining area. The husband was very lucid. If I had to guess, I'd say that he was living in the unit more to take care of his wife, who was seated next to me today. She had long nails and was always talking about getting a manicure. About once a week, the caregivers would kindly paint the residents' nails. It always did so much towards lifting their spirits.

The food today was served buffet style, with only fine china for this special occasion. Everything tasted delicious. The party had given me an opportunity to get to know some of the other residents' families. We all shared a common bond. It always saddened me to see so many without any loved ones present. I very much understood that every one of these residents had their own unique and special story.

After lunch, a woman came to the front of the room and vivaciously started singing songs karaoke style. In no time, she had complete command of the room. She also tried to engage everyone in playing some games.

At one point, I walked across the room as the song "Fly Me to the Moon" by Frank Sinatra began playing. Alexandra suddenly grabbed my hand and quickly pulled me towards her. Before I knew it, she was twirling me around and we were dancing in the middle of the hall. I looked around at some of the nearby residents as they all watched us with smiles on their faces. I noticed that Dad was grinning as well. We had the hallway completely to ourselves. It had been one of those rare and spontaneous moments that I would treasure always.

After the lunch had ended, we made our way back to Dad's room. As soon as I opened the door, a gust of hot air hit me in the face, feeling like I had walked into a sauna. It was sweltering. I could hear the unit running and immediately checked the thermostat on the wall. It was set to heat, so I quickly changed it over to a/c. "Are you hot in here, Dad?" I asked.

"Well, maybe a little," he replied.

"The thermostat was set to heat," I said. I then showed him how to turn the thermostat on and off. "I have the temperature set and it is on a/c. You shouldn't have to change that. If you get too cold, just move this switch to the 'Off' setting. When you want it back on, change it to the 'On' setting."

"That seems easy enough," he responded. I hoped that it was just a simple mix up, although I knew that he had been having trouble setting his thermostat at home for years.

While we were casually sitting in his room, I looked through his drawers. I had gotten into the habit of checking them every now and then. One day, I had found some clothes from Frank who lived across the hall. Another day, I had surprisingly found a pair of red, satiny boxers that I knew weren't Dad's. I wasn't sure how they had come to rest in his dresser.

As I looked through his top drawer, I happened to notice that his watch box was empty. I looked at Dad's arm, but he wasn't currently wearing it. I then looked through the other drawers, but to no avail. "Dad, do you know where your watch is?" I asked. He simply shrugged his shoulders which told me that he had no idea.

The residents occasionally walked into each other's rooms and took things that didn't belong to them. My dad was just as guilty of doing it as the rest of them. Had someone taken his watch or had he left it in someone's room accidentally? The only other option that I could think of was that he had given it to someone.

Dad had always been generous to a fault. I worried about him often as he would give the shirt off his back if needed. One day, he was working at his barber shop in Pensacola. One of his customers had told him that he was going through some hard times, eventually asking Dad to borrow some money. Dad really didn't know the man that well, but he gave him some money anyway, not thinking twice about it. He knew he probably wouldn't get it back and he didn't, but it didn't matter. That wasn't why he had given him the money.

Another time, someone had knocked on his front door at his home in Buford. It was a young guy who told Dad he was having car trouble. Dad could see his car pulled off of the main road. He then generously went down to his basement and got some tools for the boy who had promised to return them when he was done. The next time that Dad checked, the boy and his car were gone, as well as my dad's tools. Dad never saw the guy again, but it didn't matter. He had once again done the right thing.

Then there was the ultimate example of generosity. One of Dad's neighbors lived a few houses down from him in Buford. The man loved coming by and talking with Dad who also felt the same about him. One day, they were discussing lawn mowers and the neighbor mentioned that he would love to one day have his own riding lawn mower. My dad then took him into the basement and gave him his old riding mower. He just gave it to him. It had been that simple. The man was completely taken aback by Dad's kindness, ecstatic at this incredible gift.

To this day, my dad never ceased to amaze me. He had led by example his entire life and taught me so much about giving. I had never in my life met anyone who was as generous as he was. His kindheartedness and compassion knew no bounds.

Monday, May 9, 2011

He had always loved giving her special presents. I remembered the store that was next to his barber shop in Hialeah, the woman's boutique with clothing, perfume and jewelry. The owner always helped Dad pick out just the right gift for Mom whenever a special occasion arose. I knew that I now needed to be that person that helped him with his gifts. Yesterday morning, I had brought a bag of assorted chocolates and a beautiful card for Dad to give to Mom for Mother's Day. I knew she'd be visiting him later in the afternoon. I also knew it would make Dad feel incredibly good to be able to give her something.

He had tried diligently to sign the card, but eventually gave up. He unfortunately only managed to write a few letters and they weren't that legible. I ended up signing the card for him as close to his penmanship as possible, hoping that Mom wouldn't notice the difference.

When my mom had come up later, they went back to his room where he had given her the card and candy. She had thanked him and given him a kiss. Her happiness could only be matched by the feeling he had of once again giving his wife a special gift. Mom was thrilled with her loving card. She got confused with the chocolates, though, and thought she had brought them to Dad earlier. She actually ended up leaving them in his room.

As I entered Dad's room today, I indeed found Mom's candy sitting on top of his dresser which had concerned me a great deal. I knew Dad had a sweet tooth and the last thing he needed with his diabetes was to have a bag of chocolates in the room. I would be taking Mom's candy with me when I left later today.

At noon, Dad and I made our way to the dining area where we found Dorothy already seated at the table. Only today, she was unexpectedly seated in my usual spot. I pulled a chair over so that I was sitting between my dad and her.

As the meal progressed, I noticed that Dad wasn't eating as much as he usually did. "Dad, do you not like the food today?" I questioned.

"My stomach has been bothering me," he replied.

"Where exactly is it hurting?" I asked. He then pointed to the lower left part of his abdomen.

"How long has this been going on?" I then asked.

"Maybe a couple of days," he responded. I was very concerned as the area that he was pointing to could possibly be related to his left hernia. The thought of another operation deeply alarmed me.

"We could go back to your room and I could give you a massage," said Dorothy. I literally almost fell out of my chair at that instant. I was completely shocked as I turned to her and stared.

"I don't think my mom would appreciate that very much!" I exclaimed, my tone and glare indicating that she had clearly crossed the line. She didn't say a word after that.

I couldn't believe that she had made that comment and right in front of me no less. What the hell was going through her mind? For weeks, my dad had been telling me that she was making inappropriate comments to him, sounding so far-fetched. I couldn't believe that anyone would have the audacity to do that, especially someone her age. Now, I knew that Dad wasn't confused at all. Everything he had told me was apparently the complete truth.

Dorothy soon changed the subject. It didn't matter though as the damage was already done. I was on to her and hoped, for her sake, that she realized the error of her ways.

After lunch, I took Dad back to his room so he could lie down for awhile. Susan had given him some ibuprofen earlier. I knew that he just needed to get off his feet and give the medicine a chance to start working.

While Dad was lying down, I had him show me exactly where the pain was. I gently placed my fingers on the spot and I could indeed feel a small lump which was no doubt his left hernia. This was not good. I knew that we could pacify it for awhile with rest and pain medication. Eventually though, we would have to have it operated on. I didn't want my dad to be miserable, but the thought of losing a little bit more of him as a result of the hernia procedure was disheartening. This was one of those times when there was no good solution.

Wednesday, May 11, 2011

I scanned the many youthful faces on the field and in no time, I saw his bright yellow shirt. As soon as he saw me, he quickly ran and gave me a big hug. I felt so thankful that he hadn't quite reached the age where that type of behavior was considered taboo.

This morning was Chris' 2nd grade Field Day. The excitement on the children's faces could only be matched by the laughter in the air. The activities were divided up so that some of them occurred in the gymnasium and some took place outside. I accompanied Chris to all of the different games, capturing the priceless moments with my camera.

Before long, it was time for an activity on the basketball court. Each class was to stand in a long line, side by side. At the beginning of the line sat a bucket filled with water, while an empty bucket rested at the other end. The idea of the game was to take a sponge and immerse it into the water bucket. Then, the sponge was passed from one student to another until it reached the other end. The last student would squeeze any remaining water into the other bucket and then run to the beginning of the line to start the process again. The first class to successfully fill their empty bucket to a certain level would win.

I stood as close to Chris as I could possibly get. Unfortunately, another class was positioned between us. As the activity started, the green sponge began to make its way down the line, the children all screaming with delight and excitement. As I looked through the viewfinder in my camera, my heart suddenly sank. I lowered the camera and then saw it directly through my eyes. The boy in line immediately behind Chris was bullying him. Chris was apparently not passing the sponge quick enough to suit this boy, so he was yelling at him. I couldn't actually hear him because of all of the noise, but I could see it in his face. Then, he started making ugly facial expressions at Chris. The worst part was undoubtedly the look on Chris' face. He was trying to defend himself, but the other boy was relentless in his taunting. Chris looked so frustrated. It absolutely broke my heart.

I had coincidentally witnessed something similar with this same boy during last year's field day. There had been an activity in the gymnasium where the class was divided into groups of six. Each team had a small cart on wheels that each member had to sit on and swiftly push themselves around an orange cone using only their feet. They would go through this rotation twice and each team member would ultimately get two turns.

This same boy had been on Chris' team. He had made sure that he was first in line, while Chris happened to be last. As the game began, each team member routinely took their turn. When it neared time for Chris' second turn, a whistle blew indicating that another team had won. The remaining teams continued to take their turns. Before Chris could take his second turn, the boy grabbed the cart and maliciously sat on it. He then rudely told Chris that no one else was going because another team had already won.

Chris had been so disappointed as he choked back the tears. It wasn't about winning to him, but about the fun that pushing yourself on the cart had provided. I immediately knelt down next to Chris and tried to comfort him. I had always tried to let my children handle things on their own, but it was hard to do that when I was actually present and witnessed the abuse firsthand. "That wasn't very nice," I said, as I peered at this child. "Chris should have gotten his second turn just like you did." He had just stared at me so defiantly that day.

As I continued to watch the sponge activity, I felt torn. A part of me wanted to go pull the child away from the game and discipline him myself. Unfortunately, I knew that wasn't my place and would create some uneasy feelings with the teacher, so I held back. The game soon ended after which, I walked up to Chris and tenderly hugged him.

I continued to accompany him to each activity. My mind, however, was somewhere else. I had already decided at this point to contact one of the vice principals that I personally knew about this disturbing incident. I also needed to talk to Chris' teacher.

Before long, the whistle blew loudly and all of the children started running past me to retrieve their water bottles. I noticed that the teacher was on the complete other side of the field talking with a parent. Most of the children had already gone by. Then I saw the boy that had bullied Chris, all alone and slowly approaching. I hadn't planned on saying anything directly to him, but sometimes the heat of the moment dictated otherwise.

"I want you to leave Chris alone," I said, slowly and sternly. "If I ever see you do anything mean to him again, I'll go directly to the teacher. Do you understand?" Again, he just stared at me, not looking the least bit intimidated or scared. He actually didn't look fazed at all. I felt so angry at that moment, I could have spit nails. I could only imagine what I looked like to this little boy, but I didn't care. This was someone abusing one of my children and protecting him was all that was on my mind. He then slowly walked away.

For the rest of the field day, I kept my eyes constantly glued to this boy. Whenever he looked at me, I was looking right back at him. I had tried to let things work out on their own without interfering, but no more. It was now time that I took matters into my own hands. I had previously heard stories about him acting mean towards Chris for years. What I saw today actually made my stomach turn. As soon as I got home, I would contact the vice principal to make sure they were in separate classes from now on. I didn't want this boy anywhere near Chris and I would do everything in my power to make sure he wasn't.

When I later picked Chris up from school, he seemed to have bounced back from the earlier incident. I had no way of knowing if any emotional damage had already occurred. "How about we go see Papa?" I asked.

"Okay, Mom," he said. "We need to get a strawberry milkshake this time."

"You got it, buddy," I replied. I then took his little hand in mine and gently squeezed it. "I love you."

"I love you, too," he replied back.

When we walked through the front doors at Arbor Forest, we quickly noticed a show currently going on in the living room to the left. The room was unusually packed. As I carefully looked in, I soon found Dad sitting on a couch watching the performer. Chris eagerly made his way over to him. As soon as Dad saw him, he smiled and lovingly held his arms open for a hug. Chris squeezed him tightly and then handed him the milkshake. It was beyond me how anyone could be so mean to such a sweet little boy.

Dorothy was seated to Dad's immediate left, kindly sliding over to make room for me. The performer was singing songs karaoke style, most of them older tunes that the residents seemed to be familiar with. She was very good and everyone was enjoying the show, especially Dad.

Later that night, I got my usual call from Mom. She had eaten lunch with Dad earlier in the day. While they were seated at the table, Joseph had said something to her. Because he talks so quietly, she had to lean in close in order to hear him. "Vanessa, he asked me if I wanted to come back to his room later," Mom said.

"Are you kidding me?" I asked. She assured me she wasn't. We then both laughed for five minutes straight.

Fortunately, Dad didn't hear what Joseph said. "Whatever you do, Mom, don't mention this to Dad," I said. "He would flip out." She agreed to keep this between the two of us.

I slowly learned that despite their age or the horrible disease that these residents suffered from, one thing was for certain. Their libidos were in top, working order.

Friday, May 13, 2011

I could hear the television playing low as I walked down the hall, the only voices in the room coming from it. Even the parakeet was quiet, sitting on his perch looking out at the residents. As my eyes moved to the right of his cage, I noticed that Dad was in the chair immediately next to the bird. He had actually fallen asleep while sitting upright. I knew he must have been very tired. Susan was standing at the medicine cart and as soon as she saw me, she eagerly motioned for me to come over.

"I wanted to tell you something before you woke your dad up," she said.

"Okay," I replied. I absolutely adored Susan. She had an incredible way with all of the residents. I had especially noticed it with Dad. Susan's parents and grandparents had suffered from Alzheimer's, causing her to become accustomed to it at a very early age. She didn't know any type of life without it.

"Your dad did the most amazing thing for me the other day," she said. "It meant so much to me." I knew that Susan's father was currently in the hospital, not doing well. After working a full day here at Arbor Forest, Susan would then head to the hospital to be with her dad. She wanted to spend as much time with him as possible and so she routinely did this every single day.

"A few days back, your dad had heard me talking on the phone," she continued. "I had received some bad news about my daddy. Your dad could tell that something was bothering me. He asked me if I was alright and I told him that my father had Alzheimer's and that he was dying. As much as I tried not to, I still teared up in front of your dad. He didn't say anything more at that point, but I could tell that he was really torn up." She then grabbed a tissue from the table as her eyes had again begun to tear up.

"Well, yesterday, your dad came up to me," she said "and out of the blue, he told me that he wanted to pray with me for my daddy. He said that he just wasn't sure how." I could now feel the tears welling up in my eyes. Dad didn't go to church often, but he deeply believed in God.

"I then took your dad's hand and we walked into the dining area where it was private," she explained. "I helped him to his knees and we knelt on the floor together. Then, we held hands and we prayed for my daddy."

I looked over at my precious father as Susan told me of this incredible story. The tears began to fall down my cheeks. Here was this man who was suffering from Alzheimer's himself. He was going through the worst time in his life, sicker than he could possibly comprehend. At times, he probably had felt like he had lost everything and didn't understand why it was happening to him. Through everything that he was dealing with, all he wanted to do was lift someone else up in prayer. I was never so proud of my daddy as I was at that very moment. That was the kind of truly compassionate person he was. He had such a huge and loving heart and he always put others first. Even with the vilest disease destroying his brain, he was still the most kindhearted and caring person I had ever known. I loved him so much.

I turned back to Susan and gently hugged her. "Thank you for sharing that with me," I said. "You just gave me the most extraordinary gift." At that moment, I felt such an incredible bond with her. We both had fathers that were dying from Alzheimer's. We were both trying to be there for them as much as we could. And we both loved them so dearly.

Saturday, May 14, 2011

His excitement was evident as he placed the baseball hat firmly on his head. The season was going well except for the fact that his biggest fan had not really been a part of it. Papa had unfortunately only attended one game so far. Andrew was hopeful that would change today. The last game had gone so well and really done wonders for Dad.

When Bob arrived at Arbor Forest, he found him leisurely resting in his room, as calm as could be. "Do you feel like watching some baseball?" Bob asked. Dad immediately perked up. Today would be his second baseball game this season.

The game had again turned out very well. Monica was actually able to take a picture of Mom and Dad together on a nearby park bench. Dad had enjoyed himself so much. It had also meant a lot to Andrew. They had been special buddies for years.

For a long time, Andrew's bus had dropped him off at Mom and Dad's home after school. Dad and Andrew had ultimately spent every afternoon together. If Dad was doing yard work, then Andrew was right there helping out. Sometimes, they'd relax in front of the house on the wrought iron bench. Other times, they'd watch television together. They both loved Krystal and Dad would occasionally treat them to lunch out. Many times on the weekend, Andrew would have a sleepover with Dad. They were definitely best buds.

Later that afternoon, I visited Dad and found him in his room relaxing in his blue recliner, the room stifling hot. I checked the thermostat and it was again set to heat, with the temperature gauge moved to the high 80's. I quickly reset everything.

Before long, Dad asked me about finding a job for him again, which now seemed to occur every time he saw me. On the way in, I had run into Kevin who had mentioned that Dad had also talked to him about a job. "Dad, what about helping to hand out the mail to the residents back here?" I asked. "Or, another option would be to have you sweep the sidewalks out back in the walking area. The last idea that I had was to have you do some painting around the facility. Do any of those sound appealing?" I knew that I would have to take full responsibility for carefully watching my dad while he was doing these jobs. If it would make him happy and feel useful, then I would definitely try to make it happen.

"I might like the sweeping," he replied. "Do you think they might let me mow the back area?"

"I'm not sure, Dad," I responded. "I'll have to talk to Kevin about that." Inside, I highly doubted that the mowing would be a viable option. The liability might be too high.

"I'll keep working on it," I said. "How is your abdomen feeling?" I had already scheduled an evaluation next week with Dr. Parker concerning his left hernia. It hadn't seemed to be getting any better and I saw no reason to put it off any longer.

"It's about the same, Pootie," Dad replied.

"I think we should get that taken care of before we have you doing any type of job," I said. "Does that sound okay?" He nodded yes.

I had also debated whether I should have one of the med techs at Arbor Forest start checking Dad's blood sugar. I knew they would have to treat it like any other type of medication. They'd need a prescription for the monitor, test strips and lancets before they could actually start this process.

I knew that Dad wasn't able to check it himself. He had never successfully tested himself even when he was living at home. Doing it now was out of the question, with him becoming more forgetful every day.

When Dad first moved into Arbor Forest and I saw him every day, I had decided that it was easier for me to check his sugar level, which also gave me a record of it for his endocrinologist. Based on the psychiatrist's recommendation and my current schedule, I didn't always get to see Dad every day. Since he had started the Actoplus Met, his numbers had actually come back down, but I still thought it was important to get the daily readings. I didn't feel secure with it not being checked every day. I thought it might be time to ask Arbor Forest for some much needed help.

Tuesday, May 17, 2011

As I attentively listened to his words, the doctor confirmed my worst fears. Dad indeed had a hernia which unfortunately meant that another operation was in his future. It really was no surprise as his symptoms had closely mimicked those present with his first hernia to a tee. The decision was soon made for Dr. Parker to operate on Dad next Tuesday.

"I wanted to talk to you about the anesthesia," I said. The doctor curiously looked at me and gave me his full attention. "My dad has Alzheimer's." I then looked over at Dad to make sure he was okay. I always hated having to tell people my dad's condition right in front of him, never knowing how it made him feel. Unfortunately, this was one of those times when it was imperative that I be totally honest. "When he goes under anesthesia, even if it is only for an hour, it does damage to his brain. Not only does it put him in a bad place immediately afterwards, but once the drugs are eventually out of his system, he is never the same. Is it possible to give him a local and not put him completely under?"

The doctor paused for several seconds. "That's fine," he replied. "I don't see any problem with that. We can give him local anesthesia instead. Just make sure you bring that up at the pre-op appointment so they know what you're wanting." I happily agreed to do that.

On the way back to Arbor Forest, I felt much better. I had stopped and bought Dad a shake at McDonald's. I looked over at him and he was clearly enjoying the drive. Knowing that the doctor had listened to me and wasn't going to put Dad under made me so happy. I knew that if I hadn't asserted myself, it would have been handled exactly the same as the previous hernia operation.

Today, I had advocated for my dad and it had paid off. I felt hopeful that this procedure would be different than the others. I truly hoped that I wouldn't lose a part of my dad afterwards.

As we approached the common area, we soon found an empty couch, Dad and I deciding to leisurely relax for awhile. In no time, we witnessed Dorothy in the dining area angrily addressing one of the caregivers. "I want her to stay out of my room," she said, sounding very irate. "She came into my bathroom without asking and she peed all over the floor."

I immediately knew who they were talking about. Ruth was ninety and the oldest resident in the memory care unit. She was also probably in the best shape as she walked the halls religiously. When she would reach one end of the hall, she'd turn around and proceed back to the other end. Then, she'd routinely start all over again, probably walking over 25 laps a day.

We had also experienced the same problem with Ruth. Whenever she felt the urge to go, she would simply stop where she currently was and use the nearest bathroom. Unless your door was locked, your room was open game for her. Several times, I had to personally escort her out of Dad's room.

By now, several caregivers had gathered around Dorothy, trying unsuccessfully to calm her down. They soon sent a maintenance worker to her room with a mop and bucket to clean up the unfortunate mess. They also promised to keep a better eye on Ruth. Even with this, Dorothy remained fuming.

Dad and I eventually decided to go back to his room where it was quiet. As soon as we walked in, I felt the hot air. I checked the thermostat and wasn't too surprised to find it once again set to heat. It didn't seem to matter how many times I instructed Dad on what to do, it was always the same. I had even talked to some of the caregivers who had also found the room this way.

From now on, I would simply adjust it myself. I'd also ask the staff if they could check it daily. I was slowly learning which functions Dad could still handle and which ones he could no longer manage on his own. I knew it was the disease advancing and it wasn't abating.

Monday, May 23, 2011

As she had slowly moved her stethoscope around his chest, I saw her alarmed expression, clearly concerned about Dad's heart rate. On Friday, I had routinely taken Dad to his pre-op appointment at Parkland General Hospital. After the evaluation, the doctor had advised us to have Dad promptly see his cardiologist before the upcoming surgery. Something just didn't sound right. Late that day, I managed to get an appointment for Monday. It was at the last moment, but it was important that we get him checked before the surgery.

The plan was for Mom to go by Arbor Forest this morning and pick up Dad. They would then drive over to my house and follow me to the doctor's office. Mom had never been to this facility and I didn't want her to get confused. It had seemed like a sound idea.

By the time they pulled into my driveway, I could plainly see that Dad was very upset. This was not good. "Dad, are you okay?" I inquired.

"No, your mother can't drive," he replied.

"Dad, do you want to ride with me?" I asked.

He immediately got out of the car. "I think that's a good idea," he responded. Dad had consistently complained about Mom's driving for years. With the Alzheimer's, it seemed to bother him even more. He quickly got into my car. We needed to take separate cars anyways as I had to be at Chris' school at 12:15.

On the drive over, I tried to redirect Dad's attention. By the time we reached the doctor's office, he had calmed down considerably.

The appointment was at 10:45 with Dr. Joyce Bedford, one of the cardiologists in the practice. Fortunately, we didn't have to wait long. I tried my hardest to keep the current situation defused before it got out of hand.

After evaluating Dad, she handed me the pre-op evaluation letter necessary for surgery, feeling that Dad's numbers looked good. She was also satisfied with his current blood pressure medicine. The appointment may have been overkill, but I didn't want to take a chance where my dad was concerned.

As we walked out to the parking lot, Mom had assured me that she'd be able to get Dad back to Arbor Forest with no problems. Unfortunately, it wasn't her that I worried about. I warily looked at Dad and he actually seemed to be much better.

Chris' class was having their end of year party at 12:30. I needed to be there early to help set up. I would be hard pressed to make it there on time, especially if I drove to Arbor Forest first. I quickly kissed my parents goodbye.

I intentionally drove out of the parking lot first so that they could follow me. Once I got them back to Buford Drive, Mom would be fine. As soon as I pulled out, I looked in my rear view mirror and immediately saw Mom pull out in front of another car. My heart started racing as it was a very close call. I nervously looked back at Dad and he seemed to be fine. I truly hoped that he'd missed the incident.

Chris' party had been a lot of fun. It felt good to relax around such innocence. I was so glad that I had made the decision to be there for him. After the party, an awards ceremony took place in the cafeteria. It warmed my heart when Chris' name was called and he proudly made his way to the front of the room, the whole time looking for me. I had missed the ceremony back in January and he had been so disappointed. Never again would I do that.

Later that afternoon, I called Mom at home to ensure that everything was set for tonight. She was planning on spending the night with Dad at Arbor Forest to keep an eye on him. Because of the surgery, he wasn't allowed to eat or drink anything after midnight. I had already informed the caregivers about this requirement. Dad would also have to shower in the morning with a special Betasept solution. Unfortunately, they would need to get up by 4:30 a.m.

It was a lot to ask of my mom, but she repeatedly assured me that everything would be okay. Dad had persistently asked Mom to stay with him at Arbor Forest for months. This would actually be their first night together there. I prayed that it would go well.

Tuesday, May 24, 2011

I quietly walked into the closet so as not to wake anyone. After getting dressed, I called Mom on her cell phone. I normally didn't make calls at 4:45 a.m., but today was an exception. It was critical that I made sure that both she and Dad were up and that everything was still in order. If just one thing went wrong, we'd have to cancel and reschedule the hernia procedure. She let me know that Dad was currently in the shower. I then talked to the med tech on duty to remind her not to give Dad his normal morning meds. Today, he would only be getting Carvedilol, Lipitor, Namenda and Risperdal.

Mom and Dad promptly pulled into my driveway at 5:45 a.m. We needed to be at Parkland General Hospital by 6:15 a.m. I had offered to go to Arbor Forest and pick them both up, but Mom assured me it wasn't necessary. They would manage just fine.

Not long after we arrived at the hospital, Dad was taken back. Once he was prepped, they would let us visit him. "I need to speak to the anesthesiologist," I urgently said to the nurse. "My dad is supposed to be given a local instead of general anesthesia today. I've already talked to the doctor about it and he okayed it." She assured me that I'd have that chance once we were called back.

Mom and I patiently waited in the lobby. Thirty minutes later, the nurse came out to get us. We found Dad lying back in his bed looking very relaxed. He smiled at us as we walked in.

In no time, the anesthesiologist entered the room. I told him of my concerns and he was actually agreeable to giving Dad an epidural instead. He would just have to ensure that Dad didn't move while he administered it.

The doctor also came in and informed us that Dad's potassium level was low. It needed to come up before he would proceed with the operation. He had given him a supplement to help boost it and would recheck it soon.

A little while later, everything finally seemed to be in order. I gently kissed Dad on the cheek. "We'll be right outside, Daddy," I said. "You're going to be fine." I squeezed his hand tenderly and smiled at him. We were then escorted back out to the lobby for the long wait.

After a couple of hours, we were again called back. The procedure was over and Dad was doing fine. The nurse then led us back to his room.

Dad was sitting upright in his bed when we walked in. I always felt nervous seeing my dad for the first time after surgery, never knowing what his state of mind would be. Today, I got no smile which was not a good sign. As soon as he began to move around, he got very upset. "I can't feel my legs!" he exclaimed.

"It's okay, Dad," I replied. "Instead of putting you completely out, they gave you a local from the waist down. You'll get the feeling back in your legs as soon as it wears off. I promise you'll be fine."

"What have you both done to me?" he asked, looking frantic. I could only imagine what was going through his mind. As he continued to attempt to move his legs, he became more upset. He had that same terrified look in his eyes that he always did right after surgery. I had thought that we would avoid that by using local anesthesia, but it turned out that the after effect of the local had its own unique problems. Even though it had prevented him from going into that dark place, it hadn't stopped him from getting agitated. There just didn't seem to be any good solution when it came to anesthesia for my dad.

Both Mom and I tried unsuccessfully to calm him down. I began to slowly massage his legs and eventually worked my way down to his feet, hoping that he could feel it. It didn't seem to be helping as Dad was still irate with us. Mom and I always got the brunt of Dad's agitation when all we were trying to do was comfort him.

"It's only been a few hours since you got the epidural, Dad," I said. "Your legs are numb right now, but the feeling will eventually come back. You just have to give it some time to wear off. I promise you that nothing bad was done to your legs."

"I do not like this," he said angrily. "I'm worse off now than when I came in. You need to get me out of here."

"Daddy, you can't go anywhere until the feeling comes back into your legs," I replied. "They won't let you leave unless you can walk out on your own. You just have to be patient."

He continued to look at me with disgust. Nothing I said seemed to reach him, my frustration quickly building. I would need to dig deep to handle this the right way. I knew that the only answer was to be patient and wait it out.

I despondently sat down and allowed my dad to vent. I did not want to get into an argument over this. Before long, the nurse came back into the room. "How are you doing, Mr. Lee?" she asked.

"Not too well," Dad replied. "I can't feel my legs."

The nurse reiterated what I had said earlier. "You should start to feel some sensation in them soon," she responded. "I'll come back and check on you in a little bit to see if the feeling has come back."

After about an hour, the sensation slowly began to return to my dad's feet. It was a very happy moment, one that couldn't have come quick enough. I turned and cautiously smiled at Dad. "Do you feel better now?"

I asked. He didn't respond.

The doctor soon came into the room, briefly checking Dad's legs to ensure the feeling was indeed coming back. "Are we doing better?" he inquired. Dad nodded his head yes. The doctor then looked directly at me. "I want to keep the catheter in your dad for a few days until he has completely regained all of the feelings in his lower extremities. Right now, he may not be able to feel the urge to go."

I really wasn't prepared for this news, knowing very little about catheters. He completely caught me off guard. "How often does the bag need to be emptied?" I asked.

"About two or three times a day," he replied. "One of the nurses at his facility can do it. They'll know how."

"There are no nurses at his facility," I responded. "It isn't a nursing home. It's a memory care unit."

"Well, it's fairly straightforward," he said. "The nurse will show you how to empty it before you leave today. It can be removed on Friday. She can show you how to do that as well." Before I knew it, he was gone.

I didn't feel good about this at all. It was a lot to wrap my head around. The nurse soon came in with an instruction booklet and carefully went over the directions, which did seem easy enough. I knew that the only way this would work was if Mom were able to empty out the bag also. I'd be able to do it once or twice a day, but that might not be enough.

"Mom, do you think you can change the bag out like she just showed us?" I asked. I went over the instructions again for her. "I'll take the catheter out on Friday. I just need you to keep an eye on the bag before then. If it gets too full and I'm not there, you need to empty it." She seemed confident that she could do it.

As the day progressed, I continued to worry about the catheter. The more I thought about it, the more I felt it wasn't the best decision. I had no idea how Dad would deal with it. It couldn't feel normal to him.

By the time we were about to leave, I asked the nurse if I could speak to the doctor about the catheter. She informed me that he was already gone. "I don't think the catheter is going to work," I stated. "I think it would be better if it was removed and we just took our chance with an accident or two. Dad wears pull-ups anyways, so it really doesn't matter."

"We have to have the doctor's permission to remove the catheter," she replied, "and he is already gone." It was not the news I hoped for as I had serious doubts about this catheter.

After we got back to Arbor Forest late that afternoon, Mom and Dad went directly to his room. I needed to talk to the med tech about two new prescriptions for Dad. The doctor had prescribed Lortab 7.5 mg. on an as needed basis for pain and a Potassium supplement. The Potassium was only to be given for a week in order to get Dad's levels back up to where they needed to be.

As soon as I was done, I headed to Dad's room, not more than fifteen minutes later. I found Mom busily straightening the drawers. Looking around, I didn't see Dad anywhere. "Where is Dad?" I asked.

"I don't know," she replied. "He was here a minute ago."

"Mom, you were supposed to keep an eye on him," I said.

I nervously started searching the floor for him. He wasn't in the common or dining areas. I then hastily went down to the other end of the hall and still could not find him. Then, I came back and went to Janet's room where I found the door suspiciously locked. Alexandra immediately walked up to me. "What's wrong, Vanessa?" she inquired.

"Do you have the key to her room?" I asked. "I can't find my dad anywhere. I think he might be in here." I had a terrible feeling inside.

As soon as Alexandra unlocked the door, I quickly walked into the room. Janet was sound asleep in her bed, my dad's pants surprisingly lying on top of a chair in front of it. I then noticed the bathroom door was slightly ajar. I slowly pushed it open and was shocked at what I saw. Blood was splattered on the floor as my dad knelt down trying to wipe it up with a wash cloth.

"Daddy, what happened?" I alarmingly asked. He looked up at me with such innocence, reminding me of a little boy trying to clean up his mess before someone saw it and he got in trouble. I soon surmised that he had pulled his catheter out as he was holding the hose to it in his left hand. I quickly went inside the bathroom. This was an absolute nightmare.

"Daddy, why did you take the catheter out?" I questioned. He still said nothing, looking so confused. He had probably felt the urge to go and didn't understand why he had this strange contraption on him. It hadn't felt normal to him and he took it out. It was probably that simple.

I looked in the toilet and it had already been flushed. I then looked in the trash can where I distressingly found the catheter bag. All of the other pieces were missing. He must have flushed them down earlier. I immediately took some tissues and started gently cleaning him up. "Are you okay, Dad?" I asked.

"I'm okay," he answered. He seemed more concerned with cleaning up the blood on the floor than what he had done to himself.

"Let me get this, Dad," I said. I then cleaned up the floor and bath mat.

Afterwards, I helped him get his pants back on. "Let's get you back to your room, Dad," I said, as we slowly walked out of the room. The fact that Janet was still sound asleep astonished me. I also felt very concerned as Dad had lived here at Arbor Forest for months and apparently was still confused about which room was his.

As we entered Dad's room, Mom was still cleaning, completely oblivious to what had just happened. "Dad, you pulled the catheter out and I need to check and make sure there is no damage," I stated. I knew what the correct procedure was to remove it and I suspected that Dad had probably not adhered to it, which would definitely explain the blood.

Dad was completely calm. We went into his bathroom and I checked him for any apparent injury. Fortunately, I saw no visible wounds. "Do you think you can go pee for me right now?" I asked. "I need to make sure there is no blood in your urine."

Eventually, he managed to urinate. I felt so relieved to see no sign of any more blood. The idea that Dad had accidentally done some damage still concerned me. I had him casually sit in the recliner while I made several calls, the first one to Bob. I then tensely called the hospital. They said I could bring Dad back to ensure that he was okay, but the thought of taking him back to the hospital and having to wait around was not good. After the day that Dad had already had, I couldn't see that going over well with him. I also called Dr. Parker's office to inform them what had happened. The doctor was not currently in.

Before I could make a decision, one of the directors urgently summoned me down to her office, telling me that it was against policy to have a resident with a catheter. Since no medical personnel worked on the premises, they weren't staffed with that type of expertise. At that point, it didn't really matter as Dad was no longer wearing the catheter. Since I wasn't about to put another one in him, the point was moot.

When I returned to the memory care unit, I found my mom and dad comfortably sitting together on a couch in the common area. They were currently having a show in which two people were sitting up front, one of them playing a guitar and the other singing. All of the seats were taken as the residents relaxed and thoroughly enjoyed the music.

I knelt in front of my dad and he lovingly smiled at me, currently appearing very calm. Mom was going to stay with him another night. I decided at that moment that he needed to stay right where he was and rest. I would come back first thing in the morning and check on him. They would be eating dinner shortly. I talked to Mom before I left about keeping a watchful eye on Dad. Then, I gently kissed them both goodbye.

That night, I googled catheters on the Internet. I wanted to find out if any damage could occur by pulling them out incorrectly. I happened to run across a special type of catheter called a condom catheter or external catheter that was commonly used in nursing homes for patients with dementia. It was constructed in a way that prevented the patient from hurting themselves if they intentionally removed it. Why wasn't this used on my dad instead of the standard catheter? His doctor knew full well that Dad had Alzheimer's as I had specifically told him myself. He should have prescribed the condom catheter instead. All of the pain and confusion that my dad had gone through could have been easily avoided. The more I read, the more furious I became.

I was slowly becoming aware of the vast lack of knowledge in the medical profession where Alzheimer's was concerned. It seemed as though so many of the doctors were more concerned with their own specialty and not with the patient as a whole. Sometimes they made decisions without dutifully thinking about the consequences for a patient with dementia. I realized that I could no longer count on others to make the best decisions for my dad. I needed to become as knowledgeable about his condition as I possibly could. It was becoming more crucial every day that I advocate for him. My dad needed me to be his voice.

Wednesday, May 25, 2011

As I made breakfast for Chris, I suddenly heard the phone ring. I glanced at the caller id and immediately froze. It was my parents' home and no one should have currently been there. I had expected Mom to still be at Arbor Forest with Dad. This was probably not good news.

At 3 a.m., Dad had restlessly gotten up and turned on the overhead light as he was undoubtedly in the middle of a Sundowner's episode. Mom had asked him to turn it off and come back to bed. Instead, he got very argumentative with her, rummaging through the room, while she hopelessly tried to go back to sleep.

By 5 a.m., sleep was definitely out of the question. Dad was still very upset. After exchanging several words with my mom, he decided to head down the hall towards the common area. Jackie was on duty at the time and had heard him loudly yelling in his room.

She then saw Dad walking towards her in nothing but his pull-up. "We don't walk out of our room in our underwear, William," she stated. "Let's go back to your room and get dressed."

Jackie then followed Dad into his room and helped him with his clothes. During the entire time she was there, Dad continued to talk ugly to Mom. Jackie looked at my dad, clearly upset. "Now, that's uncalled for, William," she said. "Shirley, why don't you go down to the dining area? I'll be there in a minute." Mom quickly got dressed and left the room.

Before long, Jackie came down and made them both a cup of coffee while they sat and talked for awhile. Jackie had come to know Dad's behavior very well since she took care of him almost every night. "There's no point in me staying with him if he is going to get this upset with me," Mom said. "I might as well just go on home."

"That's probably a good idea," she replied. "You do realize that it isn't you, right? It's the disease. If he were calm, he would never treat you like this." She casually took a sip of her coffee. "When he isn't having one of his episodes, he is the perfect gentleman. I really enjoy talking to him when he is calm." She tried her best to comfort Mom. Unfortunately, Mom had dealt with this for so many years now that she was just tired. The Alzheimer's was also having an effect on her health.

When Dad eventually walked into the dining area, he was obviously still agitated. Mom went back to his room and packed her overnight bag, having made the decision to leave the facility. As she walked by the dining area, Dad looked up at her, but said nothing.

Later that morning, I drove to Arbor Forest where I found Dad asleep in his blue recliner. "Good morning, sleepy head," I said.

"Good morning, Pootie," he said groggily, as I gently kissed him on the cheek. Since eating breakfast earlier, he had calmed down quite a bit.

"How are you feeling?" I inquired.

"I'm okay," he replied.

"Do you think you can lie on the bed for me?" I asked. "I need to look at your incision."

He slowly got up and moved to the bed, after which I pulled the waistband on his pants down low enough for me to check the site. The bandage was bloody, but the staple was still intact. I carefully cleaned it up and redressed it. "Do you remember when you had your other hernia operated on?" I asked. He nodded yes. "I had to give you a shot in your stomach for a week to prevent clotting. We have to do that again." He seemed completely at ease.

I pulled the syringe out of my bag and gave him his first shot of Lovenox on his right side, having remembered the procedure from the last time. "I need to do this every day for one week," I said. "I'll make sure I come here each morning to do it." I could have conveniently arranged for one of the caregivers to do it, but I wasn't sure if they had any experience administering a shot. I certainly didn't have a lot myself, but I knew that I would be extra gentle with my dad. More importantly, he felt secure with me giving it to him.

When Dad used the bathroom a little while later, I checked his urine to make sure that no blood was in it. He also allowed me to look again for any visible damage. Everything looked surprisingly good. I was starting to feel a lot more confident that no harm had occurred yesterday.

I had noticed when I came into Dad's room earlier that the room next to him was completely empty. The pretty picture and gold name plate that normally hung on the outside in the hall were gone. Dorothy had apparently moved out. Some of the caregivers had told me that she continued to come back into the memory care unit, even though she was no longer living here.

According to Dorothy, she had made many friends back here and simply wanted to keep in touch with them. I think the truth was that she was coming back to specifically see my dad. On a couple of different occasions, she was seen sitting next to him on one of the couches in the common area holding his hand. Other than my mother, my grandmother and me, my dad hadn't held another woman's hand since he had married.

I clearly knew who had initiated this. I was beginning to feel like she was taking advantage of my dad for her own personal interest. While doing that, she was probably causing a lot of unnecessary confusion for him. The disease was already creating enough of that. He certainly didn't need any more. Unfortunately, I knew what the confusion usually led to and it wouldn't be good for my dad. I would soon have to address this issue before it got out of hand.

Sunday, May 29, 2011

Chris swiftly ran ahead of me into the garage. Before I could shut the door, I heard "Shotgun". I laughed to myself at the way he cleverly claimed the passenger seat even when it was just the two of us riding in the car. We had collectively decided to pay Dad a visit this morning as Chris hadn't seen him since before the hernia operation.

As soon as we walked into the room, Dad immediately started beaming. "Lil' Monkey!" Chris ran to Dad and hugged him tightly.

"Chris, be careful with Papa," I said. "His stomach is still healing."

After they had spent some time together, I had Dad lie down on the bed while Chris climbed up next to him. I looked seriously at Chris. "Want to watch me give Papa a shot?" I asked. His blue eyes widened. I then gave Dad his 5th Lovenox injection. "He's such a good patient." Dad and I both smiled at Chris.

I then carefully checked Dad's incision. As soon as I removed the dressing, I immediately became concerned. I didn't like the way his wound looked at all.

I had consistently kept an eye on it all week. On Friday, I had even called Dr. Parker to tell him that I was worried about the incision and the heavy bleeding that was still occurring. Every time I had changed the dressing, it was full of blood. A huge lump had also formed below the opening. Something hadn't looked right. He had called me back within the hour and said that I shouldn't worry. The lump would eventually go down and the excessive bleeding should subside as Dad continued to heal. Some people unfortunately just healed slower than others.

As I thoroughly looked at the incision today, it didn't look any better. The staple had mysteriously fallen out and the dressing was soaked in blood, with some even spreading out the sides of the bandage. The lump also seemed to be larger as it was very swollen. I gently applied some pressure around the incision to make sure that it wasn't infected. A small amount of blood seeped out. "Dad, I want Susan to take a look at this," I said. "Don't move. I'll be right back."

Within a few minutes, Susan knocked on the door. As soon as she looked at Dad's stomach, I could see the alarm on her face. "If it were up to me, I'd take him to the hospital," she stated.

I then called Bob and we both agreed that it definitely needed to be looked at. I had Susan call 911 for me.

In what seemed like no time, the paramedics had arrived. They routinely examined Dad and also agreed that he should go to the hospital to be checked by a doctor. As soon as they loaded Dad into the ambulance, I left to take Chris home. Bob and I would drive to the emergency room together.

Dad remained very calm throughout the examination. The doctor said that the incision was actually fine, just healing much slower than we had anticipated. He also informed us that Dad's age and his diabetes factored into the longer recovery time. The doctor then added another staple to the incision to help keep it closed. He instructed us to continue dressing it every day and keep a watchful eye on it.

In all the chaos, I hadn't thought to bring a pull-up or a change of clothes. Regrettably, Dad had an accident not long after the doctor left the room. Bob and I cleaned him up as best as we could. He would unfortunately have to wear some hospital pants back to Arbor Forest.

On the drive back, I thought about the many changes taking place in my dad. I then thought about the process that an infant goes through during their first years of life, having to learn how to do everything. In time, as those acquired behaviors became second nature, they gained their independence. Then they lived their life, sometimes taking even the most basic acts for granted.

Nobody ever thought that one day they would reach a point where everything would start reversing itself, the point where things they had done their entire life suddenly became foreign to them. That was what Alzheimer's did. It destroyed the brain in a very methodical manner, piece by piece. Eventually, it manifested itself by taking that person back to their infancy, where they were no longer potty trained, they couldn't talk and they didn't even remember how to swallow correctly.

With every passing day, my dad was forgetting more and more. He was slowly losing all of his independence and becoming totally reliant on others. In some ways, he was becoming very childlike. It was heart wrenching. No one deserved for their precious life to end this way. I hated this disease with such a passion. I hated the relentless manner in which it destroyed people's lives. I felt completely helpless as I watched it claiming yet another innocent victim.

Tuesday, May 31, 2011

A part of me desperately wanted to believe that I could handle everything on my own and for months, I had. As Dad's level of care had changed, I had to as well, accepting that it wasn't a sign I was weak, merely human. I had finally come to the realization that it was okay to ask for help.

As I passed the common area on my way to see Dad, I told the med tech on duty that Dad's endocrinologist would be faxing over a prescription for a blood sugar monitor, lancets and test strips. They would need to send faxes to both Arbor Forest and Collier Village Pharmacy. "His blood sugar will need to be checked four times a day, before every meal and before bed," I said. "His doctor will specify everything in the instructions that he faxes over."

I knew that no one else would be able to check Dad's blood sugar while I was gone on vacation, at least not every day. It was time to turn this over to Arbor Forest. I needed for everything to be in place by the time I left for my trip.

When I entered Dad's room, I noticed a plastic cup with some flowers sitting on his nightstand, knowing immediately who had left them. I didn't like the idea that Dorothy was coming into my dad's room.

I gave Dad his last Lovenox shot and then checked his incision. It was slowly getting better. The lump had decreased in size and there didn't seem to be as much blood on the gauze. In addition, the staple was still intact and seemed to be successfully keeping the wound closed.

After lunch, I drove Dad to his post-op appointment with Dr. Parker. I had seriously thought about cancelling it, but I wanted to get the doctor's opinion on my dad's slow healing.

When the doctor entered the room, Dad was in a good mood. He quickly examined the incision and then removed the staple. Even though the lump was smaller, it was still very much visible. The doctor didn't seem at all concerned about it.

I told him about our trip to the emergency room two days earlier. I also brought up the catheter incident, expecting some serious concern on his part or at a minimum, some type of response. I got neither.

As we left the office, I felt very disappointed with the appointment. It had been a complete waste of time as I could have just as easily pulled the staple out myself. We would definitely not be coming back to this doctor.

When Dad and I arrived back at Arbor Forest, he was visibly tired. We made our way back to his room and he lied down on the bed. I decided to lie down next to him for awhile. Before long, we both had dozed off.

As I later woke up, I noticed that Dad was still asleep. I tried not to move a muscle so he would remain resting peacefully. I looked closely at his handsome face and traced every inch of it with my eyes. He was such a good man. I felt blessed beyond words to have had a lifetime with him. He had always been an incredibly loving father.

I began to remember how independent Dad once was. He never thought twice about going somewhere alone, especially if it meant seeing one of his grandchildren. He used to casually drive over to my house all the time. When Chris was playing baseball, I would often hear the rumbling of Dad's red truck. Even if my mom wasn't able to make the game, it never stopped Dad from going alone. He would just hop in his truck and go.

One day, I had gone to Chris' school, the children all outside on the lawn enjoying several small pools set up especially for their party. As they were happily playing, I heard that familiar rumbling. Before I knew it, I saw Dad walking up to the school. He had decided to have lunch with Andrew. He had never driven to the school by himself before, but it didn't matter. I vividly remember how surprised Chris was to see his Papa that day. He had quickly run up to him wearing nothing more than his bathing suit and hugged him tightly. Dad ended up getting a little wet, but he didn't care. He got to see two of his grandchildren that special morning.

Then I remembered Dad's ultimate driving adventure. One day, my parents had received a phone call from Dyer Elementary School. Their grandson, Aaron, wasn't feeling well and needed to be picked up. Even though it was an area of town that Dad wasn't that familiar with, he didn't think anything of it. He got directions, hopped in his truck and headed out to pick up his grandson.

About fifteen minutes later, Dad reached what he thought was the school and proceeded into the building. A woman inside politely offered her assistance. "May I help you, sir?" she asked.

"I'm here to pick up my grandson," he replied. "His name is Aaron Lee."

She looked at her computer for awhile. "I'm not finding him," she said. "Does he by chance go by another name?"

Dad chuckled. "Not that I'm aware of," Dad replied.

"Well, let me try looking for him another way," she said. "What was he here for?"

Dad looked puzzled. "Uh, elementary school," he slowly answered.

The woman started laughing. "Sir, are you looking for Dyer Elementary?" she asked. Dad smiled and nodded yes. "It's across the street. This is the Gwinnett County Jail." Dad then began laughing, too.

"The last I checked, elementary school was not a crime," Dad said, as they both continued to laugh. She eventually directed Dad across the street to the appropriate location.

As I continued to watch my dad sleeping peacefully next to me, I slowly began to cry, his life so different now. It just wasn't fair. I loved this man so much. I soon closed my eyes and fell asleep once again next to my daddy.

Friday, June 3, 2011

I felt an overwhelming sense of sadness as I made my way down the hall, only intensifying the closer I got to his door. I took a deep breath as I walked into his room. Today would unfortunately be my last visit with Dad for a week as we would be leaving for Pensacola in the morning. My heart was in turmoil.

I needed to make sure that everything was in order before I left. I soon checked his incision and redressed it. It was slowly getting better. Dad had recovered so quickly with his other hernia operation in February. It was only a difference of four months. I wasn't sure why his body was healing so much slower this time around. I would need to show Mom how to care for it when she arrived later.

We decided to go out back for awhile as it was a beautiful day. We casually sat at the table and I trimmed Dad's nails for him. Then, we simply relaxed and enjoyed the peaceful atmosphere. "Daddy, we're going to Pensacola to see Randy's parents," I said. "We'll be leaving in the morning. I'm really going to miss you."

"How long will you be away?" he asked.

"We'll be gone for a week," I responded. "We're coming home next Saturday." He didn't say anything else, but remained completely calm. We were having a loving visit and he seemed to be enjoying himself. I truly hoped the unexpected news hadn't changed things.

While Dad and I were sitting together, Mom suddenly walked outside to join us. Dad seemed so happy to see her. I decided to leave them alone for awhile as I needed to check on some things inside the unit.

When I later returned outside, Dad was clearly getting tired, his demeanor definitely changing. We decided to come back inside so he could rest in his room. I sat in the blue recliner, while Mom and Dad lied on the bed.

I gave Mom a quick lesson on changing Dad's dressing, also mentioning that she needed to keep an eye on the swelling and the bleeding. I had brought several supplies and stored them in a small cabinet next to the recliner.

Dad soon started getting anxious. I didn't know if my news about not being here next week prompted it or if it was just that time of day, but he began to ask Mom about coming home. I looked at her and she was clearly uncomfortable with the conversation. Every time she would tell Dad why he couldn't come home, he would shake his head in disagreement and stop talking. Then, a minute later, he would relentlessly bring it up again. It was a cycle that we had experienced many times before.

Dad's attitude had changed completely ever since Mom had arrived. I knew that he often got agitated during their visits, especially if it was later in the day. No matter what Mom said, Dad argued with her. I wondered if what I was witnessing was the norm between them.

The conversation continued to go around in circles as Dad wouldn't let it rest. A part of me knew that I should probably go before things got worse, but I was afraid to leave my mom here alone in case they did. I hoped beyond hope that this issue would come to an end and we could leave on a good note.

Mom soon began to look to me for help. I finally decided to step in. "Daddy, Mom is just here for a visit," I said. "She isn't able to take care of you like you need. That's why you're here." He just stared at me. I had a feeling he understood me, but it wasn't what he wanted to hear.

"These people don't take care of me," he exclaimed.

"They do, Daddy," I replied.

"Who takes care of me, Pootie?" he asked.

"The caregivers back here in this unit all take care of you," I stated. "I take care of you, Daddy."

"What do you do for me?" he asked. I was dumbfounded. I knew that it was the disease talking, but it still hurt deeply.

"I do everything for you, Daddy," I responded. "I take care of all of your appointments, your prescriptions. I take care of your incision, give you your shots, make your bed, do your laundry, trim your nails, I do a lot for you." I paused for a minute to collect my thoughts. The last thing I wanted was to say something that I would later regret. "I come up here to visit with you practically every day. I'm always here trying to take care of you as best as I can. How can you say that to me?"

Mom then came to my rescue. She had been fairly quiet up to this point. "Chester, she does everything for you," she said. "You shouldn't say that to her."

Things unfortunately continued to escalate down this no-win path. When it finally became obvious that the situation was only getting worse, I decided it was time to leave. I sorrowfully gathered my things and said goodbye.

On the way out, one of the caregivers in the common area amiably wished me well the next week, her smile clearly indicating that she had heard the incident in my Dad's room. "Try not to worry," she said. "We'll take good care of him."

With that, I left Arbor Forest and my father. The visit had ended so unpleasantly. Even after everything I had seen over the past six months, I still found the way the disease could rear its ugly head on a dime shocking. I never even saw it coming. No matter how hard I tried, I could feel the tears welling up inside. A mile down the road, they began to flow freely. I cried the rest of the way home.

Later that night, I curiously called Mom to find out how the rest of her visit had gone. "Mom, I think it might be best if you plan your visits for earlier in the day," I said. "Once it gets to be 3 or 4 in the afternoon, the chance of Sundowner's increases for Dad. I don't want you both to go through another incident like today." She had completely agreed with me.

Tomorrow we would be going to Pensacola for a week, the boys so excited about the trip. I actually had mixed emotions. Part of me was looking forward to getting away as I desperately needed the break. The other part of me was worried about my dad, especially with the grim way that things had ended. I truly hoped that he wouldn't remember what had happened. Most of all, I prayed that he would be safe while I was gone.

Sunday, June 12, 2011

I had felt a nervous flutter inside of me all week. It was now stronger than ever as I thought about my dad. I'd soon be leaving to see him for the first time in over a week, having absolutely no idea what would await me. Last night, I had called Mom to let her know we were back in town. I also wanted to find out how her week had gone. We had exchanged several emails throughout the week, but I knew there was always the possibility that she had kept something from me since she wanted my vacation to be worry free.

"Your dad actually had a very calm week," she said. "He did have some confusion with his clothes though. One day, I came in and he had two pairs of jeans on with no pull-up underneath." I had also found Dad this way many times so I wasn't surprised. "We had gone back to his room so I could check his hernia incision. That's when I noticed the clothing mishap. When he took the inside pair of jeans off, I noticed that there was a little bit of blood on them from his wound. I put some new gauze on it. Then, I made him put a pull-up on."

"How is his incision looking?" I questioned.

"It's about the same," she replied. "There was also an accident earlier in the week. Don't worry. Your dad is fine. He had slipped in his bathroom and fell on the floor. I went in to check on him and he seemed to be okay. I helped him get to his feet. I couldn't tell if someone had had an accident or if the toilet had overflowed. It didn't seem to be flushing right and the floor was a little wet."

"What did you do about it?" I asked.

"I wiped it up and then went down and talked to some of the caregivers about it," she answered. "I told them that they needed to have maintenance come and take a look at the toilet to make sure it was working okay. They also needed to mop up the bathroom floor. On the way out that day, I also asked them if they would keep an eye on your father. They assured me they would."

"I have to tell you one other thing that happened," Mom continued. "It was so odd. You won't believe it. What is the woman's name that walks all of the time?" Mom then asked.

"That's Ruth," I replied.

"Well one day, your father and I were sitting on one of the couches in the common area," she said. "Your father was on the end and I was in the middle. Ruth came and sat on the other side of me. She then looks at me and says 'I know what you have been doing with him', as she nodded her head towards your Dad, 'and it makes me sick.' I couldn't believe she said that to me."

"What did you say to her?" I asked.

"I said 'Ruth, he is my husband. He has been for the past 54 years'. She just sat there and gave me the evil eye, Vanessa." I couldn't help but laugh. That was life in the memory care unit.

All in all, it was a good week, but Mom was definitely glad I was back. It had been a lot of work for her to manage everything on her own.

Later that morning, I drove to Arbor Forest. As soon as I walked through the secured door to the memory care unit, I saw Alexandra. "I'm so glad you're back, Vanessa," she said. "Your father has really missed you. I was just talking to him a little while ago and he mentioned how much he was looking forward to seeing you today."

When I walked into Dad's room, he was calmly sitting in his blue recliner. He looked up at me and immediately smiled. "Hi Daddy," I said.

"Hi Pootie," he replied. I gently kissed him hello and then sat next to him. He looked so relaxed. "I really missed you."

"I missed you, too, Dad" I said. "Did everything go okay last week?" He shook his head yes.

I then told him all about our trip to Pensacola. He had actually not returned since they had moved in 2001. We had driven by both of the previous homes that my parents had owned. The houses and the surrounding areas had changed so much since Hurricane Ivan. I closely watched Dad as I talked, seeming so lucid and engaged in the conversation.

We had a wonderful chat that morning, with absolutely no mention of how things had been left between us that previous Friday. The only good thing about Alzheimer's was that it sometimes allowed Dad to forget the bad incidents.

"Have you had any problems with your incision?" I asked. "Mom mentioned that it had bled on your pants one day."

"No, not really," he replied.

I then had him lie down on the bed. It had been nine days since I had last seen the area and it honestly didn't look that much better. I couldn't understand why it was taking so long to heal. The thought that something was going on beneath the surface that I couldn't see terrified me. Almost three weeks had passed since the procedure.

I began to wonder if Dad's active behavior in the late night hours was somehow contributing to the slow recovery. I knew that he did a lot of pacing in the middle of the night. I also wondered if he was removing the dressing. Several times the area looked like it had been disturbed. I was even starting to wonder if the staple had fallen out or if Dad had pulled it out. I didn't know the answers. It just seemed as though this wound was never going to heal.

Today, I put extra tape on the gauze. If Dad was intentionally pulling it off, I was going to make it harder for him to get to it. I would definitely know when I checked it tomorrow. I really hoped this would make a difference.

Wednesday, June 15, 2011

I was putting a load of wash in when I suddenly looked up to see Chris standing before me, quickly handing me the ringing phone. I immediately became alarmed when I saw "Arbor Forest" on the display. Apparently, Dad was very agitated last night. Around 2 a.m., one of the caregivers heard him calling out. When she hurriedly went into his room, she found him lying between the wall and the toilet. He had apparently slipped and couldn't get up. No one was quite sure how long he had lied there.

The caregiver had quickly helped Dad to his feet. "Thank you," he said. "I thought I was gonna die." He was so appreciative, continuing to thank her over and over. She then helped him get comfortably settled in his bed.

This morning, another caregiver was making her rounds. When she routinely tried to go into Dad's room, he yelled at her to stay out. He was again very agitated. She happened to notice the carpet in Dad's room upon opening the door and immediately became alarmed, seeing several blood stains. She entered the room despite Dad's objections. The trail of blood led to Dad's bed, his sheets stained as well. Because of the excessive amount of blood, the decision was made to call 911. The paramedics soon took him to Glennwood Regional Hospital in Duluth.

After I hung up with Arbor Forest, I quickly called the hospital to get an update on Dad. He was calm at the moment and was patiently waiting to be examined. I didn't like him being alone in the hospital, but with no prior notice, we were in a bind. Randy was already at work and I had to get Chris to school.

I got a call from the emergency room an hour later letting me know that nothing was wrong with Dad. They had thoroughly examined his incision, redressed it and also added another staple to help keep it closed. They desperately needed his bed and asked if someone could come to the hospital and get Dad. I was currently busy with Mom and couldn't get over to Duluth right then. I called Arbor Forest to check if someone could possibly drive their van over to pick Dad up. I knew they routinely took residents to doctor's appointments, but unfortunately, their van was already in use. I then called Bob and he agreed to pick Dad up and take him back to Arbor Forest.

I was a little upset about how they had handled the situation this morning. This was the problem with not having a medical professional conveniently on the premises. Everything was considered an emergency. They had no one with the expertise to handle something of this nature. All they would have needed to do was check Dad's incision and redress it. I think the excessive amount of blood was probably what made them panic. It wasn't nearly as bad as it looked, however, as Dad's blood was very thin. In addition, they had taken him to the wrong hospital. Parkland General Hospital would have been much closer.

Later that afternoon, I went to Arbor Forest to see Dad. As soon as I walked into the room, I saw the unmistakable trail of blood leading to the bed. While I was standing there, Susan came by. "Is it possible to have someone in maintenance clean the carpet for Dad?" I asked. She saw no problem with the request and immediately left to make arrangements. Luckily, the carpet stains were very light.

I then changed the sheets on Dad's bed. I even found some blood in the bathroom, so I took a cloth and meticulously wiped everything down. Dad had been comfortably resting in his blue recliner. I moved him to his bed and gently checked his incision. The hospital had done a good job of dressing it. I really hoped the new staple would help to keep the wound closed.

"Dad, I want you to stay off your feet as much as you can today," I said. "For some reason, this wound isn't healing. It may have something to do with you being on your feet so much." He nodded in agreement. Before long, he closed his eyes and fell asleep.

I decided to sit in the blue recliner and watch Dad for awhile. I then pulled out a book from my bag that dealt with Alzheimer's. I had probably read a dozen books from the library already, needing to be as knowledgeable as possible about this disease. If it were going to try to take my daddy from me, it was going to have to fight me for him. I would be proactive and relentless in my search for answers.

No matter how hard I looked though, I couldn't seem to find a book that provided the type of support that I desperately needed. I wanted something written from a caregiver's standpoint who had already travelled down this bleak road that I was on. I needed the emotional support and knowledge that only this type of book could provide. I knew that I could have probably found a local support group. Unfortunately, I was already spread too thin and had no time for that. A book would have to do.

Most of the publications that I had read were written by doctors and other professionals that undoubtedly knew a lot about this disease. They provided invaluable information, but I just felt as though something was missing from them. I knew from experience that unless a person was directly on the front line caring for someone with Alzheimer's, they could never completely grasp what it was like. Reading stories from someone that had seen this disease from the sidelines was just not adequate. I needed to be able to share experiences with someone else that had sat exactly where I was currently sitting.

Saturday, June 18, 2011

The boys were heavily into the video game as we came downstairs, their hands on the steering wheels and their eyes glued to the screen. The only sounds that could be heard were the racing engines of their cars speeding through the course. I gently kissed them goodbye on their cheeks so as not to disturb their concentration. "We'll be back later this afternoon, guys," I said. Randy and I then headed out the door for our trip to Arbor Forest. We'd be taking Dad to see his psychiatrist today.

We found him calmly sitting in the common area. "Hey Gump," Randy said. "How are you doing?"

"Hi Ran," Dad said. "I can't complain." Dad was dressed nicely and looked ready to go, even though he had absolutely no knowledge of the upcoming appointment. I would inform him later when it was closer to the time.

After visiting for awhile, we all then got into the truck and drove to Woodland Hospital. While we waited in the lobby, a young boy was wheeled out on a stretcher. His mother followed close behind, tears streaming down her face. One of the wings at this facility was for adolescents with substance abuse or behavior issues. I had no idea the severity of this boy's problems, but I felt certain watching his mother that his life had not turned out the way she had envisioned. I secretly looked at Dad and he had that same look of concern on his face.

Before long, the doctor's assistant called us back to a room. As we walked in, we surprisingly found Dr. Franklin already waiting for us. We all shook hands and I introduced him to Randy. He had heard many wonderful things about this man from me, but had yet to actually meet him.

The doctor asked me several questions about Dad's recent behavior. "Dad isn't sleeping well at night," I stated. "The Sundowner's seems to be getting worse. He ends up taking long naps during the day to make up for the lack of sleep at night."

"Is William having any problem walking?" Dr. Franklin asked. "I noticed when he came in that he was shuffling his feet."

"The shuffling has become a normal part of his walking," I said. "He has actually fallen a couple of times. He holds onto the hand rails in the hallway whenever he walks at the facility where he lives. When we take him out of the unit, we have to keep a close eye on him."

Dad was especially quiet during the appointment. The doctor tried to engage him in conversation a couple of times, but Dad didn't say much. Whenever we were at a doctor's office and Dad was asked a question, he usually looked to me for the answer. I had become his memory and his voice.

At one point, Dr. Franklin handed Dad a sheet of paper and a pen. He then asked Dad to write his name. Dad took the pen and slowly wrote a couple of letters, which was all he could manage. His hand was shaking the entire time. Unfortunately, it didn't resemble his name.

The doctor gave Dad a prescription for Trazodone 50 mg. to be given as needed. This was mainly for nights when he couldn't sleep due to the agitation. He also increased his Namenda from 5 mg. to 10 mg. still to be given twice a day.

"I've noticed a significant decline in William since the last time I saw him," the doctor said. "I'm also seeing what might be the onset of Parkinson's. I'm going to take him off of his morning dose of Risperdal to see if that helps. You know how to reach me if you need anything. Okay?" I smiled and nodded my head yes. The doctor's pager number was still safely programmed into my cell phone where it would remain.

When we arrived back at Arbor Forest, I took the new prescriptions to Susan and had her get them into the system. Dad went to his usual seat in the dining area to eat lunch. The caregivers had kindly saved a plate for him.

While Dad was eating, I hastily went to his room. I had brought some carpet cleaner and a brush with me from home just in case the carpet was still stained. As I walked in, I noticed that the blood had definitely lightened. Unfortunately, it was still noticeable. I got on my hands and knees and thoroughly scrubbed the rug. No matter how hard I tried, they weren't going away. The blood stains would forever be a telltale reminder of a disturbing incident that occurred late one night.

Tuesday, June 21, 2011

I smiled at him lovingly from across the room. It was lunchtime and he was seated in his regular spot at the dining table, seemingly very calm. His hair was combed back neatly and he had the blue and white striped shirt on that I loved seeing him wear. It was by far his favorite shirt, one I had fondly seen him in for many years. I remembered the day I had come in to find it unexpectedly folded up on the couch in the common area. The caregiver had told me that Dorothy had placed it there. I immediately took it back to his room and put it in one of his drawers. That was one item I definitely wasn't going to allow to just walk off. It was sentimentally special to me.

"Hi Daddy," I said as I walked up to him. I tenderly kissed him on the cheek as he smiled back at me.

Most of the other residents had already finished eating and left the room. Dad was still diligently working on his dessert. "Are you doing okay?" I asked. He nodded his head yes. As I carefully watched my dad, something didn't seem right.

Alexandra soon came up to me and said hello. "Do you want some iced tea, Vanessa?" she asked. "What about a piece of cake?"

"I'm good," I replied. "Thank you anyway." When I looked back at Dad, he seemed very dazed. I realized at that moment that I hadn't heard him say one word since I had come in. "Dad, are you feeling okay?" He just looked at me, still saying nothing. No matter what I said to him, I couldn't get him to talk. This wasn't like him.

I then began to wonder if it was somehow related to the recent change in his medications. Dad looked like a zombie, which had me deeply concerned. He literally couldn't talk. To anyone else watching him, he probably appeared completely calm. To me, something was definitely wrong.

After lunch, I walked Dad back to his room and he eagerly lied down. I nervously sat on the bed next to him. He looked at me and finally said his first words. "Something doesn't feel right," he said. My heart absolutely sank.

"I knew it," I replied. "Wait right here, Daddy. I need to talk to Susan about this. I'll be right back."

I quickly ran down to the common area. Susan was standing in front of the medicine cart.

"Susan, has Dad been given any Trazodone yet?" I asked.

She swiftly opened up the log book and found Dad's section. "Yes, he has," she answered. "It looks like he has actually had a couple of doses already. One was last night and the other was the night before."

"Susan, he doesn't look good," I said, beginning to panic. "He can't seem to formulate any words."

"It's just his body getting used to the new medicine," she said. "I've seen it before. I promise you that in a couple of days, he'll be fine. It's just going to take some time for him to adapt."

I was completely torn. I trusted Susan implicitly as she had lived on the front line with Alzheimer's her entire life. I still deeply worried about my dad though.

I walked back to his room feeling so disturbed. Dad was still resting in his bed, but was wide awake. I lied down next to him and told him what Susan had said.

As he continued to rest, I tried to talk about different things to help take his mind off of it. "Shawn is taking Driver's Ed," I said. "He is actually out driving with an instructor right now. I'll pick him up later this afternoon. I have to admit that I'm a little nervous." Dad smiled at me.

I continued to talk to Dad for over an hour, after which he slowly started to come back to me and eventually began talking. Within a few hours, he miraculously appeared to be his normal self. I felt so relieved. Maybe Susan had been right. Even so, I knew that I would be watching him very closely from now on. I didn't ever want to see him in that state again. It had really frightened me. That was no way for someone to live.

Friday, June 24, 2011

The unit seemed unusually hectic as I walked in the door. One of the directors was currently giving a tour to some people dressed in suits. As I made my way past them, I amiably smiled and said hello. I then found

Dad eating lunch with the other residents. He was actually sitting at a different table today as his usual spot was already taken. I greeted him and then made myself comfortable in the common area while he finished his meal.

When Dad was done eating, I watched him stand up, only to notice that he had accidentally dressed with a pull-up on top of his pants. No one around him even batted an eye at this. I had seen other residents do this from time to time, but it wasn't quite as humorous when it was happening to my dad.

I knew this wasn't the first time he had inadvertently dressed this way. I had actually been told by several caregivers that it had happened before. "Dad, let's go to your room and change your clothes," I said. As we walked down the hall, he smiled at me. "You're so silly, Daddy. What am I going to do with you?" He then laughed.

Later that afternoon, Dad and I were relaxing together in the common area. It was a very good day, Dad seemingly very lucid and in a great mood. I had mentioned to him earlier that his brothers were in town and would actually be visiting him soon.

Before long, I pleasantly looked up to see my Uncle Shelby and Uncle Ronnie. Dad immediately smiled. It seemed as though whenever the two of them entered a room together, everything brightened up, including Dad.

They soon pulled some chairs over and the four of us sat together. The other residents soon became very interested in the new visitors, continually coming over to talk with us. At one point, I looked up to find that Margaret had cornered my Uncle Ronnie. We couldn't refrain from laughing as we watched the two of them interact.

The residents continued to curiously make their way into the common area. Alexandra even joined in for a quick visit. As if on cue, Dorothy suddenly appeared in the hallway carrying a cup of flowers that she had probably picked herself. As she slowly walked by us, she flirtatiously eyed my uncles. In fact, she couldn't seem to take her eyes off of them. She quickly took the vacant seat on the other side of the room, but continued to look our way. As I occasionally glanced over at her, she seemed completely mesmerized. The interruptions eventually reached the point where we couldn't talk privately, causing us to move out back.

Not long after we sat down at the wrought iron table outside, Mom joined us. The five of us freely laughed for what felt like hours, talking about anything and everything. A lot of special reminiscing took place.

I carefully watched my dad throughout it all, looking so completely relaxed. The smile never once left his face as he was clearly enjoying life. At that moment, there was no Alzheimer's. There was no Sundowner's. There was not a trace of dementia. There was only my precious father, the oldest of three brothers, who looked like the ultimate picture of happiness. I wanted to freeze this moment in time so that he could remain like this forever.

Saturday, June 25, 2011

One of my fondest memories of growing up in Hialeah was the Royal Castle on 49th Street. It was conveniently located very close to my Dad's barber shop on Palm Springs Mile. He had always loved their hamburgers and would occasionally go there for lunch. When we moved away, we left many things, including Royal Castle. The closest establishment that we had found to it was Krystal, which Dad also loved to eat. He actually hadn't had a Krystal burger since he had moved to Arbor Forest.

My uncles had mentioned to me awhile back that they wanted to take Dad someplace special the next time they came to town. They had asked for my input and I honestly couldn't think of anything more appropriate than a Krystal burger and a walk down memory lane.

Later that afternoon, Dad and I were in his room. I was helping him get dressed when we suddenly heard a knock on the door. My uncles and my cousins, Jeanneen and Johnny, had all excitedly come into the room as I assisted Dad with his shoes. My uncles had decided to take Dad out of Arbor Forest today. It would be a welcome break for him. While they were out, they'd planned on surprising him by going to Krystal. I knew he was going to absolutely love it.

Jeanneen soon asked me if she could take her little dog out back. I entered the secret code and as soon as I opened the door, I shockingly found myself face to face with a huge black snake coiled up right in front of me. I quickly shut the door. "Jeanneen, you can't go out right now," I said. "There's a big snake out there." I then asked one of the caregivers to let maintenance know.

Before long, Kevin entered the unit. When he boldly opened the back door, the snake hadn't moved, so he decided to approach him from the outside. A few minutes later, I saw Kevin smiling through the window with the snake hanging from the handle end of a rake, at least 2 - 3 feet long. Apparently, it was a rat snake and was actually helpful around the facility. I was just glad he hadn't surprised my dad and me on one of our usual outings.

Once Dad was ready, everybody slowly started making their way down the hall. One of the caregivers stopped in her tracks and stared at my uncles. "These are my dad's brothers," I said.

"I can tell," she replied, looking shocked. "All three of you look so much alike. It's amazing."

As we continued our way to the door, Shelby lovingly held Dad's arm. He moved a little slower these days, shuffling as he walked. I knew as I watched them that Dad was in good hands.

As we opened the front door, we met Susan coming in. "You have fun, Mr. Lee," she said, as Dad leaned forward and hugged her. She was definitely one of his favorites.

The walk from my Dad's door to the rental car was very slow, feeling easily like thirty minutes had elapsed. They had talked with practically everyone they saw on their way out. Anyone watching this scene from afar would have rolled on the floor with laughter. It then took another five minutes to get everyone situated in the car. It was tight as Shelby drove, Dad sat in the passenger seat and Ronnie, Jeanneen and Johnny all squeezed into the backseat, joking with each other nonstop. I couldn't refrain from laughing as I observed the humorous interaction between them.

I happily watched them as they finally drove away, wishing I could have been a fly in that car. I knew without a doubt that they were going to have a great time this afternoon. It would be so good for Dad. No medicine could have ever been as therapeutic as this visit.

Later that evening, Randy and I took the boys to Provino's for our anniversary. Normally, we would have gone out by ourselves. However, the five of us had not eaten out together in months and I missed our family time so much. Tonight, we would celebrate together.

While we were eating dinner, our waitress came by and delivered a message to us. It was an anonymous note wishing Randy and I "Happy Anniversary". I suspected who was behind it. The waitress later confirmed that one of my uncles had secretly called the restaurant and asked for a special message to be delivered to us. I loved them so much.

Our families were always very close growing up in Miami. We lived five minutes away from my grandparents in Hialeah, fifteen minutes away from my Uncle Ronnie's family in Carol City and an hour away from my Uncle Shelby's family in Tamarac.

Every Christmas Eve, we would alternate the party between one of the three brothers. Christmas dinner was always held at my grandparents' home. It was such a special time as everyone would come dressed in their new Christmas clothes. There was more food than any of us could ever eat, my favorite being the ambrosia. My grandmother would sit in the kitchen for hours peeling and cutting up the fresh oranges, to which she'd add maraschino cherries, coconut and pecans. It was always delicious and something I looked forward to every year. The get-togethers had been our family tradition for as long as I could remember. Looking back on all the precious memories, I now had so much more appreciation for these special gatherings.

Our lives were so intertwined back then. Curtis had played baseball for my Uncle Ronnie for years. His daughter, Wendy, and I were very close, spending many summers together. We even stayed with Uncle Shelby and Aunt Annette a couple of summers to help take care of their twin boys. My Uncle Ronnie had worked at my Dad's barber shop for years. The shop was conveniently located a couple of miles away from my grandparents' home. My dad would leave the shop every Saturday and eat lunch with his parents, my grandmother always having a spread waiting for him. The connections between us were endless. Our families were very close indeed.

When Curtis graduated from high school, he was awarded a football scholarship to Tulane University in New Orleans. Mom had pressured Dad to move for a long time as Miami was changing and she desperately wanted to move away. Dad eventually agreed to move to Pensacola. It would be close enough to New Orleans to visit Curtis and also allow us to remain in Florida where my dad's barber license would still be valid.

I felt so brokenhearted when we moved. I was born in Miami and lived there for fifteen years, having the most incredible childhood possible. It was there that my roots would always remain. As unhappy as I was, it probably didn't compare to what Dad experienced. He left his mother and father and both of his brothers. He left his barber shop that he had spent years building up. He left friends that he had had since high school. He left his hometown. If anyone had a right to oppose this move, it was Dad, but he didn't. Not once did I ever hear him say one negative word about leaving.

He had ultimately made the move because he felt it was the right thing to do for his family. He was probably heartbroken. I never once stopped to think how hard that move must have been for my dad and he never brought it up because that was the type of selfless person that he was. He always put everybody else before him.

Tuesday, June 28, 2011

As I walked through the lobby, I noticed several residents congregated on the couches to the left. A special service was currently underway and the large room was crowded. I carefully glanced around to make sure my dad wasn't in there and then continued on to the memory care unit. Before I reached the door, I heard my name called by one of the directors who needed to talk with me. I immediately became alarmed.

A meeting had apparently been held a few days back concerning Dorothy having access to the memory care unit. She had repeatedly gained entry into the unit despite not having the special code. Invariably, they'd find her sitting in the common area holding my dad's hand. It was very confusing to him. After she would leave, he'd become extremely agitated, not understanding why he wasn't allowed to leave freely like she was. The caregivers would inevitably find him yelling and banging loudly on the front door trying to get out.

Dorothy was officially informed of the latest decision. She was no longer allowed back in the memory care unit. Needless to say, she was not happy about this. In fact, she had written an angry letter vehemently stating her dissatisfaction with this matter. The director had instructed me to refuse access to her if she ever tried to cunningly follow me into the unit.

A few of the caregivers had mentioned to me that some other residents in the assisted living section had to be monitored closely when they were inside the unit. One of the women back here was named Christine, a petite woman who no longer talked much. She did, however, laugh a lot. It was not uncommon for her to be looking at you and simply break out in uncontrollable laughter. It was infectious. We had both found ourselves giggling together at times and had absolutely no knowledge of what we were laughing at.

Christine had an older sister that lived in the assisted living section. She was always coming back to visit Christine. Apparently, one of the caregivers had caught the sister trying to brush Christine's teeth one day, being extremely rough and causing Christine to wince in pain. They had to force the sister to leave the unit that day. Even though she was still allowed in the unit, she was strictly forbidden from going into Christine's room.

When I came into the common area today, I found Dad casually sitting on one of the couches in such a good mood. I sat next to him with Margaret sitting on the other side. The husband of one of the residents walked past us headed towards the front door, their small, white dog trailing behind him. The man continued to walk down the hall, never realizing that his dog had suddenly stopped in the common area.

I looked at Dad and he had a huge grin on his face. He looked directly at Margaret and said "Your dog just peed in the living room." He then started laughing, which in turn got Margaret doing the same. There was no way I could refrain from joining in. Dad was obviously very confused, but he seemed happy and content. This was his new world.

Inside these walls, I was surrounded by Alzheimer's. Once I left, whether it was to go to one of the boys' schools or to the grocery store or even to the library, it was easy to feel like I was returning to a different world, one not affected by dementia.

Even though it may have seemed that way, I knew that was far from the truth as Alzheimer's was everywhere. It was estimated that 5.2 million Americans currently had this horrid disease. By 2025, the number of people with Alzheimer's was expected to reach 7.1 million, an increase of 40 percent in just twelve years. By 2050, that number could nearly triple to 13.8 million.

The worldwide numbers were even more astounding with approximately 44.4 million people having dementia. That number was projected to almost double every twenty years, to 75.6 million in 2030 and 135.5 million in 2050. That was, of course, unless a medical breakthrough to prevent, slow or stop this terrible disease occurred. Not a day went by that I didn't pray for that miracle.

The other day, I shockingly read that every 68 seconds someone in America would develop Alzheimer's. That was almost one person every minute. I was astonished as the numbers were reaching all time highs. By 2050, that number would increase to one person every 33 seconds. Soon there would be but two kinds of people in this world: people that had Alzheimer's and people that knew someone that had Alzheimer's. It could no longer be viewed as something that happened to other people. This devastating disease would eventually touch everyone. It was a very alarming thought.

Friday, July 1, 2011

The tense look on their faces clearly told me that something was amiss. As soon as I walked into the memory care unit, I noticed Lauren and another woman nervously leaning against the wall in the hallway. They were in the middle of a serious conversation and their expressions were not good. Were they perhaps talking about my dad? They soon stopped me and let me know that he was having an extremely rough morning, refusing to take his meds. "Could you try talking to him?" Lauren asked. "Just be careful. He's very agitated."

As soon as I walked into the dining area, I found Dad sitting in his usual spot, his clothes looking a mess. He had a long-sleeve, red t-shirt on, inside out. His jeans looked fine, but his shoes were mismatched and he had no socks on. His hair was completely unkempt and he looked very disheveled, almost like he had just crawled out of bed and come straight down to eat. As he was talking to the med tech, his voice louder than usual, he was obviously very agitated.

He suddenly looked up at me as I walked to his table. "Hi Daddy," I said. He didn't smile at me which was definitely not his normal greeting. "What do you say we get out of here? Do you want to go back to your room with me?" He still didn't say anything, but slowly stood up and walked back with me willingly.

Once we made it to his room, I shut the door and helped him change into some clean clothes. I put some water on his hair and gently combed it back. He looked like a new man and I could tell that he felt completely different. Then, we leisurely sat in his chairs for awhile, Dad in the blue recliner and me in the burgundy Queen Anne chair. The med tech had earlier given me his morning pills in a cup and I successfully got Dad to take them, eventually dozing off.

Later that afternoon, Dad and I went out back, amazed at the transformation in his demeanor. He had calmed down completely since his disturbing episode that morning. I had successfully managed to redirect him out of an agitated state and I had done so without any medication. I was finally getting it.

"Why don't we sit on the couch?" Dad suggested, as we later walked back inside and found an open seat. I had Dad take the spot next to Helen while I conveniently pulled up a chair. With Helen, you never knew what kind of mood she'd be in, always one of two extremes.

While several of the residents were talking, I noticed that Helen was looking directly at my dad. It looked like she was getting agitated with him, even though he was doing nothing but sitting there. "What are you doing?" she asked, continuing to stare at him. Then, she took her hand and tried to swat at him.

I immediately stepped in as I had gone through a lot of hoops to pull him out of his earlier agitation. I was not about to have her put him right back there. Plus, I didn't like watching anyone be mean to my dad. "Helen, that's not very nice," I said. She then turned her gaze to me, her expression blank. I had no idea whether my stern words had impacted her or not.

Before I knew it, she swatted at Dad again. "Helen, do not hit my dad!" I said firmly. Dad just sat there like such a gentleman. As if on cue, a nurse came into the room and knelt in front of Helen to check her blood pressure. Helen then unleashed her fury on the nurse.

It was a very uncomfortable feeling when one of the residents was upset. I had to admit that I always felt a sense of respite when the source of agitation was someone other than my dad. I knew that he had his fair share of episodes, but I felt a tremendous relief that this afternoon was not one of them.

Tuesday, July 5, 2011

My stomach had growled intensely ever since I pulled into Mom's driveway to pick her up. I had managed to do three loads of laundry, bills and clean my house earlier, but I had somehow forgotten breakfast. On the ride to Arbor Forest, we had decided that we'd eat lunch with Dad today.

We ended up having a very calm and pleasant lunch, just the three of us. All of a sudden, Dad looked behind me as someone had obviously walked up. I turned my head to surprisingly find Dorothy standing there. "They won't let me in here, so I have to make this quick," she said. "I wanted to give this to you." She then handed my dad a small, yellow envelope.

"Why aren't you allowed back here?" I asked, curious whether she truly understood why she was banned from the memory care unit.

"They think I'm a bad influence on your father," she replied. "They say that he gets very upset in the afternoons and starts banging on the door. He's still my friend."

One of the caregivers walked into the common area about that time and Dorothy quickly turned to leave. "I better go before I get in trouble," she said. "I'll try to come back, Bill."

I shockingly watched her scurry off before turning back to Dad. He rolled his eyes as he handed me the card. "Do you want me to read it,

Dad?" I asked. He shrugged his shoulders as if to say he really didn't care one way or the other.

The envelope was addressed to Mr. Bill Lee. It appeared as though it was originally going to be mailed to Dad as it was completely made out to his Arbor Forest address. I carefully opened up the envelope to find a thank you card which I then read out loud.

Dear Bill,

The powers that be have decided that I can't come down there anymore because it agitates you too much. The powers are Lauren and Cynthia. I'm cut to the quick. They think we have been too cozy. Our friendship is still ON no matter what. They say it will be at least two weeks before I can visit you. Be careful what you say to them. I'll still say my prayers for you. Take the vitamins. You are still my best friend.

Dorothy

I looked up at Dad and he had no reaction to it whatsoever. A part of me thought that he was oblivious to what Dorothy was doing. Dorothy, on the other hand, seemed completely coherent as was obvious from her letter.

I had previously talked to Mom about her several times. Mom actually thought she was very nice and wasn't the least bit threatened by Dorothy. She trusted Dad implicitly.

That night, I got an unexpected call from one of the caregivers at Arbor Forest as Dad was highly agitated. They couldn't get him to take his evening meds. I could hear Dad yelling in the background. "Why should I trust you?" he asked. "I am not going to take anything from you."

"Can you put my dad on the phone?" I asked.

"Sure, here he is," she replied. I could distinctly hear her hand the phone to Dad, but he didn't say a word.

"Daddy, this is Vanessa," I said. "Are you okay?"

"No, I'm not," he answered, the tone of his voice clearly indicating he was very upset. I knew that I had to remain calm and somehow redirect him. "I told you. I am not gonna take that," he said to the caregiver.

"Daddy, would you take the pills for me?" I asked. "I promise you. It's okay. They'll help you to calm down."

"What is wrong with you?" he asked the caregiver. He was talking to me and yelling at them simultaneously. He finally handed the phone back to the girl.

"Hello? Is anyone there?" I inquired.

The caregiver soon came back on the phone. "I think he is finally going to take the pills," she replied.

"Alright, go take care of him," I said. "Will you call me back afterwards and let me know if he calms down?"

She agreed to return my call. After about an hour, I still hadn't received a phone call, so I called the memory care unit. They had finally managed to get Dad to take his pills, after which he had gone to his room. He was currently lying down in his bed and seemed calm. They were going to keep an eye on him and would call me back if things got out of hand again.

I remained on pins and needles all night, worrying incessantly that my dad would wake up and again return to an agitated state. I knew that if it got too bad, I would have to go to Arbor Forest myself. Fortunately, that phone call never came.

Thursday, July 7, 2011

It was sometimes so hard to pinpoint the exact cause of his agitation, at times seeming to come out of nowhere. I knew that was the disease, hard at work. As I walked into Arbor Forest this morning, I hoped to find Dad in a calm state. He had been very agitated for several days now, more so than usual. One of the directors had talked to me about Dad possibly having a urinary tract infection. "They are very common with Alzheimer's patients, especially when they start to suffer from incontinence," she explained. "The UTIs can cause a lot of agitation. If I had to guess, I'd say your dad probably has one. He has all of the signs."

We had decided to take Dad to see Dr. Soham R. Patel, a general practitioner who specialized in internal and geriatric medicine. The director was successfully able to get us an appointment with him late this afternoon.

Most of the residents in the memory care unit were patients of Dr. Patel, whose office was conveniently only a mile away. In addition, he visited the facility a couple of times a month. He also was on call whenever an emergency occurred. I had held off seeing him because I wanted Dad to remain with his own doctors who already knew him well. Lately, I was having second thoughts. The convenience of having a doctor nearby and one that made house calls was becoming very enticing. It would also be nice to be able to consult him whenever an unexpected crisis arose, regardless of the time of day.

Late this afternoon, I left Arbor Forest to pick Shawn up from driving practice. The plan was that Mom would drive Dad to Dr. Patel's office. I had already given her the directions. Once I dropped Shawn off at home, I would hurriedly meet them there. It was going to be close timing for me already. I absolutely couldn't get to the appointment on time if I had to pick Dad up also.

As I pulled into the parking lot, I looked around for Mom and Dad, not finding them anywhere. I waited and waited. I had no idea what could have happened to them, but I was starting to get a little nervous. Finally, I saw them pull up, hoping they hadn't run into any problems.

As I walked to their car, I opened the passenger door and soon noticed that Dad wasn't talking. I helped him out of the car and had him stand up after which he froze. I could not get him to take a step as he stood there looking terrified. It was almost as if he had forgotten how to walk. "Daddy, can you walk up to the door with me?" I asked. "I'm not going to let you fall. I promise."

I firmly held him up and he slowly started taking steps. I successfully managed to get him to the front door before he again stopped in his tracks. He had both hands strongly holding on to the door frame and wouldn't budge. "Dad, it's okay," I said. "I've got you." I didn't understand what was happening as I had never seen him like this. He had no problem walking when I saw him earlier today.

I eventually got Dad inside and helped him take a seat. It had actually taken almost ten minutes to walk about ten steps. I then checked him in and filled out the necessary paperwork.

After about fifteen minutes, the nurse called us back. Dad was again very hesitant while walking. It took a major effort to even get him to step up on the scale to get his weight.

We eventually made our way back to an examination room. When Dr. Patel came in, Dad was very quiet, the doctor directing most of his questions towards me. Dad just watched as we went over his current medications and his medical history in detail.

Dr. Patel then had Dad lie down on the exam table where he checked his stomach area very thoroughly. After his examination, the doctor felt certain that Dad had a UTI. He was able to tell simply by the way Dad's abdomen felt. He would need the urine sample though to be absolutely sure. The doctor then brought a wheelchair in to help us get Dad next door to the restroom.

Dr. Patel ended up prescribing an antibiotic for Dad who definitely had a UTI. It would explain the increased agitation recently. I would need to bring a urine sample back in a week to ensure the medicine had worked.

After the appointment, we actually had to use the wheelchair to get Dad back into the car. I closely followed my parents back to Arbor Forest. It couldn't have been more than five minutes.

By the time we had arrived, Dad was visibly upset. Mom had pulled up to the door to quickly let Dad out. As soon as he stepped out of the car, he slammed the door. "Dad, what's the matter?" I asked.

"Your mother couldn't figure out how to use the a/c in the car," he said. "I was burning up." He was clearly agitated, but it had seemed to take his mind off of his walking. He was moving right along, with absolutely no hesitation. I then took him by the arm and led him back inside the memory care unit.

As soon as we made it to the common area, I noticed that all of the residents were casually seated around Alexandra as she was reading them a story. Dad was apparently getting more agitated with every step. "Shirley, let's go!" he said angrily. Alexandra suddenly stopped reading as she looked up at Dad. He had actually snapped at me, only I think it was intended for my mom.

"Daddy, it's me, Vanessa," I remarked. "I'm the one that has been walking with you, not Mom." He looked strangely at me, but didn't say a word. I then led him down the hall towards his room.

I had Dad sit in his recliner and I made sure the a/c was on. Then, I quickly got him a glass of iced water. He was slowly starting to relax. Mom soon joined us in the room, looking flustered by the earlier incident. I had no doubt that she knew how to operate her car, especially the a/c. Something else must have caused Dad's agitation.

An hour later, I felt comfortable that Dad was in a calm state, so I decided to leave. I saw the medical director on the way out and gave her the new prescription for Dad which she promised to take care of immediately. The sooner he got on the antibiotic, the sooner his UTI would go away and the less agitated he'd be.

Later that evening, I got a startling call from Mom. Not long after I had left, Dad had gotten upset again. He was very hot and decided to take his pants off. When Mom tried to get him to put them back on, he got very agitated with her. It seemed as though all he wanted to do was argue. She eventually decided to leave.

As she walked by the common area, Alexandra came up to her. "He is very agitated, Alexandra," Mom said. While they were talking, they saw Dad walk out into the hall, still dressed in his pull-up.

"I'll take care of him, Shirley," Alexandra replied. "Why don't you go home and relax?" She then led Dad back into his room to help him get dressed.

I thought about how my dad had snapped at me so easily when he had mistakenly thought I was Mom. Once he realized that it was me, his whole demeanor had changed. It seemed that had been the norm between my parents for years. Dad didn't seem to be able to control his temper around Mom like he could with the rest of us which was one of the reasons we never suspected anything was wrong with him. We thought they just argued a lot.

As I studied the latest of my dad's afflictions, I became very disheartened with the UTI. It sounded as though the threat of one occurring in my dad was something we would have to be cognizant of from now on. Several factors made my dad a high risk for contracting it, most importantly his incontinence. The diabetes and enlarged prostate also made him susceptible. Unfortunately, I knew those conditions would not be going away.

The part that really struck me as I carefully read was one of the specific symptoms in older individuals, that of mental changes or confusion. That one statement explained so much. Dad had been extremely agitated for days. It seemed to mysteriously come on without any warning and at times of the day when he was normally very calm.

It also explained my dad's temporary inability to walk. It had literally manifested itself in the short ride over to the doctor's office. I hadn't expected it to come on so suddenly as Dad had walked out of the facility and sat in the car with absolutely no problems. Something had happened to him on the ride over that had left him powerless to take even one step.

Today, he had managed to bounce back for which I was very grateful. I knew that there would eventually come a day when he would no longer be able to remember how to walk. The disease would make sure of that. Sometimes reading ahead in the life of an Alzheimer's patient was difficult. The future was bleak.

Saturday, July 9, 2011

I felt a sense of panic as I nervously roamed the halls, unable to find Dad anywhere. He wasn't in the common or the dining areas. I then quickly went to his room, but to no avail. I thought maybe I had missed him, so I went back to the common area. Still, there was no Dad. I ran to the other end and started walking down the hallway once again, looking scrupulously in each room as I passed it. After checking all of the rooms that I thought he might be in, I began to get very worried. I didn't know where he could be. "Susan, have you seen my dad?" I asked. "I can't find him anywhere."

Both Susan and the other caregiver began anxiously looking for Dad. The terrifying thought that he might have gone out the back door entered my head. I became frantic as I ran down the hall towards the back entrance. As soon as I turned the corner, I suddenly saw him sitting on the floor leaning against the wall, his eyes closed. I had absolutely no idea what was wrong with him.

I immediately knelt beside him. "Daddy, are you okay?" I asked. He slowly opened his eyes, seeming a little disoriented. Susan and I gently helped him to his feet. I looked at the caregivers, feeling very disturbed. "How did no one notice him?"

"I don't think he was lying there that long," the caregiver said. "I saw him just a little while ago."

We then walked Dad to his room and got him comfortably seated in his recliner. He seemed so tired and eventually dozed off again.

The more I thought about it, the more upset I became. What really struck me as unusual was that nobody else seemed to be as concerned as me.

Susan soon came down to check on Dad, finding me still visibly upset. "Vanessa, he does this a lot," she explained. "It's not the first time we've found him sitting on the floor. Sometimes, he sits by the back door. Other times, he sits near the front door. I think he is waiting for his family to come."

As she walked away, I thought about her insightful words. I tenderly looked at my dad as he slept so peacefully, tears soon filling my eyes. All he wanted in this entire world was to see his loved ones. None of this was fair.

Dad had started taking his antibiotic yesterday. By now, he should have already had a couple of doses. I knew that with antibiotics, that was sometimes all it took to make a positive difference. He was definitely calm today as the medicine seemed to be making a huge distinction.

From now on, whenever an unusual increase in Dad's agitation occurred, I would immediately suspect a UTI. Based on his condition, it was very probable that this would not be his last one. I knew that the longer the UTI went undetected, the more agitated Dad would get and hence, the more potential damage to his brain. Allowing an Alzheimer's patient to remain in an agitated state for an extended period of time was very dangerous, not just for the patient but also for those around him. Even though no cure for this terrible disease currently existed, I felt that keeping Dad as calm as could be would go a long way in prolonging it.

Monday, July 11, 2011

She looked up and smiled at me as I casually passed the dining hall. Dorothy was seated at a round table with several other women, seemingly enjoying herself. I waved to her after which she returned to the conversation at hand. I felt a tremendous sense of relief knowing she wasn't currently in the memory care unit. As soon as I entered the secret code and opened the door, I startlingly found Dad lying on the floor against the wall. Beneath him was his red, heart-shaped pillow. I immediately became alarmed as I knelt by his side. "Daddy, Daddy?" I said, trying to wake him up. He slowly opened his eyes. "Daddy, are you alright? Do you need something?"

"I'm really thirsty, Pootie," he replied.

"Hold on one second," I said. I hurried to the common area and found Alexandra. "Alexandra, my dad is lying on the floor at the end of the hallway. He needs something to drink." She got me a cup of water and I quickly took it back to Dad. I managed to get him to sit up while he drank every bit of the water. "Is that better?" He slowly nodded his head yes. I then helped him to his feet and walked him down the hall to one of the couches in the common area.

I realized after we sat down that I forgot Dad's red pillow, so I went back down to the end of the hall where Dad had been sleeping. His favorite pillow was lying on the floor just as we had left it. I picked it up and then returned it to Dad's bed. I knew he was very fond of that pillow and I wanted it safe and secure in his own room. When he eventually went to bed tonight, I wanted it waiting for him.

Alexandra would later tell me that my dad had begun regularly walking to the end of the halls, sitting down and taking a nap. I had assumed when he was doing this that he was uncomfortable on the floor, that he must have fallen. As I was finding out, that was not the case at all. He was simply resting where he'd be sure to see his family when they came to visit him.

My dad was steadily declining. For awhile, it seemed that all he did was sleep. When he was awake, he was sometimes very disoriented. Since taking the antibiotic, he seemed a lot more lucid, but unfortunately with that came the agitation. I longed for the day when he became stabilized with his medication. I just wanted him to be peaceful.

Later that day, Dad and I went out back, thinking the fresh air would do him good. He absolutely loved sitting outside. After about thirty minutes, he was ready to come back in. As soon as I entered the code into the back door, I respectfully held it open for him. After I shut the door and turned around, I saw Dad kneeling down to take a seat on the floor right inside the door at the exact same spot where I had found him on Saturday.

"No Daddy, you don't need to sit on the floor," I said. "Let's go to your room. You'll be more comfortable there." He got up with no objections whatsoever, reminding me of a little boy minding his mother. We slowly walked together to his room where I got him seated comfortably in his blue recliner. I then made sure the a/c was on.

Dad looked up and caught me secretly watching him. He smiled and lovingly scrunched his nose at me after which I smiled back at him. I knew that if I hadn't been there today, he would have lied down on the floor at the end of the hall and taken his usual nap. What I slowly realized was that he would have been completely content in doing so.

Tuesday, July 12, 2011

No sooner had I cleaned the dirty dishes than Shawn wandered into the kitchen wanting some pizza. It was the one room in my home that seemed to stay operational 24 hours a day. All I could do was smile at him. As I pre-heated the oven, Mom routinely called on the phone to let me know that she was back home.

She and her friend, Frances, had met this morning at Arbor Forest. Frances had been a dear friend to my parents for years, coming to their home in Buford once or twice a month to witness to them. They had developed a close relationship. When Dad moved into the memory care unit, Frances had begun visiting him there. It was not uncommon for me to walk into the common area and find Frances and several of her friends amiably chatting with Dad.

The main purpose of today's visit was to get Dad to sign a power of attorney. Frances was a lawyer and had prepared the document as a favor to Mom. Unfortunately, Dad wasn't able to sign his name. He never even came close.

Later that afternoon, I came to Arbor Forest to visit Dad and found him leisurely sitting in the common area. Dad didn't seem to talk much anymore. Sometimes, he would look intently at me and clearly want to say something, but he just couldn't seem to form the words. I would then try to help him out and start guessing until I would eventually say what he couldn't.

Today, we were sitting on one of the couches when he suddenly looked over at me and gave me that look, obviously trying to tell me something. "Do you need something to drink?" I asked.

"Noooo," he replied slowly.

"Do you need to use the bathroom?" I questioned.

"Yes, yes," responded Dad. He then smiled at me as we stood and walked to his room. As the disease was steadily advancing, I needed to learn Dad's new language.

Later that afternoon as we were leaving his room, Dad turned and picked up his red heart-shaped pillow and carried it out of the room with him. I watched him as he intentionally started walking down the hallway towards the back door. He placed the pillow down on the floor and carefully leaned it against the wall. He then turned around and began walking back down the hallway towards the common area.

"Do you want to leave your pillow there, Daddy?" I asked. As he nodded his head yes, it suddenly hit me. "Is that in case you want to take a nap there later?" He again nodded yes. I smiled at him lovingly as we continued walking down the hall.

For the first time, I looked at the situation through the eyes of Alzheimer's and it made perfect sense. The old me would have picked the pillow up and carried it back to his room. The new, wiser me left it on the floor where Dad had specifically placed it so that it would be there when he later decided to take his nap. I could now see the logic in his thinking.

For so long, I had wrestled with wanting to pull my dad back into my life, but I now undeniably understood that was no longer possible. Instead, I had to join him in his Alzheimer's domain. I finally had to accept that he would not be leaving that world. I would no longer try to get Dad to see things my way. From now on, everything would be viewed through his eyes. Today had been a major breakthrough for me.

Monday, November 30, 1953

6351ST MAINTENANCE SQUADRON
6351ST MAINTENANCE AND SUPPLY GROUP
APO 235

30 November 1953

Dear Mr. and Mrs. Lee:

I am happy to inform you that your son, William, was named "Airman of the Month" for this organization for November, 1953. He was chosen over numerous other airmen for this honor.

The "Airman of the Month" is selected on the basis of job performance, character, military bearing, leadership, attitude, in fact all qualities that make an outstanding airman both on and off the job.

Is is gratifying to have airmen of his caliber in my command.

Sincerely,

JOHN M. PATTON
Lt. Col., USAF
Commander

Tuesday, December 15, 1953

6351ST MAINTENANCE SQUADRON
6351ST MAINTENANCE AND SUPPLY GROUP
APO 235

15 December 1953

SUBJECT: Appreciation

TO: A/1C William O. Lee, Jr.
        6351st Maintenance Squadron
        APO 235

1. During the period you have served under my command your devotion to duty has been such to reflect great credit upon you as an airman.

2. I wish to express my appreciation for the loyal service rendered by you as airman in charge of the Hydraulic Shop during your overseas tour. It is realized that the conditions under which you have been required to serve have not always been ideal. There have been many times when you have been called upon to work long hours and many instances in which you have been required to perform duties outside your primary career field. The cheerful and co-operative manner in which you have accepted and performed these additional duties are indicative of your ability and character.

3. I would like to congratulate you for being chosen Wing Commander's Orderly and Airman of the Month for November, 1953.

4. Thank you for a job well done. I hope that we may have the opportunity to serve together in the future.

JOHN M. PATTON
Lt. Col., USAF
Commander

Thursday, July 14, 2011

He didn't move a muscle as the clippers slowly glided through his hair. I smiled at him in the mirror. The image brought back so many precious memories of my father cutting Chris' hair over the years. Eight months had now passed since my dad had given him his last haircut. Some memories never faded.

Chris and I had decided to visit Dad afterwards, planning on arriving right after lunch. As we walked in, we saw Dad casually seated in the dining area. Both Dad and Joseph were relaxing at their table. "Well, hello there you two," said Alexandra. "Your dad was just finishing up his meal." Chris and I both kissed Dad hello, after which I greeted Joseph.

"We'll wait for you in there," I commented to Dad. "Just take your time."

We then found a couple of vacant spots on a loveseat in the common area, the couches almost completely full. It was a very relaxed day and everyone seemed to be in a good mood after lunch.

While we were comfortably seated, Margaret intentionally walked over to us. She had been staring at me for awhile with a very serious look on her face. "If I see you do that one more time, we're gonna have words," she said, looking back and forth between Chris and me.

I knew that Margaret was, at one time, an elementary school teacher. I had a feeling that her current behavior had something to do with that. She must have mistakenly thought I was being mean to Chris. I apologized to her and she soon walked off. I felt like I was attending grade school and had just been reprimanded by the teacher. I then turned to Chris and we both started chuckling. Sometimes, that's all you could do.

I then looked up to notice some new visitors to the unit. Seeing Christine's older sister and Dorothy nonchalantly walking down the hall left me utterly shocked. Dorothy had walked into the common area as if nothing was more natural and then even took a seat on one of the couches. I nervously looked back towards the dining area and saw that Alexandra had also seen her. This would not be good.

I had spoken privately to Alexandra several times about this issue. She was very fond of Dad and some of Dorothy's recent behavior had really upset her. She definitely wasn't going to let Dorothy anywhere near my dad on her watch.

She immediately walked up to Dorothy. "Now, Miss Dorothy, you know you are not supposed to be back here," she stated. "You need to leave right this instant." Dorothy watched her intently as she talked, but didn't move a muscle. After Alexandra finished, Dorothy continued to sit on the couch defiantly, completely ignoring Alexandra's words.

Another caregiver immediately took a seat on the couch right next to Dorothy and they talked confidentially for awhile. I overheard her trying to reason with Dorothy and convince her to leave on her own. After about ten minutes, Dorothy got up and decided to come into the dining area, intentionally making a beeline right for my dad.

Alexandra quickly blocked her path and stood directly in front of her. "Miss Dorothy, you need to leave right now," she said sternly. "Do I need to go get one of the directors?" I felt very uneasy as it was getting ugly. Dorothy had always been very nice to me and I didn't like seeing this unfold in front of us. I had to remind myself that this wasn't about her. It was about my dad and what was best for him. The truth was Dorothy had no business coming back here.

I looked over at Dad and he was just sitting there. I didn't know if he realized what was going on or not, but I wanted very much for this to end without him getting agitated. If she didn't leave soon, I would need to intervene and take Dad back to his room.

Finally, Dorothy turned around and slowly headed back towards the front door as one of the caregivers escorted her out. During the entire time Dorothy was back here, she wore an insolent look on her face. I started to understand why some of the caregivers were so leery of her. She could be very manipulative.

I looked back at Alexandra as she rolled her eyes and shook her head exasperatingly. Today, Dorothy had managed to sneak into the memory care unit by cleverly following another resident in. I was convinced that her sole purpose was to see my dad. Fortunately, she had been stopped. I wondered though how many other times she hadn't.

Thursday, July 21, 2011

The ride over was extremely hot. I had finally resorted to putting the windows down as the a/c was not working well. It had a small leak and couldn't seem to hold a charge for long. The mechanic had informed me that the system was very outdated and needed to be completely replaced, but since it was so costly, I'd put it off for awhile now. I worried about driving Dad in my car later. I was accustomed to the heat, but I didn't know what it would do to him.

I arrived at Arbor Forest just in time to eat lunch with Dad. Lately, he didn't seem to have much of an appetite. It had actually gone on for a couple of weeks now. Today, he had eaten some of his vegetables and his roll, but wasn't really interested in his meat. I had even cut it up for him thinking that might help, but unfortunately it didn't. This wasn't like Dad at all.

When his dessert arrived, he hungrily ate the entire piece of cake. "Do you want another piece, William?" Alexandra asked. Dad smiled and she immediately knew the answer.

After lunch, we decided to go back to Dad's room for awhile. He lied on his bed and peacefully stared out the window. It was such a beautiful day and the serene view from his room was very picturesque with lots of trees and greenery. He was completely relaxed and seemed to be enjoying himself. Before I knew it, he had fallen asleep.

While Dad was resting, I busied myself in his room, quietly straightening things up. When I looked in his top dresser drawer, I surprisingly found a stack of envelopes. Several were from his brothers; one was from his cousin, Jeanneen. Amidst the stack were two small, yellow envelopes that had not been delivered through the regular mail. I immediately recognized the envelopes as looking the same as one that I opened for my dad weeks ago. I inevitably knew who had sent the letters without even opening them. When I pulled the cards out, they were both identical to the thank you card that Dorothy had previously given my dad.

The first card was addressed to Bill Lee and was fairly short. She had apparently given it to Dad awhile back.

HAPPY FATHERS DAY PAPPY! YOUR FRIEND DOROTHY

The second card that I found was more involved. It was addressed to Chester Lee and was definitely the more recent of the two cards.

Good morning Fair Bill!! The sun is shining, birds singing, but there is no joy in my heart, Friend. I hope you are feeling good and your spirits ringing. I'm praying for you every day – so smile. Some day we will meet again.

Have a good day blue eyes.

Dorothy

Dad hadn't mentioned receiving the cards. I doubted that he had read them by himself. Sadly, he didn't seem to be able to do that anymore. I assumed Dorothy had personally delivered them to my dad. I wondered curiously if she had also read them to him.

When Dad woke up, I informed him that we needed to go to Dr. Martinez's office to have his blood taken for some routine tests. Hopefully, it would be a short appointment.

Unfortunately, even with no traffic, it still took about 45 minutes to get there. The car had turned unbelievably hot. "I'm sorry, Dad," I said. "I know my car is hot. Are you okay?" He nodded yes, but his pink cheeks clearly said otherwise. My sweet father just didn't want to burden me.

After the appointment, Dad asked if we could rest for a little bit. I assumed that he just wasn't ready to drive back in the sweltering heat. We conveniently sat in the two seats nearest the door for about ten minutes after which I helped Dad to his feet and we again got into my oven of a car.

On the way back, I stopped at McDonald's and got Dad a vanilla milkshake which definitely helped. Every time I looked over at him, he was slowly sipping it. By the time we got back to Arbor Forest, it was completely gone.

When we walked into the common area, some caregivers that I hadn't seen before greeted us. One of them apparently knew Dad very well. "I usually work the nights," she said. "I spend a lot of time with your Dad. He gets up in the middle of the night and we watch movies together." She was so bubbly, her dimples showing with every grin. Dad smiled at her as she talked so effervescently. It always warmed my heart to meet a caregiver that was so respectful towards Dad. It was extra special when those feelings were reciprocated. Dad's interaction with her clearly told me they were friends.

I soon got Dad seated at one of the dining tables and fixed him a glass of iced water. One of the caregivers was seated at the same table, painting one of the female resident's nails. I knew they would be eating dinner shortly and since Dad looked so content, I decided it was a good time to say my goodbyes.

On the way home, I stopped by Chris' elementary school, the class lists for next year supposedly posted near the front entrance. As I soon found his name, I looked through the rest of his class. I then looked through the other classes until I found the boy's name that had been so mean to Chris. I felt so relieved as I found him in another class. I had taken matters into my own hands by contacting one of the administrators. She had done what she had promised. For the first time in awhile, I felt a ray of hope.

Sunday, July 24, 2011

As I steadily made my way down Camp Perrin Road, I felt rejuvenated. The sun was shining bright and the heat was invigorating. Unless someone intentionally pulled up beside of me, I knew the run would be free from any bad news. It was my special time to unwind free from any stress with the music blasting in my ear.

Not long after I had returned home, I was drinking a bottle of water in the driveway when the phone suddenly rang. Mom was currently at Arbor Forest visiting Dad. "Vanessa, your father is very agitated," she said. "He won't listen to a word I say. I don't know what to do." She sounded so frustrated. "I've talked to the caregiver. I thought they had some medication to help calm him down. She says that Dad is all out."

I could hear Dad yelling in the background. "Mom, can you put Dad on the phone?" I asked.

As soon as he picked it up, I could distinctly hear his breathing. He never said a word though. "Daddy, what's wrong?" I questioned. "Why are you so upset?"

"Your mother doesn't care a thing about me," he said.

"That's not true, Daddy," I responded. "She wouldn't be there if she didn't care."

"Why don't you just go," he said to Mom. "I know you don't want to be here." I could hear Mom in the background telling him otherwise, but it just seemed to make him more upset.

The conversation with my dad was split between me on the phone and the people in his room. He was clearly agitated with Mom. I had no idea whether anything specific had happened or if it was just that time of day.

"Daddy, can you try to calm down for me?" I asked, raising my voice in order to get his attention. I wasn't reaching him. He eventually set the phone down as our conversation was over. I could hear him walking away, his voice continuing as he strode determinedly down the hall.

Mom then picked up the phone. "Mom, can you give your phone to the caregiver?" I asked. "I need to talk to her about Dad."

Before long, the caregiver got on the phone. "This is William's daughter," I said. "My mom said something about my dad not having any more medication for his anxiety."

"He doesn't," she explained. "I've looked in the medicine cart and he is out. I'm trying to get it refilled, but it won't arrive until later this afternoon."

"That can't be," I responded. "I checked just a few days ago and the prescription had just been refilled. There should still be plenty. You can check the log to verify it. He should have some Trazodone available." She assured me she would check the cart again.

In less than ten minutes, I got another call, this time from the caregiver. She had actually found Dad's Trazodone in the bottom of the cart and he indeed had plenty. They were going to try to get him to take one. Hopefully, a nap would ensue.

A little while later, Dad lied down in his bed as Mom lied down next to him. The caregiver had managed to get him to take something for the agitation and he had calmed down completely. He soon fell asleep.

About an hour later, Dad awoke. Mom was reading a book, but was still lying next to him. She slowly closed it and looked at him as he was staring at her so lovingly. He then told her he had always loved her and had never wanted anyone else. This was the man she had fallen in love with. This was why she stayed.

No one hated the agitation more than Dad. It absolutely wasn't him. He simply had no control over it when it occurred. Unfortunately, it wouldn't be the last time today.

Mom and Dad ate dinner together later that evening. She eventually decided to leave so she could get home and let Barron out before it got too dark. Dad didn't want her to leave and soon got agitated again. It seemed like an endless cycle.

That night, I sorrowfully thought about my dad. As the Alzheimer's progressed, his agitation only seemed to intensify. Some days it was so unbelievably hard to deal with. I had always felt strongly that God never gave us more than He knew we could handle. I had watched so many people go through so much heartache in their lives and felt such relief that I wasn't going through similar despair myself. I assumed that I wasn't strong enough to handle something like that or God would have definitely placed it in my path.

I remember one afternoon I was in Michaels. A mother was standing in front of me in line with a little girl that had Down's Syndrome. The mother was so loving towards the little girl. When she smiled back at her mother, it was obvious they had a special bond. As I closely watched the mother, she impressed me with the way she handled everything so perfectly.

I then thought about my own children. Why was I blessed with three healthy children and this woman was given a special needs child? It didn't seem fair. Maybe that wasn't the right way to look at it. Was this God's way of telling me that I wasn't strong enough to handle a child with special needs?

As I now looked back on that day, I thought about how much my life had changed since then. I had no idea why God would give the most incredible man I had ever known such a horrid disease. I might not ever know. What I did know was that I was exactly where He wanted me to be. He wanted me taking care of one of his special children that just happened to be my father. I think God was trying to tell me that maybe I was a lot stronger than I thought.

I believed with all my heart that we were supposed to take care of our parents. It was as basic as "Honor thy mother and father." I may not have always handled things correctly. I may have made mistakes along the way, but I would never desert my daddy. If he was forced to go down this terrible road, then I would be by his side holding his hand the entire way.

Tuesday, July 26, 2011

I casually sat on the deck watching Riley, marveling as nature slowly came to life. The birds were singing and the squirrels were running about, trying to dodge the dog. She had just completed her morning security patrol around the perimeter of the backyard when I unexpectedly heard the phone ring from inside.

Someone from Arbor Forest was calling. Dad's caregiver was very concerned about his increased agitation. "Vanessa, I've never seen him quite like this," she said. He had actually snapped at her a couple of times which had never happened before. "There is definitely something going on with your father lately. He may need to have his meds adjusted or he may have another UTI."

I had also noticed the recent increase in agitation in my dad. Something definitely wasn't right. I promptly made an appointment with Dr. Franklin for 12:30 on Saturday. I had mentioned Dad's agitation on the phone, but the doctor wouldn't change his meds without first seeing him. He wasn't that type of doctor.

It just so happened that my Dad's brothers were coming into town this weekend. They had previously expressed an interest in meeting his doctor. Unfortunately, the timing had never worked out before. I wanted them to be able to meet Dr. Franklin and openly ask him any questions that they had. Mostly, I wanted the doctor to determine what was causing the sudden change in my dad.

Later that afternoon, I went to Arbor Forest. When I arrived, I found Dad sitting in the common area. He had just eaten lunch and seemed very relaxed, smiling when he saw me. "Hi Daddy," I said, as I sat on the couch next to him, several residents sitting nearby. We talked freely for awhile. Dad then suggested we go to his room.

We both sat together at the foot of his bed. He was calm, but had a very apprehensive look on his face, something obviously bothering him. "How is your mother?" he asked.

"She's fine, Dad," I responded. "She'll probably come up to see you tomorrow."

"What does she do all day?" he then asked curiously.

"She's been trying to get the bonus room cleaned up," I explained. The bonus room at one time was extremely neat and well organized. The room was huge and took up half of the top floor. It was a combination spare bedroom, office, home gym and TV room. In time, it had become the repository for all projects, paperwork and anything that basically couldn't be placed in any other room. It was currently a mess.

"She stays at home all day, Daddy," I replied. "Believe me. You have nothing to worry about." The concerned look on his face clearly said he was troubled over this. "Mom isn't interested in anyone else. I promise you that." His elbows were resting on his knees. He then put his hands up to his eyes and gently rubbed them. He looked like he was crying.

"This is not the way I pictured my life turning out," he said. He turned and pleadingly looked straight into my eyes. "I want to go home."

It was these times when he was so lucid that were often the hardest. "I know you do, Daddy," I replied. "You can't. You just can't." I then began to cry, my response obviously upsetting him.

He slowly stood up and moved to the top of his bed where he lied down. "I feel like I have no control over anything anymore," he stated. "I have no say over what happens to me." His voice was quivering, sounding as though he was on the verge of breaking down. I hadn't seen him this distraught in awhile.

He then got up and suddenly left the room. In a flash, he was gone. I stayed there on his bed and cried. He was absolutely right. Every single thing he said had been right. When he was coherent like he currently was, everything that he said made perfect sense. I could think of nothing to say that would possibly make him feel better. It was a no-win situation for all of us, but especially for my dad.

After about fifteen minutes, I secretly poked my head out and looked in the common area. Dad was quietly seated on one of the couches next to another resident. He clearly wasn't coming back to his room. Part of me felt like that was his way of telling me to go and leave him where he belonged. I didn't fit in here, at least not today. I would respect his wishes.

I soon gathered my belongings and dried my eyes. As hard as it was, I knew it was best that I leave. I had unfortunately only made things worse by coming.

As I walked out to the common area, Dad looked up at me, appearing very calm. I leaned over and gently kissed him on the cheek. I then whispered in his ear "I love you, Daddy". He said nothing. With that, I slowly walked away.

Wednesday, July 27, 2011

Contrary to what we all hoped for, Dad's anxiety wasn't getting any better. In fact, it was getting worse, much worse. Today was very much a repeat of what had happened on Sunday. Mom arrived early this afternoon to visit Dad. He was fine for awhile. As the conversation veered towards him coming home as it always seemed to do, he eventually got upset with her. They had to again give him some medicine for his increased agitation. As was the usual case, it put Dad to sleep.

The difference today was that when he awoke, he was still highly irritated. After arguing with Mom for several minutes, he suddenly left his room to go to the common area. Mom gathered her things and followed him out. She didn't seem to be helping the situation, but was afraid to leave Dad in his current state. Mom finally decided to sit in the dining area out of the way, pulling her book out of her bag and trying to read. Her hope was that her mere presence would eventually help to calm Dad down.

"Move over there so I can sit down," Dad said to one of the other residents. He was acting rude which was not like my dad at all. His agitation had escalated to a very high level. He clearly felt like he was in charge, almost as if he needed to prove something. None of the other residents said a word. Dad was being very intimidating and they weren't going to challenge him today.

It soon became very hard to ignore the increased anxiety as Dad began to get louder. "Do you see that woman in there?" he asked. "She doesn't care a thing about me."

"Well, sure she does, Mr. Lee," said one of the caregivers. "That is your beautiful wife, Shirley. She loves you."

"Oh no, my wife wouldn't leave me in here if she loved me," Dad replied.

Mom continued to quietly sit in the dining area, trying to let Dad's remarks go by the wayside. It was becoming harder to do every second. He was baiting her and she knew it was futile to respond. It would only make matters worse. Inside though, her heart was breaking.

Eventually, Mom realized that her staying was pointless as she had inevitably reached her limit. She reluctantly picked up her purse and book and began walking down the hall towards the front door. Dad didn't try to stop her this time.

Whatever was happening to my dad was clearly getting worse. I began to wonder if he'd be able to make it until his appointment on Saturday. This was definitely one of those times where having a doctor or nurse on the premises could have possibly made a huge difference. As much as I loved this place, maybe Dad needed more specialized care. Maybe he needed a skilled nursing facility. I didn't want to admit what that meant. He was possibly advancing into another stage. The disease was winning.

Thursday, July 28, 2011

Being a mother of three boys was such a blessing for me. I remembered a time when I desperately wanted a little girl, but that feeling had long since gone away. Boys provided a protective love that was like no other. I felt truly blessed to be able to take care of them. I was downstairs in the laundry room folding their clothes when I got an alarming phone call from Arbor Forest. Dad had been very agitated during the night. Unfortunately, it had escalated through to the early morning. They were calling to inform me that there had been an unfortunate accident.

At about 6 a.m., Dad had walked directly across the hall to another room which currently had two men living in it. One of them was waiting for another room to open up. They were both sleeping at the time.

Dad began yelling at one of the men to get out of the bed. Frank had occupied that room ever since my dad had first come to live there. He was recently moved to another facility. I didn't know whether Dad thought the men were in the wrong room or whether he thought they were in his room. Either way, he was clearly confused.

He then grabbed the corner of one of the bed sheets and started vigorously pulling. Where Dad's mental faculties suffered, his physical strength more than made up for it. He had a firm grip on the sheet and wouldn't let go. "Get out of this bed right now!" he yelled.

A male caregiver currently on duty was trying his best to calm Dad down. Unfortunately, it wasn't working. The male resident in the bed was terrified as Dad continued to yell at him. Before anyone could stop the incident, Dad lost his balance and fell backwards onto the floor, yelling out in intense pain.

The caregivers gently helped get Dad to a couch in the common area where he began complaining about his ankle. At that point, they weren't sure what damage had occurred as they were trying to get Dad to pinpoint exactly where the pain was located. They would keep a watchful eye on him and call me back when they knew more.

A little while later, the phone rang again. "Vanessa, your dad is in a lot of pain," the caregiver said. "We think that he may have broken his hip. We called 911 and the paramedics are here right now. They are getting ready to take him to Parkland General Hospital." My heart absolutely sank.

I quickly drove to the emergency room. As soon as I arrived, I was taken back to a room where I found my dad. He was lying in a bed in the middle of a huge room filled with every type of equipment imaginable. His eyes were closed. "Daddy, Daddy?" I said. His eyes didn't flutter at all. I gently took his hand in mine and caressed it. "Daddy, can you hear me?" Still, I got no response. He was apparently heavily sedated.

I bent down and tenderly kissed his cheek. My poor father had endured so much already and now he had to go through this. I closed my eyes and deeply prayed that God would see him through this nightmare. We needed his miraculous touch now more than ever.

I nervously sat in a chair directly opposite my dad. A doctor soon came in and introduced herself. She then confirmed my worst fear. "Your father fractured his right hip," she said. "He needs to be operated on as soon as possible. He is in a tremendous amount of pain."

I looked over at my precious father. This was so unfair. All I wanted to do was take away his suffering. "He also has a UTI," the doctor continued. "My suggestion is that he be put on a low-dose antibiotic permanently to help stave off any future infections. Based on his condition, they will probably continue to occur. It might be better to be proactive." She then left the room.

I thought about the increased agitation that my dad had experienced this past week. Now I found out that he had another UTI. It was just three weeks ago that he had his first one. I knew that he was highly susceptible, but I honestly wasn't expecting another one so soon. It was probably responsible for the adverse episode that had caused him to fall and break his hip. I just stared at my dad, feeling completely numb.

For so long, I had heard nightmares about people breaking their hips. It was the dreaded turning point, the one that usually marked the beginning of the end. Everything inevitably went downhill after that. Most people never completely recovered from hip surgery.

Randy had been telling me this for years. His grandfather had a bad hip that had caused him a lot of pain. He had elected to have hip replacement surgery, the anesthesia leaving him with a lot of confusion. While in the hospital one night, he attempted to walk to the bathroom on his own instead of calling a nurse. He accidentally fell and broke his new hip, requiring a second operation. The anesthesia from back to back hip surgeries was just too much for him, causing a lot of damage to his brain. He was never quite the same afterwards.

I silently sat there in a stupor. It had actually happened to my dad. He was at that dreaded point that I had been warned of so many times. Was this the beginning of the end for my father? Hadn't he gone through enough already? What more could possibly happen to this poor man? I sat there and watched him as he occasionally moaned in pain. I had feared this moment for so long and now, I was here. I closed my eyes again. "Lord, please give me hope," I whispered.

Another doctor soon came in needing to take an additional x-ray of Dad, only this time, with Dad on his side. As the doctor and nurse carefully tried to move him, Dad screamed out in intense agony. It was so hard to watch. I quickly looked away, but the sounds of my dad's misery continued. At that point, they gave him some more drugs to ease his pain.

The doctor talked to me about the upcoming surgery which was planned for this evening. "My dad has Alzheimer's," I said. "He doesn't do well with anesthesia. Every time he goes under, a little bit less of him comes back." I had delivered this same speech so many times. With the type of surgery we were looking at, I wasn't sure it would make a difference this time.

"He is in a lot of pain," the doctor remarked. "I doubt we can move him to his side to give him an epidural. You just saw how much it hurt him when I tried to get an x-ray. It would be much worse than that. He would have to remain on his side and be completely still for at least a couple of minutes. Honestly, I can't see that happening. We may have no choice but to give him general anesthesia."

As soon as the doctor left the room, I returned to my dad's side. "Daddy, it's me," I said. "It's Vanessa." He was now fully awake. He looked at me, but didn't say a word. I truthfully couldn't tell if he knew it was me or not. What I did know was that he was hurting, the painful look in his eyes clearly indicating it was excruciating for him.

Dad was operated on later that night. They indeed had to put him out with general anesthesia. I didn't want that, but I wanted him in pain even less. The operation was a success. Everything had gone fine. He was resting comfortably and probably would remain that way throughout the night.

I had absolutely no idea what would await us when Dad finally woke up. The thought of losing any more of him terrified me. I hated Alzheimer's with such a passion. How much more of my father did this vile disease want? When would this hell end?

Saturday, July 30, 2011

The intense feeling of apprehension hung in the air all around me. I tried to be positive, but just couldn't seem to shake the worrisome mood. It was a very frightening time for my dad. As I got ready to go to the hospital, I truly hoped that Dad would be awake at some point. When I had visited him yesterday, he was still heavily sedated from the hip surgery. I had gently kissed him on his cheek and whispered his name, but ultimately got no response. I stayed with Dad for several hours, but he never woke up. Later that afternoon, Dad also received a visit from his brothers and cousins. Unfortunately, he remained asleep during their visit as well. When I had called the hospital and spoken to Dad's nurse late yesterday, she had informed me that he was still out. It wasn't that surprising as he was the exact same way after his heart surgery.

In the middle of the night, Dad finally came out of the anesthesia. He had no idea where he was and got very agitated, eventually requiring his arms to be physically restrained. It wasn't safe for him or anyone else. The drugs had really had an effect on him.

This morning, Shelby and Ronnie drove to the hospital to visit with Dad. Mom had already arrived an hour earlier. Dad was awake and seemed to recognize everybody, occasionally smiling at his brother's jokes. Everything seemed fine.

The physical therapist soon came into the room. Dad was currently wearing compression boots to help keep the blood circulating and lessen the chance of him getting a blood clot. As she carefully tried to change his right sock, he cried out in extreme pain. By the time she was done, Dad had regrettably become very agitated.

It then turned extremely ugly, the situation escalating fast as Dad began yelling. Ronnie stood to the left of him and firmly held his hand. Shelby stood on the other side holding his other hand. "Gump, it's me, Ronnie," he said. "I'm your brother." Dad had a crazed look in his eyes. Everyone was a stranger at that moment.

Dad was a very strong man, but with his adrenaline surging, he was even more powerful. His brothers couldn't control him. He was squeezing their hands so tightly, their knuckles were white.

By now, several nurses and orderlies had quickly run into the room to assist. Staff members were positioned on all sides of the bed trying vigorously to hold Dad's legs down and prevent him from kicking. The last thing they wanted was for him to accidentally pull the needle out of his arm or even worse, to re-injure his hip. My dad was out of control. Mom just sat there watching this horrific scene unfold, helpless to do anything.

I had seen Dad in this state so many times in the past. This was a first though for his brothers. In all the times they had come to visit him, he had never been agitated to the level he was now.

The head nurse was eventually able to give my dad a shot which calmed him down almost instantaneously. He lied there peacefully, completely sedated once again. The room then went quiet as the hospital staff slowly left, the commotion finally over. Ronnie looked at my mom, shaking his head all the while. He wasn't surprised as what was happening to Dad had seemed inevitable. Shelby, on the other hand, was not at all prepared for this. He quietly walked away towards the foot of the bed, keeping his back to everyone. His older brother had never in his life treated him that way. He was devastated.

I understood only too well how he felt. We were repeatedly told not to take this type of behavior personally, but it was so hard not to. The aftereffects were scarring, the painful memories forever engrained in our minds.

I was convinced that there was a reason why today happened the way it did. My uncles had been sympathetic with what we were going through from the very start, but they had never witnessed it firsthand. They had never seen the disease take control of my dad. Today, that had happened. For some inexplicable reason, God had wanted them to experience it for themselves.

Later that day, I came to the hospital. My dad remained sedated as I made myself comfortable on the small couch in front of the window. I wasn't going anywhere.

Before long, my Uncle Shelby walked into the room. He immediately came to my side and we hugged each other tightly. As I closed my eyes, I could feel the tears streaming down my face. Nothing was said between us as no words were necessary. There was a new dimension to our relationship that had not existed before today. We had now both witnessed someone that we deeply loved turning on us and treating us with hostility. We had now both seen a side of Dad's disease that we would never forget.

Dad was going through a living hell and we were powerless to change it. So much was said in that silent hug with my uncle. He had now gotten a glimpse into what life on the frontline was like.

My dad's mind had yet to recover, the anesthesia changing him once again. The hospital staff wouldn't allow Dad to stay in his bed all day because of the serious threat of bedsores and blood clots. So, once a day, they carefully moved him to a recliner. Later in the day, they moved him back to his bed where he would remain for the rest of the day. Every time they moved him, he cried out in intense pain, eventually causing him to get agitated. They had to keep him in physical restraints and on medication because he was so combative. With so many narcotics in his system, he was very confused. The drugs were changing him once again. It was an endless cycle.

He still had a urinary tract infection which was only adding to the agitation. He also wasn't eating. I didn't know how long his body could survive without any nourishment.

Today, my mom made an offer on a house directly behind my home and across the street from Bob's, her offer actually accepted an hour later. My mother needed to be looked after as this ordeal had been very hard on her. Having her next door would undoubtedly make it much easier for us to take care of her.

It would have been a dream come true to have had both of my parents living so close to us. Nothing in the world would have made my dad happier than to be right next door to his children and his grandchildren. Barring a miracle, he would probably never step foot in this new house. I knew I should be happy about this purchase and perhaps, one day, I would. Today was not that day. I thought about my father lying in the hospital and my heart absolutely broke. I was left with an overwhelming sadness over the future.

Sunday, July 31, 2011

As I cautiously walked into his room, he suddenly looked up at me. It was the first time I had seen him awake since his hip surgery. There was unfortunately no smile, actually no recognition of any sort. I was simply a stranger. I missed my dad so much.

"Hi Daddy," I said. "It's me, Vanessa." He still showed no signs of knowing me. I couldn't even kiss his cheek for fear of upsetting him.

At first, he was very calm. A tray of food was sitting at the foot of his bed, untouched. Over three days had passed since he had eaten anything. It had to be taking a huge toll on his body.

I found a container of apple sauce with his lunch. I opened it up and proceeded to give my dad a small bite. He didn't want anything to do with it. "Can you take a bite?" I asked. He eventually opened his mouth a little bit and allowed me to put the spoon in. I then tried another bite. In all, I successfully got three spoonfuls in before he completely lost interest.

Then, he got very upset. He started moving around anxiously, pulling the restraints as he did. He appeared to be looking for someone and it wasn't me. "Daddy, you're going to hurt yourself," I said. "Please calm down." He looked at me funny, almost as if he was wondering why this stranger was calling him "Daddy". He was getting more upset with every passing moment.

"Shirley, where are you?" he yelled.

"Daddy, Mom isn't here," I said. "I'm your daughter, Vanessa. Do you remember me?"

"Shirley!" He continued moving his head back and forth, looking around the room. He didn't know me and he didn't want anything to do with me. It felt as if I was doing more harm than good.

After about five more minutes, I finally gave up. I gathered my belongings and quickly walked out into the hall. His nurse was sitting at a desk writing something down. She looked up at me. "I need to leave," I said, my voice quivering. I tried with all my might to keep it together. "He is getting really upset. He doesn't seem to know who I am. I think I may be making it worse. Can you check on him?" She got up and quickly went into his room. As I despondently walked down the hall away from my dad, I could hear his angry voice. It was the voice of a stranger.

I ran out to my car and locked myself inside. Then, I lowered my head into my hands and I cried. All of the pain inside came out at that very moment.

I had experienced so many operations with my dad. I knew the routine only too well. After every operation, we would wait until all of the drugs were out of his system. Then, we would look for the inevitable change, never failing to come. He was never the same afterwards. Each operation took a little more of my dad away from us.

This time was much worse as I had never seen him so agitated. I had also never experienced him not recognizing me. That was by far the most painful part of today. I had been a complete stranger to him. I felt like I had lost my father.

Tuesday, August 2, 2011

As the doctor stood next to me in the room, his serious expression told me how dire the situation was. Testing had shown that his blood counts were dangerously low. As a result, Dad received a blood transfusion yesterday. I prayed that it had done some good as I was really worried about him. He didn't seem to be bouncing back from this operation.

At times when I was here, I felt like I was doing far more damage than good. I just couldn't seem to connect with my dad. When I would stay away, I felt like I was deserting him. There was simply no good solution. Inside, I felt like I was losing it. I didn't know what I was supposed to do anymore. With every passing day, I felt like I was losing more and more of my dad.

Today, Randy and I brought him a milkshake which he normally loved. I was curious whether we would be able to get him to drink it. When we saw Dad yesterday, he only managed to eat a couple of small spoonfuls. I knew that wasn't enough to sustain him. He was now going on six days without any food. They were giving him fluids intravenously, but I knew that his body couldn't take much more of this before it started having serious repercussions.

When we walked into his room, we found him sleeping peacefully. He woke up soon afterwards and looked up at me. "Poot," he said. It was the sweetest word I had ever heard. He knew me. My dad was back.

I immediately went to his side and gently kissed his cheek. "Hi Daddy," I said smiling. He smiled back at me.

Randy soon joined us on the other side. "Hi Chester," he said. He tenderly ran his hand through Dad's hair.

Dad didn't say much, but his smile and demeanor spoke volumes, a certain comfort reflected in those blue eyes. I held up the milkshake for him to see. "Look what we brought you," I said. His eyes soon brightened.

Randy and I managed to get him to take a sip which he thoroughly loved. It was written all over his face. He continued to try to suck the shake through the straw. We were only able to get a couple of ounces in him, but it was definitely a start.

After about an hour, a woman came by and politely introduced herself as Dad's case manager. She handed me some paperwork that listed several rehabilitation facilities in the area. She was trying diligently to find a location for Dad to get the therapy that he needed in order to successfully walk again. Unfortunately, a lot of them would not take Dad because either they were not set up to handle an Alzheimer's patient or they didn't want someone that suffered from Sundowner's. That, in and of itself, could pose a huge danger. All of the facilities also had the requirement that Dad be free from the physical restraints for 24 hours. So far, he had not reached that milestone.

This news was very disheartening. I was getting scared. I was also extremely sad as none of these places knew my real Dad. They were basing their decision solely on his behavior at its worst, looking at the disease and not the man. What did a person do when facing this life changing dilemma? What were we supposed to do?

Wednesday, August 3, 2011

I gathered the necessary paperwork and some snacks on our way out the door, hoping I hadn't missed anything. Shawn smiled at me as he got seated in the truck, his MP3 player already in place. As we slowly backed out of the driveway, I glanced over at Randy. I was so thankful they were both by my side. I had a bad feeling that it was going to be a long day ahead of us as we had decided to do our own facility searching. I didn't like the idea of my dad's future being held in a stranger's hands.

Based on the paperwork that the case manager had previously given us, I had called all of the facilities on the list beforehand. Unfortunately, most of them couldn't accommodate my dad's needs. From the remaining ones on the list, we had mapped out our route for the day.

The first location was in Gainesville. It was very fancy and looked more like a country club than a rehab facility. Unfortunately, the doors to the outside were not locked and residents were free to come and go as they pleased. The biggest negative, though, was that they didn't take patients with Alzheimer's.

The second place was not far from my parents' home in Buford and was very easy to get to. When we walked inside, it was very chaotic, the halls busy with patients, employees, equipment and carts. As I looked around amidst all the mayhem, the patients seemed happy which was a big advantage.

One of the directors soon gave us a tour of the facility. Everyone that we met seemed so nice. When we got back to her office, I decided to ask her about Sundowner's. It was usually at this point that the type of facility I was dealing with came out. "Do you have any patients with Sundowner's?" I asked.

"Actually, most of our patients have Sundowner's," she replied. "We're very accustomed to dealing with it." The answer gave me hope as I knew that at some point in the future, Dad's Sundowner's would invariably surface. I needed to know that the facility we chose would definitely be able to handle it when it did. I felt optimistic that they had the experience that we needed.

The third facility that we looked at was in Lilburn where we were also given a tour. It was simply okay. It wasn't great, but I also didn't notice anything bad about it. It was just okay. At this point, I didn't want to settle for okay as far as my dad was concerned.

The biggest negative with this place was its location as it was a little too far away. I needed a facility that I could get too often and quickly in case of an emergency.

The fourth location was very close, but they regrettably had no openings. It was unfortunate because I really liked this place. It seemed ideal.

By the time we had gone to all of the facilities on our list, we were all exhausted. Throughout the day, I found that you could get a very good feel for what a place was like by simply walking in unannounced. The sad truth was that most of these places were very depressing, making me want to give up and just bring Dad home with me. However, I knew that I couldn't provide him with the care or rehabilitation that he needed.

What we had found today was that there just weren't that many facilities for us to choose from. We not only needed a place that would provide rehabilitation. It also had to be a secure environment that catered to Alzheimer's patients, more specifically Alzheimer's patients with Sundowner's. When you added in the fact that Dad had to be tied down with restraints after the hip surgery, it severely limited our options. We would unfortunately have to make a decision soon with what we had.

I would have loved it if Dad could have remained at Arbor Forest. Unfortunately, they could not provide him with the extensive rehabilitation that he needed. Their inability to keep an eye on Dad as closely as he needed to be watched also concerned me. I didn't want a repeat performance of the incident where he broke his hip.

We had ultimately made the decision to move Dad's things out of Arbor Forest tonight. Mom had already boxed everything up earlier in the day. Randy, Bob and the older grandchildren carried the heavy furniture out, with the younger grandchildren carrying the lighter boxes.

I filled out the necessary forms to get the medical technician to release all of Dad's medications to me. It was very tedious as she had to inventory all of them. The moving was done long before the meds were ready.

"How is your dad doing?" the med tech asked.

"He's not doing too well," I replied. "He's had a rough time since he fell. It's going to be a long road ahead."

"I'm really sorry to hear that," she said. "You know that your Dad was in charge back here." I intently looked at the caregiver. In some ways, her words were shocking. In other ways, they were expected. "He was. He was a strong and determined man. He was clearly in charge." I didn't know if that was a good thing or bad. Dad had always been a leader. Some things were hard to change. Being in charge back here was probably the only control he had felt for months.

While she was busy getting Dad's meds ready, I carefully looked around to make sure that I hadn't forgotten anything. As I slowly walked down the hallway, I looked at the bulletin boards. Then I saw it, a picture of my dad sitting next to Dorothy. He was wearing his favorite blue striped shirt.

I was completely torn. In the picture, Dad was smiling and looked so handsome. I very much wanted the picture of Dad, but not of Dorothy. I thought about it for several minutes and finally decided to leave it. It inevitably belonged at Arbor Forest. I wanted them to remember my precious father.

As I continued to look around, I suddenly noticed something red on the book shelf in the common area. I walked over to find Dad's red, heart-shaped pillow sitting before me. I picked it up and held it close to my heart. It had been here with Dad from the very beginning and had no doubt provided countless hours of comfort for him. It would definitely be coming home with me.

While I continued to wait, I noticed several family members coming down the hall. There had to be over twenty of them as they all walked past me. I turned to see them eventually walk into the last room on the left. I knew the woman that lived in that room. She was dying. Hospice had already been called in. Her family was saying goodbye to her, wanting to spend as much time with her as possible. For her, the end was near. It was very somber in the memory care unit tonight.

Friday, August 5, 2011

We were all deeply feeling the uncertainty of Dad's plight, having only found a couple of places that could actually handle all of his needs. Bob, Randy, Mom and I had all exhaustively discussed our limited options and agreed that the best facility was Rising Meadow Rehabilitation Center. It was also the closest location to my mom which was an added bonus.

This morning, I went to see Dad in the hospital for the last time. He was going to be discharged sometime this afternoon. While he slept soundly, I gathered his clothes, dentures and other belongings. I had had too many of his personal things go missing during previous hospital stays. It would have been especially difficult to get his dentures replaced if something unfortunate happened to them. I decided to take everything to the new facility myself.

Dad's mind had still not completely recovered from the hip surgery, but the hospital felt that his body ultimately had. It was their professional opinion that he was ready for rehab. Just last night, they had to give him drugs to settle him down. While I was in his room, Bob had texted me letting me know that he and Andrew were on their way up. Unfortunately, Dad was not in a good mood. It was that time of day and he was starting to get very agitated. The last thing that Bob wanted was for Andrew to see his beloved Papa upset. I quickly met Bob outside of the elevator and I took Andrew down to the gift shop with me. Bob then went into Dad's room and helped the nurse get him settled down. Not long after that, I received another text indicating that everything was okay. Andrew and I then headed back upstairs. By the time we got to the room, Dad was sedated once again.

Dad had been totally free from the restraints for 24 hours now. He still regrettably was not eating well. Nine days had now elapsed since he had eaten anything substantial. The hospital was still medicating Dad periodically for his agitation. I had serious doubts as to whether Dad was really ready to attempt any type of rehabilitation. Unfortunately, the decision wasn't up to me.

At noon, I picked Mom up and we went to a meeting at Rising Meadow Rehab Center. A lot of necessary paperwork needed to be reviewed and signed, actually taking more than two hours to complete. The director informed us that Dad's bed in the 2-bed room was not currently available, but would open up on Monday. Until then, he would be temporarily moved into another room with 3 beds.

As we finished up with the required documents, I looked out into the hall. I then coincidentally saw my dad pass by on a stretcher, his eyes closed. They had no doubt drugged him for the ride over which seemed to be customary when transporting a dementia patient from one facility to another.

After the meeting was over, Mom and I immediately walked down the hall to see Dad. When we walked into the room, we found him sleeping soundly. As I looked around, I noticed how incredibly small the room was. It had that same cold, sterile feel of a hospital room, nothing like his comfortable room at Arbor Forest. Dad was in the middle bed with curtains separating him from the other two beds. I couldn't see the man nearest the window as his curtains were pulled out. I had actually passed the man nearest the hall as I walked into the room. He was a small, Indian man that was very quiet, but very polite.

Dad was in and out of sleep the entire time we were there. As we continued to talk to him, he tried to open his eyes, but was still so tired from the drugs. He was undoubtedly too weary to realize that he was somewhere new, eventually falling back asleep.

I placed Dad's personal belongings in his designated area. The three closets were positioned consecutively in a row, with Dad's located in the middle. I had originally thought that three beds were currently in this room because of circumstances beyond the facilities control. I thought they had to move an extra bed into the room temporarily. Now as I stood looking at the closets, this room was obviously designed to house three patients all along.

Mom and I stayed with Dad for a little while longer, but he never woke up again. We eventually decided to leave, unknowing whether he would remain sleeping the rest of the night or not. I also had no idea the level of drugs currently in his system. I had watched Dad come out of sedation so many times before. I prayed that this transition would be a calm one.

When I arrived at home later, I noticed a message on my answering machine from one of the physical therapists that worked at Arbor Forest. The woman had always been very friendly towards Dad and me. She wanted to let us know that she was thinking about my dad and praying that he was doing well. I would return her call tomorrow morning. I had also received a phone call a few days earlier from the caregiver that had originally called to let me know that Dad had fallen. She was also worried about Dad.

On this journey through Alzheimer's, I had met some of the most incredible people that I had ever met in my life. It took an extremely dedicated and loving person to be a caregiver to someone with dementia. I had learned from some of the best. I felt truly blessed to have met such angels along the way.

Saturday, August 6, 2011

Runners tediously stretched and warmed up as I rapidly made my way to the starting line, soon seeing him walk by with his friends. Regardless of how many times I had seen him race, I still got butterflies inside. Today was the annual Dennis McCormick 5k Road Race. I felt so excited and appreciative to be able to watch Shawn run. Since Bob and Mom were going to visit Dad later today, I had made the decision to spend the entire day with Randy and the boys. It would be the first time I had done this in quite awhile.

At 7:50 a.m., Mom received an alarming phone call from Rising Meadow. Dad had accidentally slipped out of his bed and fallen on the floor. He was fine, except for some slight agitation.

"When we were there yesterday, one of the nurses had tried to put the rail on the side of the bed up, but couldn't get it to stay," Mom said to the caller. "My husband has brittle bones. He needs the rail up at all times." The woman assured her that someone in maintenance would take care of it today.

We had noticed yesterday that a large piece of navy blue carpet was lying on the floor next to Dad's bed. Located underneath the mat were sensors that notified the attendants whenever the patient stepped on them. The bed was very low to the ground to prevent any injury if Dad happened to fall out of it. However, nothing would stop him from getting out of the bed on his own as this facility did not use any form of restraints. Dad did have access to a button on the wall that he could press whenever he needed assistance. Whether he would actually use it remained to be seen.

When Bob and Mom walked into Dad's room, he was lying in his bed and seemed very calm. One of the staff had already helped him get dressed. Mom had brought several changes of clothing for Dad which she neatly placed in the middle closet.

Before long, Dad's lunch was delivered, his appetite still not having returned to normal. Dad eyed the food intently as if he were interested. Bob helped him sit up and Dad actually managed to eat a small portion of his meal. It was definitely a start.

The television was conveniently located in the middle of the room against the wall. Since Dad's bed was in the middle, he had a perfect view. Unfortunately, it was on whether he wanted to watch something or not. The man near the window currently had the remote to the TV and was controlling it. The curtain was again drawn most of the way, so he could not be seen. Regrettably, he could still be heard, and very loudly at times.

The current setup was far from ideal, but since it was only temporary, we were biding our time. It was not conducive to visitors and definitely not personal conversations. Hopefully, everything would change on Monday when Dad was moved into a more private room. That was also the day that his rehab was scheduled to begin. So far, Dad's recovery was moving very slowly. I truly hoped that he would soon start making some much needed progress towards getting better.

Monday, August 8, 2011

As I drove by the street where I normally turned off for Arbor Forest, I felt an immense sadness. My new route would be several miles further up the road. Dad had now moved into another stage of the disease and another facility as a result. As I cautiously walked into his new room, he immediately looked up at me and smiled. I was very nervous on the drive over as I never knew what to expect. Now that I was here, I felt so relieved. Dad was slowly returning to his old self.

Only a couple of chairs were in the room and some family members of the patient near the window were currently sitting in them. Dad was comfortably seated in a wheelchair, so I casually sat next to him on his bed. I told him all about what was currently going on with the boys, knowing how much he loved hearing about them. He sat and listened so attentively, occasionally saying one or two words in response. For the most part, I did all of the talking.

Before long, a young girl brought his lunch into the room. She set the tray on his table and carefully wheeled it in front of him. "Hi there, Mr. Lee," she said. "I hope you're hungry."

"How did he do with his breakfast?" I asked.

"He actually ate about half of it," she replied. That news left me feeling ecstatic, knowing it was key to giving him the energy that his body ultimately needed for the rehab.

As Dad looked over his tray, he immediately chose the dessert which was Strawberry Shortcake. I didn't care what order he ate things in, just as long as he ate. The main entrée was fish. I sampled it and several other items on the tray. Everything tasted delicious. Dad ate almost his entire lunch. He finally had his appetite back and it was a wonderful sight. "You have no idea how good it is to see you eat, Daddy," I said.

When Randy and I had visited Dad yesterday, all we could get down him was about eight ounces of Glucerna and six bites of mashed potatoes. Today was definitely much better. It seemed as though every day, he was making substantial progress with his eating.

This afternoon, Dad officially started his rehabilitation therapy. The physical therapy room that he used was conveniently located right next to his room. It actually took two therapists to help Dad stand. He invariably had a long way to go before he could attempt walking. I knew this was one of those scenarios where we needed to concentrate on baby steps.

So many people had told me that this was a critical time for a dementia patient attempting physical therapy. The most important factor was not necessarily their physical strength, but it was their mind. They had to want it. Sometimes, the patient just didn't have the drive to get better. Where Dad went after this stint would clearly depend on how well he did in rehab.

Dad still got very agitated in the late afternoon and evening, for which I had had several conversations with the staff. They were currently tweaking his medications. I truly hoped they could get him to the point of remaining calm 24/7. It might be the determining factor in whether his rehab was successful or not.

November, 1972

Dad had thought about his mother's special Christmas gift for some time now. She loved listening to music on the small radio that sat atop her dresser in her bedroom. Unfortunately, that didn't allow her the ability to play her favorites whenever she desired. Dad wanted so much to buy her a stereo system for the living room so she could then play her music and have it be heard throughout the house. To be able to watch her face as she opened it on Christmas morning would be priceless.

He soon approached Mom with the idea. It was a lot of money, but Mom could tell how much it meant to Dad. He loved his mother very much and wanted more than anything to do this for her. They had always had a very close relationship as he was her firstborn. In the end, Mom gave her blessing.

Dad then told both of his younger brothers about the gift. The stereo Dad had picked out came complete with an 8-track player. Everyone decided to join in on the present and buy Grandma some of her favorite music for Christmas. She would be so surprised.

Monday, December 25, 1972

On Christmas Day, all of the children and grandchildren came to Grandma and Grandpa's house to celebrate the special day as had been our tradition for years. The house smelled incredible. Grandma had started cooking first thing this morning, the turkey already in the oven.

Everyone soon gathered around the Christmas tree to watch as Grandma started opening up her many presents, several of which were suspiciously the exact same size. As she unwrapped each 8-track tape, she graciously remarked about how much she loved the artist, the look of confusion obvious on her face. Grandma never once said anything about how she had nothing to play them on. She was too goodhearted for that. She simply thanked each person genuinely from her heart and moved on to the next present.

By the time all of the presents had been unwrapped, Grandma had a nice collection of her favorite music. Our hearts were beating as the anticipation for that special unveiling moment built up. We then watched as Dad brought out her final gift. "Mom, I think you forgot one," Dad said. Everyone remained silent with their eyes glued to Grandma.

As she opened up the last box, she surprisingly saw the new stereo system. She then began to cry. They were tears of joy. "I wondered why everybody was giving me 8-track tapes," she said laughing. Dad knelt down and gently kissed his mother on the cheek. "Oh, Chester, why did you do this?"

"Because you deserve it," Dad replied. "Merry Christmas, Mom."

My dad had picked this gift out completely out of love for his mother. It wasn't about the price and it wasn't about the status. It was about bringing a smile to the face of someone you dearly loved. Being an impressionable eleven-year old, it moved me beyond words. As I watched my father and grandmother tenderly hug each other, I truly hoped that one day I could give my dad a special gift from my heart like I had just witnessed him do.

Tuesday, August 9, 2011

I could see him in the hallway as I casually came around the corner. He was looking down and hadn't seen me as I slowly approached him. I passed several carts on my way in, having to maneuver my way around them. The atmosphere was very different than what I was accustomed to. I soon knelt beside his wheelchair and smiled lovingly at him. "Hi Daddy," I said. He seemed so happy to see me. He was dressed neatly, but his hair was in complete disarray. I reached into my purse and pulled out my yellow comb, gently fixing his hair for him as he sat completely still. I imagined it felt very soothing to him. I also knew it would do wonders for his disposition. He had always taken great pride in his appearance.

I then wheeled Dad down to the end of the hall where he could conveniently look out the glass door. It was a sunny day and I knew how much he loved being outside. He was in such a good mood. While we were there, an attendant thoughtfully brought Dad some peanut butter crackers. He hungrily ate every single one of them. The attendant also mentioned that Dad had eaten a good amount of his breakfast this morning. It thrilled me that Dad was eating better.

I soon saw the metal lunch cart in the hall coming towards us. I eagerly took Dad back to his room to get ready for lunch. I remained by his side throughout the entire meal. He managed to eat and successfully use the utensils without any assistance from me. I was so thankful that he had not lost this ability.

The television in the middle of the room was currently on and the volume was unbearably loud. I knew that Dad's hearing was getting poor, so it probably didn't bother him, but it was fast getting on my nerves. The man near the window again had the remote control. I saw absolutely no reason for it to be so loud. I determinedly walked over to the television and manually turned the volume lower. The man never said a word.

Dad didn't talk too much today. The truth was he hadn't talked much at all since the hip operation. I had yet to have a conversation with him that consisted of more than a couple of sentences. I missed talking to my dad.

About an hour after lunch, Dad started getting tired so I carefully helped him back into his bed. I casually sat on the edge and continued to talk to him. I soon looked up to see an attendant entering the room, quickly walking past us to the patient near the window who had apparently paged her. "What can I do for you, Mr. Whitmire?" she asked.

"I need to be changed," he said gruffly. He had to be one of the grumpiest individuals I had ever encountered. The nurse proceeded to clean him up.

"That hurts," he yelled. He had complained the entire time. "Watch what you're doing!"

"Mr. Whitmire, I'm trying to be as gentle as I can," she said. "I have to move you in order to do this."

"Well, be careful," he ordered.

A little while later, the attendant walked past us again. As she looked at me, I could clearly see the frustration on her face. Some patients could be exasperating and this was definitely one of them. All week, I had witnessed him treating his mother terribly. She would relentlessly come to visit him every day and he never had a kind word to say to her, always so demanding. Some days, I seriously had to bite my tongue.

All I could think of was how much I wanted my dad out of this room. This man's demeanor couldn't have been good for him. Was he partly responsible for my dad's outbursts at night?

Dad eventually fell asleep and I gently kissed him goodbye. As I walked out the door, the Indian man looked up at me. I hadn't heard one word from him the entire time I was here. He was the complete opposite of the man near the window. "Have a good day," I said to him. He then smiled at me.

On the way out, I briefly stopped by the director's office. We were promised that Dad would be moved into a more private room yesterday. As of yet, that still hadn't happened. I was very upset. "Did something happen with the new room?" I asked. "I thought my dad was going to be moved yesterday."

"We're still working on it," she replied. "The other patient has still not left. Until that happens, we can't move your dad. Hopefully, it will happen in a day or two."

Later that evening, I got an unexpected phone call from one of the nurses on duty at Rising Meadow. Dad was still getting very agitated at night with the staff. They were having to give him medication to calm him down. They unfortunately still hadn't found the right combination, but wanted me to be aware of what was happening. The medicine that he took at Arbor Forest was no longer strong enough to handle his agitation, evidence that the disease had progressed since the hip surgery.

"Can the doctor test my dad for a urinary tract infection?" I asked. "My dad is very prone to them. When he gets one, it makes him very agitated. That needs to be ruled out before he is given any more drugs." She assured me that the test would be done tomorrow.

As I slowly hung up the phone, I began to feel sick to my stomach. I had a bad feeling this was not going to end well. I absolutely hated that my dad was going through this on top of everything else. When was he going to catch a break?

Thursday, August 11, 2011

I nervously took my seat at the large conference table, with Mom sitting directly across from me. Before long, three of the directors and the head nurse also sat down. At 11:00 a.m., the meeting at Rising Meadow officially began with the primary purpose to discuss Dad's progress. I had a strong feeling that his increased agitation would also be brought up.

Dad's actual progress was insignificant. His appetite had thankfully returned and he was now eating regularly which was a very good sign. He had started his rehab on Monday. Unfortunately, he hadn't made much stride in that area. It was a very different scenario for Dad than for someone who was simply trying to walk again. With a dementia patient, it was all about the mind and its ability to direct the legs.

The financial director went over the time frame that my dad's insurance companies would cover him to receive physical therapy. There was a definite limit. I felt a little concerned that it might soon become an issue.

The nursing director then asked me several questions about Dad's agitation, some of the questions delving into very painful areas. While talking, my voice soon started to break up. I stopped for a moment and looked down to get my composure. The director got out of her chair and walked over to me. She then bent down and gently hugged me. This clearly wasn't just a job to her, her loving actions so genuine. Afterwards, I looked directly at her and said "Thank you" which was all that was needed.

Dad had a follow-up visit scheduled for this afternoon with the surgeon that had performed his hip operation. I didn't see the point in going so soon, but the financial director informed me that it was necessary in order for his insurance to continue paying for the therapy. Unfortunately, I had a scheduling conflict today. It would be the first doctor's appointment that I wasn't able to take my dad to.

The rehab facility had a van that was equipped to handle a wheelchair. The driver accommodatingly drove both of my parents to the appointment. When they got there, the driver got Dad out of the van and settled in his wheelchair. He then surprisingly informed my mom that he'd be back in a couple of hours. We were under the impression that he would remain with my dad the entire time to assist.

My mom ended up having to handle my dad totally by herself. Not long after they sat down, Dad let her know that he needed to use the bathroom, so she wheeled him into the facilities. Dad wasn't able to get out of the wheelchair and Mom definitely couldn't lift him by herself. He was dead weight. She had no choice but to ask someone at the desk for help.

A staff member soon came in to assist Mom, managing to lift Dad up and firmly placing him on the seat. He told Mom to call him when Dad was done. Unfortunately, Dad had diarrhea. Mom did her best to take care of him.

Not long after that, Dad and Mom were seated back in the waiting area. Before she knew it, Dad again had to go to the restroom. Mom ended up having to get the same person to invariably help her again. The staff looked at Mom as if they couldn't understand what the problem was. This was clearly not something that they were accustomed to dealing with on a regular basis.

By the time my dad was called back, nearly two hours had passed. It was a miracle that Dad had not gotten agitated over this. Having to wait this long could have easily upset anyone. Fortunately, he was very tired. I wondered if he had preventively taken some type of drug for the ride over which would have explained his demeanor.

When the doctor eventually came into the room, he noticed the wheelchair that Dad was sitting in and immediately looked at my mom. "Why isn't he walking yet?" the doctor asked. "He should be walking by now."

"He just started physical therapy three days ago," Mom replied. "He can't begin to walk yet."

The doctor never addressed my dad directly. Dad just sat there, seemingly oblivious to what was going on.

This doctor may have excelled at his specialty, but he didn't seem to have a clue when it came to Alzheimer's. I had specifically brought up my dad's condition to him prior to the surgery. The response I got back was one of indifference which was usually the case. Most doctors that I had dealt with greatly underestimated the impact of Alzheimer's. Only two weeks had passed since my dad's surgery. It was beyond me how this doctor could have expected Dad to be walking so soon.

The common lay person like me took for granted that people in the medical profession had some basic knowledge of dementia. I was finding that there was a lot of ignorance. How could they treat a patient when they had no knowledge of what was happening in their brain? How could they possibly know that they were making the right decisions for someone if they weren't familiar with the disease? Some of these doctors could be so frustrating. I was infuriated with this one.

Whether my dad ever walked again wasn't dependent on the success of the surgery. It wasn't even based on how strong his legs were. The determining factor would be whether his brain still had the capacity to deliver the correct messages to his legs. A lot would depend on the extent of damage that had occurred as a result of the anesthesia. We still didn't know whether walking was going to be possible for my dad or not. Only time would tell.

Friday, August 12, 2011

The trying incident at the doctor's office yesterday was not handled well at all. I wished so much that I had been there to help, the thought actually running through my mind all night long. I imagined how difficult it must have been for my mom who was a very tenacious woman. I never knew just how strong she was until this past year. Still, I didn't think the reality of what was happening to Dad had totally registered with her yet.

I read something the other day that Mom had sent me in an email called "The Long Goodbye". Alzheimer's was such a cruel disease, turning your life upside down for so many years. It would slowly steal everything until eventually, nothing was left. In the end, it would inevitably win. For this reason, it was sometimes called "The Long Goodbye."

I had never really imagined what my mom was going through. To have your husband of more than fifty years forget a little more of you and your marriage every day must have been heart wrenching. The worst part hadn't even occurred yet. One day, there would be absolutely no memory left at all. There would be no sharing of their past together as Alzheimer's would make sure of that. I didn't think Mom had prepared herself for that time. I guess none of us really had. It was just too painful.

When I arrived at Rising Meadow today, Dad was not in his room. He wasn't in the hallway either. I curiously walked next door and peered into the rehabilitation room. I then found Dad sitting in his wheelchair, not looking well at all. In fact, he looked like he was about to fall asleep.

I quickly walked up to him and knelt by his side. "Daddy, are you okay?" I asked. He just looked at me, his eyelids so droopy. He was completely lethargic.

One of the therapists soon walked over to me. "We haven't been able to get him to do anything today," she said.

"Daddy, do you think you're up to rehab right now?" I asked. He didn't respond to me in any way, not even to shake his head. He just sat there.

I looked back at the therapist with deep concern. "This doesn't even look like my dad," I replied. "He's been given some kind of drug that's made him this way. There's no way he can do any type of therapy in his current condition. This is a waste of time." It was beyond me why they had even attempted the therapy. How long were they going to keep him sitting here? They should have consulted one of the nurses or the doctor instead. I was very upset at this point.

"He could hurt himself like this," I stated. "Can you help me get him back to his room?"

We then wheeled Dad back to his room and gently put him in his bed after which he quickly fell asleep. I devotedly sat by his side for three hours and still couldn't get him to wake up. I spoke to the doctor and she agreed to take him off of the a.m. dose of one of his medications. They were also going to put him on an IV for some much needed fluids.

I didn't know whether today was completely a result of too many meds or if it was partly due to the disease progressing. Either way, I was very upset about Dad's current state. I was even more upset that it took me to bring it to the attention of someone in charge. I was hastily losing faith in this facility.

Sunday, August 14, 2011

I was absolutely shocked as I walked through the doorway. He was restlessly lying in bed naked from the waist down with no covers on him, his pull up sitting on the bed next to him. Randy and I alarmingly looked at each other, assuming he had taken it off himself and no one had seen him yet. Regardless, it was still very disturbing. As he continued to lie there, his hands were extremely fidgety. Even after we put his underwear back on him, he continued to pull on them.

The behavior had really frightened me. I remembered a woman that lived in the memory care unit doing the exact same thing not long before she passed away. As I mindfully looked at Dad lying in his bed, he reminded me of a child with such a look of innocence about him. My strong, virile father had changed so much.

We got Dad to sit up and then helped him get dressed. He remained very calm through it all. Afterwards, he again lied down in his bed. "Daddy, how do you feel?" I asked.

"I feel really good," he replied, his response clearly indicating to me that he had taken something. He definitely appeared to be drugged. I knew the doctor was working on getting Dad's medications fine tuned for him. I had hoped that he would be closer to his old self when we saw him today. He was definitely better than the other day, but he was still not there yet.

Dad's lunch soon arrived. We tried to get him to sit up, but he was just too tired. I then adjusted his bed so that he was sitting more upright. Randy managed to give Dad several spoonfuls. Eventually though, he had enough. Dad may have been hungry, but in his current state, it was hard for him to eat. Something had to change soon.

While Randy tried to get Dad to drink some iced tea, I went in search of the doctor on duty. I found someone sitting at the nurses' station down the hall. "Is there a doctor currently on the premises?" I asked.

"He hasn't come in yet," she responded. "Can I help with something?"

"I need to leave a message for him," I said. "I know they've been trying to come up with the right combination of meds for my dad, Mr. Lee. Whatever he's being given is still too strong. I can't even get him to eat. He can hardly keep his eyes open."

"I'll definitely let him know your concerns," she replied.

The line between agitation and over drugging was sometimes a tough one to manage. You didn't want the patient combative because then they could be a danger to themselves or others. The agitation also seemed to make the dementia progress more rapidly. On the other hand, you didn't want the patient so drugged up that they looked comatose and couldn't even function. It was imperative that they find the right balance for my dad.

I then sought out one of the directors. She had promised us that Dad would be moved to a more private room six days ago. Every time I asked about it, she invariably told me the same thing, the move would happen in one to two days. I again heard the same thing today. I hopelessly felt like they were giving me the run around. Dad was still in the middle bed of the small, cramped room with virtually no privacy. I had little hope that it was going to change.

Tuesday, August 16, 2011

As I routinely drove to Rising Meadow, I thought about the daily condition that I had found my dad in ever since his rehab began, every day being different. I honestly had no idea what to expect. It was not at all a good feeling. When I warily walked into his room today, he was lying in his bed appearing very tired.

I had actually found him much the same way yesterday, except he was lying directly on the floor. As soon as I had seen Dad, I hurried to his side and knelt down. "Daddy, are you okay?" I had asked. He had apparently fallen out of his bed. The attendant was standing over him, waiting for someone to come in and help him get Dad up. I looked up at the attendant, feeling very disturbed. "So, you just left him on the floor?" He had no response, at least not anything that carried any weight. I turned towards Dad and gently helped him sit up. Then the attendant helped me get Dad back into his bed.

The more I thought about the incident, the more upset I became. I would have attempted to get Dad back into his bed on my own before I would have left him on the floor. This guy was a lot bigger than me. He couldn't help Dad up on his own? At least he could have knelt down beside Dad and talked to him comfortingly while he was on the floor. The incident had left me furious.

I sat on the edge of Dad's bed and tenderly took his hand in mine. He lovingly smiled at me. "Are you doing okay today?" I asked. He shook his head yes. "Do you want something to drink?" He again nodded yes. I got a cup and poured some ice water from the pitcher on Dad's table. I then put a straw in the cup. Dad managed to successfully take several sips.

Soon after, a woman came up to me and amiably introduced herself as the psychiatrist at the facility. She asked me several questions about Dad's history. I gave her the complete rundown, talking for about twenty minutes. I reiterated all of my current concerns with Dad and his medications to her.

The attendant from yesterday soon walked past us towards the patient near the window. "Mr. Whitmire, how are you doing?" he asked.

"I'm not doing well at all," he replied. "I need to be changed."

The attendant proceeded to take care of him, but it was not going well. Within five minutes, Mr. Whitmire had begun yelling loudly. Another attendant soon ran into the room to help as things had escalated fast, the man near the window now in a full blown rage.

I cautiously looked at Dad and his eyes were closed. This was one of the few times that I was thankful that his hearing was failing him. I hoped that the yelling wasn't nearly as loud to Dad as it was to me. It was getting very uncomfortable.

One of the attendants then assertively ushered the doctor and I out of the room. I didn't want to leave Dad in there by himself, but I unfortunately had no choice. I truly hoped that he would remain asleep.

While continuing our conversation in the hallway, the screaming from inside the room persisted. Even with the door shut, his voice remained excessively loud. I hated the thought of this happening in my dad's room every day.

About fifteen minutes later, the door suddenly opened and the attendant said that I could return inside. Dad was still sound asleep. It was beyond me how he had managed to remain that way. I think it was the combination of hearing problems and medication that had helped this to happen.

On the drive home, I thought about my dad's current state. Nineteen days had now elapsed since his hip surgery. It had been eight days since he had started his rehab. I didn't think he was any closer to walking now then he was on day one. He wasn't doing well at all. The only progress that he had made was that he was eating, at least when he wasn't too drugged. Other than that, he had made virtually no other advances.

Yesterday, Mom officially closed on her new home behind us. It should have been a very happy day for all of us. Would there ever be a time that my mom and dad would enjoy it together? I prayed that one day Dad could live there, too. I knew at this point it was probably just wishful thinking. It was hard to be so hopeful when everything about my dad's future seemed so dismal.

Wednesday, August 17, 2011

I watched him step out of the truck as the breeze blew his hair ever so gently, the gray beginning to frame his face endearing him to me even more. It seemed like just yesterday he had chased me in the shallow water of Pensacola beach and kissed me for the first time. As I prepared our sandwiches, I knew that I would never tire of having lunch with my husband. It was the only part of the day that we could openly talk, just the two of us. For years, we tried to make it happen at least a couple of times a week.

About midway through our lunch, I received an alarming phone call from the case manager at Rising Meadow. They had made the crucial decision to send my dad to a psychiatric hospital to be re-evaluated. He was not doing well at the rehab facility. He was highly agitated and they couldn't seem to get his meds right. They either overmedicated him which left him too doped up or they under medicated him which left him agitated. They had ultimately decided that he needed his medications adjusted before he could continue with his rehab. Since they were not the best facility to be doing this, they were transferring him elsewhere.

At this point, I agreed with the decision. I had felt skeptical about his ability to do the rehab from the very beginning. I just wished that he had been evaluated immediately after the hip surgery. I wished that someone at the hospital would have realized that his current meds were no longer working and stepped forward to make the suggestion then. This entire stint at the rehab facility was a complete waste of time and money, not to mention the anguish that Dad endured. The worst part by far was that all of the agitation may have even done additional damage to Dad.

The case manager then gave me the name of the hospital that they typically used. It unfortunately was not one that I was familiar with. When I looked it up, it was actually a good distance away. My dad's psychiatrist practiced at Woodland Hospital. He had already been there once and was used to their routine. What sense would it make to send him somewhere new?

I then called the case manager back and convinced her that it was in Dad's best interest to send him back to Woodland Hospital. She agreed to change his orders if a bed was available.

Later that afternoon, Dad was sent to the emergency room at Parkland General Hospital to be physically cleared. After that, he would once again be transferred to Woodland Hospital.

I began calling Parkland General an hour later. They would not tell me if Dad had transferred yet due to privacy issues. Since I was not the one to bring Dad into the hospital, I was not privy to any information about him. At that point, I called the case manager back at Rising Meadow. I needed her to find out what Dad's current status was. She wasn't able to come to the phone, but would return my call later.

I then called Parkland General back. This time, they did give me an update on Dad. He was currently doing fine. He was also tested for a UTI which came back negative. However, they still would not tell me when he was scheduled to be transferred.

Not long afterwards, I called Parkland General again. This time, the girl told me that Dad was indeed gone, but she wouldn't tell me where. Fortunately, I already knew that answer. I felt like I was putting a complex puzzle together. It should not have been this difficult to get a status on my dad.

The next step was to move on to Woodland Hospital. I knew from experience that they would absolutely not release any information on a patient without the patient number. The gentleman that I spoke with also confirmed that. "How am I supposed to get my dad's patient number?" I asked. He then transferred me to the nurses' station in the geriatric wing.

When she looked up Dad's information, my name was surprisingly not listed as a contact. I had no idea how that could be as I was the primary person that had overseen all of Dad's affairs for months.

Apparently, the contact name came from the emergency room. She then told me that their contact was my brother, Bob. They had actually made several calls to him already. Unfortunately, they had called his home phone and he was currently at work. I felt so unbelievably frustrated.

I finally decided to call Dr. Franklin's office, his assistant answering the phone. I quickly explained the situation to him. Unfortunately, I had hit another brick wall. He wouldn't give me Dad's patient number either.

At this point, I paged Dr. Franklin. I had tried everything else and I was at my wits end. Within a couple of minutes, Dr. Franklin called me back. l told him about the dilemma I faced and how I couldn't get any information on my dad. He promised to look into it and call me back when he knew something.

Within ten minutes, the doctor returned my call, giving me Dad's new patient number. He also let Dad's nurse know that I needed a current update on Dad. She would be expecting my call. Dr. Franklin had once again come through for us. He was truly one of a kind.

Friday, August 19, 2011

I knew the routine only too well as I had already become acclimated to it once. I dialed the phone number and soon after the woman asked for his patient number. After the necessary preliminaries, she then transferred me to the geriatric unit. The nurse informed me that Dad was very peaceful, leaving me immediately relieved. I felt comfortable with Dad being at Woodland Hospital. I wasn't sure what it was about this facility, but other than a couple of times on his initial visit, Dad seemed to remain calm there. I knew it wasn't because of excessive drugs as Dr. Franklin always seemed to err on the side of caution, overmedicating just not his style. I felt confident that if anyone could regulate my dad's medicine correctly, it would be Dr. Franklin.

Mom and I later drove to Rising Meadow to pick up Dad's personal belongings. The financial director had called Mom earlier, actually wanting her to pay a deposit of $160 a day to hold Dad's bed. We had briefly discussed it and decided against it as I really didn't want Dad going back there. It had not turned out to be the place we were led to believe it was. I had not been impressed at all.

We had no idea what the outcome of Dad's re-evaluation would be or how long it would take. Holding the bed could get very expensive. In addition, the bed we were holding was never the one we were originally promised. It would have been crazy to have given this facility any more money. We would just take our chances.

As we walked into Dad's room, the Indian man was currently lying in his bed. I assumed that the man near the window was also in his bed. His curtains were pulled and separating the beds as usual.

I gathered some of Dad's miscellaneous belongings on the table. Then, I made my way to his closet. All of his clothes were still there, along with his toiletries. I quickly gathered his things and placed them in a bag.

It would have been the easiest thing in the world for me to simply turn around and finally get a glimpse of the man near the window, Mr. Whitmire. The closets were directly in front of his bed. I had spent so much time in this room and as of yet, I still hadn't seen the man. I knew his voice. I knew it only too well, but I had never seen the face that went with it.

I decided at that very moment that my vision of him would be best left to my imagination. No good would ever come of me being able to remember his face. I slowly turned and walked out of the room for quite possibly the last time.

Tonight I got an unexpected phone call from Bob. Earlier today, he found out that Monica had scheduled an interview on Monday for a high ranking position at a car dealership in Arkansas. It was her dream job and if she got it, they would be moving.

Nothing could have prepared me for this news. I was completely in shock. A million thoughts began running through my head, none of them good. This couldn't have come at a worse time. How would we manage everything without my brother? What would this do to my mom and dad? I was absolutely heartbroken, unable to even wrap my head around it. It was just too much to deal with at the moment.

I tried hard not to dwell on it. Whatever was going to happen would happen. It was out of my control. At this point, there was still a slight possibility that they wouldn't be moving. It might have been a small chance, but it was one that I held onto nonetheless. I had already lost one brother. I couldn't bear the thought of Bob leaving.

Saturday, August 20, 2011

We talked about Mom and Dad as I drove us to Woodland Hospital, intentionally trying to keep the conversation light. The proverbial elephant was in the room and I needed to avoid it, the latest news still a little sensitive for me. Bob and I ended up making it to the facility in time for the 12:30 visitation. Only two opportunities to visit with Dad each week existed and we made sure that between us, we never missed one. Dad was so happy to see both of his children. He knew exactly who we were and even called us by name. It was such a special time for all of us.

Dad didn't do an abundance of talking, but did manage to answer most of our direct questions. When he did, he seemed somewhat coherent. It was definitely a good sign. At one point, I asked him if he remembered my nickname. "Pooterooni," he replied.

"Hey, not so loud," I said. He then smiled. This was the absolute best that I had seen him since the hip operation. He was calm, yet not falling asleep. He stared at me several times and even reached his hand out to caress my hair. At one point, he looked at me so intently. "You are so beautiful." I would remember that precious moment forever. He had treated Bob, or Bobby as Dad sometimes called him, the exact same way. Dad was so affectionate towards us both today, creating a special memory we would treasure always.

The next visitation would be Tuesday night which would be interesting. That was during normal Sundowner's time. If Dad remained calm throughout that visit as well, then I would feel confident that his meds were finally right.

I hoped that Dad could eventually return to doing rehab and one day possibly walk again. That was my ultimate goal and my dream. I didn't know if Dad was up to it or whether he even wanted that any more. If he did, I wanted to give him that opportunity.

After that, we would have to decide what type of facility would best fit Dad's needs. It was quite possible that it would be a skilled nursing facility. His disease had progressed significantly since his stay at Arbor Forest. That type of caregiving would no longer suffice.

I had learned that I couldn't plan too far into the future with Dad, never knowing what to expect from day to day on this tragic road. With every moment that passed, I felt like I was changing. This journey had changed me. I no longer looked at life in the same way, having seen a devastating side of it that I would never forget. My prayers for my dad were changing as well. I used to pray for miracles, wanting the disease gone completely. Now, I settled for so much less. I just wanted my dad to be peaceful.

I watched an interview the other night with a famous country music singer which was so incredibly sad. Throughout the program, he kept looking to his wife for the answers. She had become his memory. His demeanor was still very happy as he was currently on his last tour. So far, he had not forgotten any of his music. He even commented that he hadn't felt the effects of Alzheimer's as of yet.

To an outsider watching him, many of the symptoms were very obvious. I could see so much of my dad's earlier behavior in him. My heart broke as I watched his daughter. The road ahead was going to be a hard one for her. I had never met this woman, nor did I know much about her, but it didn't matter. I already knew what her future looked like. I was living it.

Monday, August 22, 2011

I remained sitting in the chair feeling heartbroken long after I hung up the phone. I couldn't move. I had just found out that Bob and his family would definitely be moving. He sounded so distraught as he told me the news. I couldn't imagine what my brother was going through, knowing that he must be so torn between his family and his dying father. It was a position that no one should ever be put in.

I was going to miss him so much. I may not have seen him every day, but I knew he was always there. Now with him living so far away, I seriously doubted that we would get to see each other that often. For the most part, my dad would be losing contact with his only living son and two of his grandchildren. He might not have a lot of time left as his health during the past ten months had deteriorated so rapidly. He was already going through so much. This move would break his heart.

I would also be losing a major part of my support system. The thought of what lied ahead for me was daunting, the bulk of my dad's care already falling on my shoulders. It would mean that much more that I inevitably had to pick up. I was already stretched too thin as it was. I didn't really have any more of myself to give. Something else would suffer as a result.

In addition, my mother had just purchased a second home with so much work still needing to be done to it. Her other home needed work as well. The biggest obstacle by far was that we would somehow have to condense the three floors from her old home into two floors in her new home. I honestly didn't know how Randy and I would manage it all by ourselves. The pressure was overwhelming.

My family was going through hell right now. Out of all the times for something like this to happen, this was absolutely the worst possible time. I honestly couldn't imagine things getting any worse. Sometimes the hardest decisions in life involved doing what was right for others. My parents had always been there for me and now I would be there for them. At the end of the day, I could sleep knowing that I did everything I could to take care of them. It was the right thing to do. Today was indeed a dismal day.

Tuesday, August 23, 2011

He smiled at us lovingly as they slowly wheeled him in. I never tired of the sight. It not only meant he was happy, more importantly, he knew who we were. I knelt down and gently kissed his cheek. Dad seemed calm, but fairly alert. They had just eaten dinner in the geriatric wing. For most of the visit, Dad just stared, doing very little talking tonight. The disease had made carrying on basic conversations nearly impossible.

At one point, I stood behind him and tenderly gave him a neck rub. He seemed to be in Heaven, although it soon got him very tired. The past month had really taken a toll on Dad. As I intently watched him, he looked like he had aged so much. I could see such a difference in him just since the hip accident.

Towards the end of the hour, Dad began looking at me, trying to tell me something the only way he knew how, with his eyes. I had seen the look before and knew from experience what he was trying to tell me. "Daddy, do you have to go to the bathroom?" I asked. He nodded his head yes, rapidly losing the ability to communicate with words.

Dad's doctor was satisfied with his current medications. Based on his demeanor, they definitely seemed to be better regulated. I hadn't witnessed or even heard of him getting agitated since he was initially transferred. If everything continued as it had, the doctor was planning on discharging Dad this Friday where he would continue with his rehabilitation. Whether he would ever be able to walk again was still an unknown.

My mom tried to always be there for Dad, but she sometimes had a hard time connecting with him. Tonight, she had asked him a couple of questions to attempt a conversation. One was the year of one of his first cars; the other question was the name of one of his barbers in Pensacola. They were both questions that he normally would have had no problems answering. Today, he wasn't able to reply to either of them.

The disease had now started taking away some of my dad's long term memory. I already knew what the future stages would steal from him, his past memories by far one of the worst things that he would lose. That was one of the major differences between dementia and other fatal diseases.

As our lives often changed, the thing we always held onto was the fact that we still had our memories, firmly believing that nothing could ever take them away. With Alzheimer's, that simply wasn't true.

The disease already caused so many different problems that in turn created other serious ramifications. Getting lost, forgetting how to do things that you had routinely done for years, incontinence and unlimited confusion were but some of the many issues that someone with Alzheimer's faced on a daily basis. Unfortunately, that wasn't enough for this horrific disease. It wanted to take my dad's precious memories away as well. At least with other illnesses, the mind was left intact, but not with Alzheimer's. It would continue to wipe away every single memory that my dad held dear until he just existed with absolutely no knowledge of family or any type of past.

We took it for granted that no matter what happened to us, we would always have our memories. They kept us going when so many other things were failing us. Without them, it would be like we had never lived. What was happening to my daddy wasn't right. It wasn't fair. Memories should last a lifetime.

Friday, August 26, 2011

As I casually walked through the store, I grabbed the various items and set them inside the cart. I had no list, but was simply biding my time while the pharmacist filled Mom's prescription. I had a few more errands to run and wanted to have everything out of the way early as today was the day. Anticipation was rising as I eagerly waited for news about the move. Several days had passed since I had received any information from Dad's case manager. He was supposed to be discharged today. I had assumed that everything was in place, but as of this morning, I still hadn't heard anything.

As soon as I arrived home, I quickly called Woodland Hospital only to be told that Dr. Franklin had decided to monitor Dad a little while longer. He was delaying his discharge. Then, I received the bombshell. The rehab facility that my dad was previously at wouldn't accept him back. When the case manager had contacted them with Dad's original discharge date, they informed him that they no longer had a bed available. I was furious and didn't believe it for a minute. They didn't seem like the type of facility to ever turn down a paying customer. I think that the real reason was a combination of us not paying them the extra money that they wanted to hold the bed and not wanting to deal with Dad's agitation anymore.

The main reason we chose that facility was because we believed they knew how to handle patients with Sundowner's. During the initial tour, they had known exactly what to say to convince us of this. Since then, I had seen firsthand what their strategy was in dealing with a patient's anxiety. They simply upped the medication until the agitation was under control. Oftentimes that left the person incapable of functioning at all, as was clearly the case with my dad.

I was so upset at this latest development. I honestly wasn't thrilled about my dad returning there, but at least I wanted him to have that option. Now, I felt like they were washing their hands of him. How could they wait until the last minute to tell us? This wasn't just a bed number. It was a person's life.

The case manager then let me know that he had sent my dad's information to several different facilities trying to find a place for him. As of yet, he hadn't found one. From the sound of things, he didn't seem to even have any leads. I felt very nervous, already discovering when we searched for the last rehab facility that we didn't have a lot of options. I hoped that the case manager had more connections and would soon find an acceptable place for my father.

Sometimes, I felt as though this world was not at all prepared for Alzheimer's. Out of the top ten fatal diseases that currently existed, Alzheimer's was the sixth leading cause of death in the United States. It was the only one that had no possible cure or prevention. Some drugs currently on the market were believed to slow its progression, but as of yet, I hadn't seen any evidence of that with my father. On the contrary, it seemed to be progressing at a rapid pace.

It was estimated that one out of every three seniors would die from Alzheimer's or another dementia. It was mind-boggling. How could there not be more awareness for this disease that would ultimately touch everyone in some way? How could there not be more facilities to help care for those that were given this death sentence? It was a scary thought when you didn't know where else to turn.

Thursday, September 1, 2011

As I carefully looked through the brochure, it was hard to imagine him living at any of them. The colorful ads and enticing words painted a picture that was difficult to accept so easily. I had learned the hard way that things were not always what they seemed as a depressing tone fell upon me this morning. In the midst of this, I received a phone call from Dad's case manager at Woodland Hospital, wanting to let me know that he might have found a rehabilitation place for Dad. The only caveat was that it was thirty miles away. On top of that, the area was a highly congested one, easily taking an hour to drive just one way. That was unacceptable. "That is too far away," I said. "It would affect how often we are able to visit my dad. I was really hoping to find something closer."

The case manager had never consulted me as far as what type of facility we were looking for or even how far away we were willing to drive. I honestly didn't know how much legwork he was actually doing to find a place. My dad had been back at Woodland Hospital for fifteen days now and all the case manager had so far was one facility thirty miles away. I was not happy with his meager progress at all.

I decided that it was time I took matters into my own hands. I was already researching skilled nursing facilities for when Dad's physical therapy was over. Now, I would put that aside and concentrate my efforts on rehab facilities once again.

I started thoroughly searching the Internet and several brochures that I had, eventually coming up with a new list. I then began making phone calls and surprise visits.

The first facility that I found that seemed promising was actually within a mile of Woodland Hospital. I had decided to drive there myself this afternoon. As I soon pulled up to the building, it was eerily deserted, a lone truck parked out front. I cautiously got out of the car and peered in the front door, the entire place completely dark. It was obvious that no one was currently living here. I would later find out that the roof in the dining area had collapsed awhile back. Fortunately, no one had been hurt. All of the residents were promptly sent to other facilities which explained why so many of them were currently full.

On the way home, I stopped by a facility that was just a few miles from my house. It was definitely my number one choice as far as location. It had a rehab section and a memory care unit with a nurse on the premises 24/7. It would have been perfect had they had any openings in the memory care unit.

The director that spoke to me had asked me several questions about Dad's need for rehab. She had also asked me where he was coming from. Maybe it was my imagination, but it seemed as though her entire demeanor changed once I said that Dad was currently at Woodland Hospital. I already knew that the case manager had contacted her and that she had previously turned him down. I imagined at this point that she was putting two and two together. She told me that they'd call me if an opening developed. Inside, I knew they wouldn't.

Most facilities were scared to have someone with Sundowner's, but Dad was facing even more of an uphill battle. He wasn't simply a patient that had hip surgery and was now in need of rehab. He was a patient that had already attempted rehab at another facility and then been transferred to a psychiatric hospital to be re-evaluated. The first rehab had not been successful and it didn't bode well for my dad. I truly hoped that one of these facilities would show their human side and give my dad a chance.

Through all of my visits, my observations seemed to run the gamut, finding some very poor facilities and some really good ones. However, a lot of them were full right now or at least that is what they were telling me. I hoped that by visiting these locations in person and making a lasting impression, they'd now put my face with my dad's chart and it would make them much more likely to accept him.

I was so sad when I thought of the current situation. They were judging my dad based on a disease and not the real man. If they could have seen him before the dementia, they would have fallen in love with him. Dad was a true gentleman. He had always been such a kind person with a loving heart. Some people didn't trust others until they proved they could be trusted. Dad was just the opposite as he trusted everyone until they proved otherwise. I started to get seriously worried that we wouldn't be able to find a suitable place for him. He deserved so much better than this.

Later this evening, Shawn had a cross country meet at Mill Creek. He did really well in his race. As he crossed the finish line, he victoriously raised his arms straight up. I had seen him do this during several other races and it always made me smile. It was now his signature trademark. I imagined Dad standing next to me watching the race. It was the kind of move that would have made him smile, too. He would be so proud of Shawn right now.

Friday, September 2, 2011

As I leisurely drove down the winding road, I was taken aback at its picturesque setting, nestled in the middle of so many beautiful trees. From the outside, it was beautiful. The rehabilitation facility was almost twenty miles away which was a little further than I would have liked. However, the drive over was an easy one. I sadly realized that my options were dwindling.

I was very pleased as I walked inside, so much nicer than the previous rehab location. I soon met one of the directors and asked for a tour. She was very amiable and immediately took me around.

The first thing that I noticed was that the halls weren't completely blocked. Even with residents walking or sitting in their wheelchairs, there was still ample room to get by, everything seeming so organized.

As we slowly walked down the hall, the director showed me the different room layouts, having both private and semi-private, which housed two patients. Based on some of the rooms, they clearly had some openings, at least in this wing. She also showed me two different rehabilitation rooms that had several therapists currently in each. I was very impressed. It would definitely be worth the extra drive to get Dad into this place.

Before long, the director curiously began to ask me about my dad. I already knew that she had previously turned the case manager down. I had hoped that by meeting me and hearing my side, she would change her mind. I carefully explained the dilemma we were currently facing. When I told her the name of the previous rehab facility that Dad was at, she smiled and uttered something about them being in it for the money. Apparently, that facility even had a poor reputation amongst caregivers.

By the time we walked back to the director's office, she had graciously decided to accept Dad into their rehab unit after all, his story touching her compassionate side. The visit had been successful. I felt both thrilled and relieved.

Unfortunately, once the rehab was over, we would have to find another place for Dad to be moved as they did not have any openings in the long term care section. I would worry about that issue later as a lot could happen between now and then. It was quite possible that they'd have another opening by that time. The truth was I hoped to move Dad closer to us anyway. I already knew this stint might just be temporary. The primary objective right now was to get Dad the physical therapy that he needed in order to walk again. If it didn't happen now, it never would.

When I got home, I tried to call Dad's case manager to let him know that I had managed to get a place that had previously turned him down to actually change their mind. Unfortunately, I couldn't get in touch with him, seemingly the norm these days. It was so frustrating.

Later this evening, Preston came home from college. I very much needed his visit. He was doing so well. He had started working on campus last week part time for UGA Housing in the maintenance department. It was usually easy work and he really liked his boss. The money would also help a lot with his college fees, which were so expensive. With his new job, I would probably not see him as much as last year.

Preston was happily living in Oglethorpe House this year, loving his room and enjoying all of his classes. The best part about this school year was that he had a great roommate. They had been friends since the beginning of last year, actually having lived next door to each other in Lipscomb Hall. It was going to make all the difference in the world. After everything that he had gone through as a freshman, he deserved some happiness this year.

Monday, September 5, 2011

As I hung up the phone once again, the feeling of exasperation grew stronger, a part of me inclined to drive to the facility and find him in person. It shouldn't be this difficult to reach someone. I had called relentlessly, but couldn't seem to get through. I left numerous messages and got no return calls. I had even done a lot of the legwork in finding rehab facilities for him to contact. Still, he couldn't seem to do his part. My dad had been cleared for discharge for several days now and still, he wasn't set up to transfer anywhere. I was furious with his case manager.

Yesterday, I had reached my limit. Dr. Franklin had given me the name of the director of patient advocacy back when I initially had problems getting information on my dad. I had frustratingly called her and left a lengthy message, not knowing where else to turn. She definitely needed to know what was going on. The case manager was not doing his job. He was clearly not taking care of my dad.

Early this morning, I received a call back from the director of patient's rights. She was very understanding of the situation and promised to look into it. My dad wasn't able to speak for himself, so I needed to advocate for him.

The last operation had definitely caused the dementia to progress. Dad sometimes said things that didn't make any sense, almost like he was going back in time. When Mom and I had visited Dad on Saturday, he was excitedly talking about going to a parade earlier that morning, even describing it in detail. The mind was a powerful tool. I wondered if my dad was having flashbacks. At one point, he started talking about different types of weaponry. Was he possibly thinking about his time in the military? I was very concerned at what was currently happening to my dad.

I had read an article awhile back about how the brain functions for a person with Alzheimer's. The statements First In, Last Out and Last In, First Out accurately described how their memory was processed. It was very different from how a healthy brain functioned. Current events, even ones occurring the same day, were oftentimes not remembered. Whereas memories from years before, even childhood, were still present.

When a person with a healthy brain created a memory, it was first registered in the hippocampus and then stored separately in another part of the brain for later retrieval. Unfortunately, the hippocampus was one of the first parts of the brain to be damaged by Alzheimer's. As it became impaired, it lost the ability to store new memories. If it couldn't store the memory, then it definitely couldn't retrieve it later. Memories stored before the hippocampus was damaged, however, were still intact, at least for awhile. They were still able to be retrieved. This explained why my dad could remember his military days and not what he had for breakfast.

My parents' first grandson, Chad, and his wife Alanna were in town. We had mentioned to Chad that a special visitation with Dad had been planned for tonight. Due to the holiday, Woodland Hospital had generously scheduled an extra day. I didn't know whether he felt comfortable seeing his grandfather in his current state or not. Either way, I would have understood completely.

Today I found out that Chad had ultimately made the decision to visit Dad. I was so happy to hear this, saying so much about his character. I imagined Curtis looking down on the situation and feeling so proud of his son. I knew it would mean a lot to Dad as well. It might very well be the last chance he'd ever have to see his Grandpa Lee.

Later that day, we all conveniently met at Woodland Hospital. Unfortunately, only two visitors were allowed in at a time. My mom and Chad would visit during the first thirty minutes. Randy and I would take the second shift.

During the first half of the visit, Dad had surprised Chad by asking him when he was going to have a baby. The question was completely out of the blue, making both Chad and my mom laugh. Dad was nothing if he wasn't completely honest. He always had been. Sometimes his mind was so unbelievably crisp. Unfortunately, those times were becoming few and far between.

The second part of the visit was a very emotional one. I found it so hard not to cry. Randy and I had both hugged Dad as soon as we walked into the room. I had never seen him so happy to see us. He had a huge smile on his face and seemed so content. "I miss you all so much," he said.

My eyes soon filled with tears. I hadn't prepared myself for those genuine words. Sometimes I felt that God gave my dad temporary moments of clarity to allow him to give us words that we could hold on to and treasure long after Dad was gone. "We miss you, Daddy, more than you can know," I replied. I gently took his hand in mine and slowly caressed it.

All I could think as I stared at my precious father was that this man once had everything. Over the past year, I had watched it slowly being taken from him, little by little. Through it all, he still managed to be so incredibly loving. I learned that it took a very special person to rise above the disparity. I was in the presence of one of those amazing people. My dad could still smile even in the midst of his life crumbling down around him, even in the face of such adversity. As the tears slowly ran down my cheeks, I wondered why God created such a terrible disease. I didn't know if I would ever understand.

Wednesday, September 7, 2011

I was awestruck as I thought about their many years together, through good times and bad. It said so much about their love for one another. I knew that these past years had been extremely difficult. Alzheimer's had made sure of that. Today was a very special day for them, their 55th wedding anniversary. It would also sadly be the first time that they had ever spent it apart from each other.

Last night, Mom had gone to see Dad during his normal visitation, carrying with her a special anniversary card. He was so happy when he opened it. In all of their years together, he was never so thrilled to receive a card as he was this year. He soon began excitedly showing the card to all of the other patients and their visitors, not letting it out of his sight.

Dad was in such a good mood, talkative and outgoing during the entire visit. Even in the geriatric wing of a psychiatric hospital, his infectious personality had still managed to come out. Dad had always had that type of aura about him. People loved him. I had always felt that it was one of the reasons he was so successful at barbering. Not only could he cut hair exceptionally well, but people loved to come in and simply talk to him.

This place was clearly no different. Dad had talked to everyone in the room and they had all responded happily to him. The patients, as well as their visitors, were all laughing and having a good time. Dad had made that happen. I felt nervous about my mom going to the facility to visit Dad alone, but it had actually ended up being the most enjoyable visit that she had experienced with him since his initial diagnosis.

I began thinking about how different Dad's stay at Woodland Hospital was this time. When he had gone there initially, he was still so coherent. Even though he didn't have direct access to a phone, it hadn't stopped him. At least once a day, I would get an unexpected call from one of the nurses informing me that Dad wanted to talk. In time, the nurses got to where they'd just give the phone to Dad instead of interceding. When I would answer it, Dad would invariably be on the other end of the line, usually wanting to verify something. It was simply a time for me to reassure Dad that we were handling things for him. It was his only connection to the outside world.

This time was much different though. I hadn't received the first phone call from Dad. He could no longer initiate that type of request. He no longer had the words, his progression now beyond that stage.

Later that afternoon, I got a call from the facility that had agreed to accept Dad into their rehab unit. The case manager at Woodland Hospital was previously notified about the opening. They needed for him to immediately fax over Dad's progress reports, for which they had now been waiting over 24 hours. I couldn't believe it. I had never dealt with such incompetence. I ended up calling the patient advocate again and asking for her help. The case manager had really let the ball drop on this one. He was close to useless. I had already done all of the necessary legwork for him. Could he not seal the deal?

Thursday, September 8, 2011

As he stood grinning in front of the large bird cage, he was mesmerized with the parakeets, seemingly talking directly to him. I could see his sweet face as he talked back to them, trying to get them to mimic his words. He looked back at me and smiled. Fortunately, I was able to see Chris from my chair in the director's office. The birds would keep him entertained while I took care of the necessary paperwork.

I had needed to fill out some forms at Village Green of Georgia before my dad was admitted. One of those forms listed all of his current medications. By now, I could easily write them from memory. When I curiously asked about the form, the director told me that it would be used to verify that the medication list from Woodland Hospital matched. It definitely gave me a comfort feeling, everything finally coming together. Dad should be transferred sometime tomorrow.

Later that evening, I received a phone call from Dr. Franklin. We had a very honest conversation about my dad. I asked him the tough questions and he gave me truthful answers. "Your father is currently in the last stage of dementia," he said. I knew Dad's condition had progressed, but somehow hearing those words of finality hit me hard.

"How long do you think he has?" I asked. The last time I had asked this question, his doctor had said 5 – 10 years. I knew that was no longer in the realm of possibility.

"With no complications, he could possibly live 3 - 5 years," the doctor replied. "If he falls again and has to have another surgery or has a heart attack or develops pneumonia, then he will probably go downhill fairly rapidly and die within a year. At this stage, these are all distinct possibilities."

It was so difficult to hear this news. I knew that Dad wasn't doing well, but the thought of him dying in less than a year was inconceivable. I absolutely couldn't imagine my life without him, so hard seeing my father perish right before my very eyes. Life could change on a dime...and so drastically.

"Do you think that he'll ever be able to walk again?" I inquired.

"He will probably never be able to walk like he used to, but it will be possible for him to get around," he responded. "A lot will be dependent on how the rehab goes. He is not currently in any pain, so that shouldn't prevent him from doing the therapy. It will really depend on his mind." The doctor paused for a few seconds to let this information sink in before he continued.

"The disease has definitely progressed a lot since he was last here," he said. "Your dad has trouble communicating. He wasn't really able to have any meaningful conversations with me this time. We talked at every meeting. Unfortunately, I had a hard time understanding him."

"Do you think that his agitation is under control?" I questioned.

"He didn't show much anxiety while he was here," he replied. "Once I adjusted his medications, he remained fairly calm. I actually didn't have to use his PRN much at all."

"What should I do if he gets too agitated at the new facility?" I then asked. "What if they decide they can't handle him like the last place did?"

"They have my pager number," he answered. "If your father gets too upset, I will work with the staff at Village Green. If necessary, your dad can always come back to Woodland Hospital." I truly hoped that wouldn't be necessary, but it made me feel good to know that Dad had the option.

"They will only take Dad for the rehab," I said. "I have to find another facility for him to move to once it's over. Do you think he could ever go back to a memory care unit?"

"No, I don't," Dr. Franklin replied. "He needs too much care and he needs to be watched very closely. It's my opinion that he needs to be in a skilled nursing facility where he has access to medical professionals at all times."

The doctor had patiently answered all of my questions, never once rushing me or making me feel pressured. This was a very painful conversation for me. I felt overwhelmed with this latest information. "You know how to get in touch with me," he said. "If anything comes up, don't hesitate to call me."

"Thank you, Dr. Franklin, for everything," I said. I then hung up the phone with undoubtedly the most compassionate doctor I had ever met. I meant it from the bottom of my heart. He truly cared about my dad. I loved this man and would forever be grateful to him.

Friday, September 9, 2011

The drive into the facility was still as serene as the first time I had experienced it. I wondered if he would feel the same. The emotions inside of me were very mixed. I was ready for him to move forward with his rehab, but felt nervous at the same time with memories of the last stint leaving a bad taste in my mouth. Late this afternoon, Dad was finally transferred to Village Green for his 2nd rehab attempt. As soon as Shawn got home from school to watch Chris, I quickly made the drive over, wanting the transition this time to go as smoothly as possible.

As I approached Dad's new room, I noticed that the nametag in the hall said "Willy Lee". I was a little taken aback. At first, I thought I had the wrong room. I had never heard anyone call Dad that name in my entire life. What would make them put that on his nametag?

I then remembered seeing one of his pictures from his time in the Air Force, his signature on the front of the photograph reading "Willy". It was extremely odd. The only time that I knew Dad to go by this name was when he was in the military. I had also noticed during the past few weeks that Dad sometimes talked about his days in the Air Force as if he were still in it. He had surprisingly told me things that I had never known about that time. Had someone asked him what name he wanted on his nametag? I found it hard to believe that that had actually happened. The typical thing to do would have been to use the name currently in his file. Nowhere in it would it have said "Willy". What were the odds of this happening?

As I walked into Dad's new room, he was lying upright in bed. I walked to his side and gently kissed his forehead. "Hi Dad," I said. He smiled lovingly back at me. The nurse was seated next to him going through some paperwork. I introduced myself and she then began asking me several questions.

I noticed two plastic bags lying on the floor with Dad's personal belongings, sent over from Woodland Hospital. In addition, I had brought some miscellaneous things for dad. The nurse soon handed me a form to inventory everything. Afterwards, I neatly arranged Dad's things in his new closet.

Dad was very calm and definitely knew who I was. He soon began talking about random things that made no sense...racehorses, military days, hair tonic, pictures on the wall. Everything that he talked about was coincidentally in his past. He had changed so much in just one month, the last surgery being very hard on him.

After the nurse left, I noticed that Dad had a roommate. Fortunately for them, the room only had two beds in it. It was definitely much quieter than the last place. His roommate was currently sitting in his wheelchair on his side of the room and had been staring at me for several minutes. "Hello," I said to him. He said hi back to me, but didn't smile.

After a couple of hours, Dad started looking extremely tired, having a difficult time keeping his eyes open. I tenderly kissed him on the cheek. "I'll come back tomorrow, Daddy," I said. "You get some rest now." I prayed that his first night in this new facility would go well. He had appeared so calm at Woodland Hospital once his medications had changed. I truly hoped it would continue through tonight.

On the way out, I noticed that several patients were congregating peacefully at the end of the hall across from the nurses' station, most of them being women. They smiled at me as I slowly passed them. I smiled back at them. They were simply sitting together in their wheelchairs watching the action. I wondered if in time Dad would be joining them.

Monday, September 12, 2011

She closely followed me through the unfamiliar halls, passing several patients on our way. I pointed out the rehab rooms and the dining hall to her, periodically looking back to make sure she was still with me. It took a few minutes to get there as his room was on the complete other end of the facility. Mom had never visited Village Green before today, but her expression told me she definitely liked it.

As we soon approached his room, we surprisingly saw that his bed was empty. His roommate was again seated in his wheelchair by the window. "Hi," I said. "Do you know if my dad is in therapy?"

"I think so," he replied. I still couldn't get a smile out of him.

While I was there, I decided to check Dad's closet. A bag with dirty clothes in it was sitting on the floor. He still had several clothing items hanging up which was good. The last thing I wanted was for Dad to have to wear a stranger's clothes.

Mom and I then walked down the hall towards the nurses' station which was right across from one of the rehabilitation rooms. A couple of patients were currently doing therapy, but Dad wasn't in the room. We continued down the hall until we came to the other rehab room where we found Dad sitting down doing some arm exercises. The therapist was standing next to him urging him on. He looked completely different from the last time I had seen him in therapy. It was a welcoming sight.

We decided to patiently sit in the waiting area down the hall. It was actually a beautiful room with several couches, a door off to the side leading outdoors. Everyone that passed by was so friendly. We casually sat and took in the busy environment while we waited. It was easy to understand the wheelchair congregation by the nurses' station. It was simply human nature to watch other people.

"How is the packing going?" I asked. Mom had started the arduous task of boxing up the bonus room. Twelve, huge standalone closets had been moved over to her new home. Randy and I had arranged ten of them in the basement and the remaining two in the garage. As Mom slowly packaged her belongings, we would move them over for her. It was going to be a long process.

"Well, it's keeping me busy," she said. "There is certainly plenty to pack." She then looked me straight in the eyes. "I don't know how we're going to get it all moved."

"Don't worry, Mom," I said. "Just do a little bit each week. It'll add up. You'll see." She was apparently deep in thought and very worried. "Right now, our number one priority is Dad. We need to put him first. If it means that nothing gets packed or the new home doesn't get worked on, it's okay. Dad has to come first."

About an hour later, the therapist wheeled Dad up to the couch where we were sitting. "Hi Daddy," I said, as I kissed him on his cheek. Mom gently took his hand in hers and also greeted him. He was alert, but very quiet. He looked at us so seriously with not a trace of a smile. I soon noticed that he didn't have his upper denture in. I decided to let Mom and Dad have some time alone while I went back to his room.

When I got there, I began to carefully look through his closet and drawers for his teeth, knowing he would definitely need them for lunch. Otherwise, he would be restricted to a soft diet. I soon found them in his top drawer next to his bed.

When I got back, I found Mom and Dad sitting just as they were a few minutes earlier when I had left them. "Daddy, do you want me to put your teeth in?" I asked. He nodded yes. I then tried to put the denture in, but it was not fitting correctly and I was leery about forcing it. Dad was visibly starting to get a little agitated. He then tried to get it in himself, but wasn't having any more success than I had. Mom decided to give it a go and actually managed to secure it in his mouth. I really hoped he wouldn't take them out. We had no more backups and it would be extremely difficult to get him to a dentist right now.

We then wheeled Dad outside to a nice covered patio located immediately beyond the door. It was a beautiful day and once outside, Dad's demeanor completely changed. As he got more comfortable, he began to smile. The transformation in him once he got out in the sun left me amazed. He still didn't talk much, but paid attention to everything that was said. Sometimes, he would say something really off the wall that was so funny. It was hard not to laugh, especially when he was already laughing. The three of us spent an hour outside in our own little world acting silly. It didn't matter what we looked like. It was all about Dad.

That night, Mom got an alarming phone call from the rehab facility. Dad's wheelchair was positioned next to his bed. In the middle of the night, Dad had tried to get in it. He ended up accidentally falling out of the bed instead. The nurse found him on the floor lying in front of it. Fortunately, he wasn't hurt. They just wanted Mom to know about the incident.

All I could think of when I found out about it was what Dr. Franklin had said to me. "If there were no complications, Dad could live another 3 – 5 years. If he had another fall that required surgery, his health could digress and he could die within a year." I began to realize just how fragile my dad was. It was so easy for him to fall, even from a sitting position. In order to prevent that from happening, he would have to be watched nonstop. I knew the chance of that happening in this type of facility was very slim. An hour later as I finally drifted off to sleep, I did so with a very uneasy feeling inside.

Wednesday, September 14, 2011

No matter how hard I tried, the ride over was still rough. I looked over at Chris as he attempted to do his homework, the math worksheet and notebook resting on top of his lap. Every tiny bump seemed to be magnified as he tried to hold his pencil still. I had intentionally tried to drive as smoothly as possible, but I could only do so much. The terrain was out of my hands. He looked up at me smiling and I knew exactly what he was thinking. "I'm sorry," I said. "Just do your best, sweetie." With that, he continued on.

Before long, we made our way through the now familiar halls. As soon as I turned the corner, I suddenly saw him, the image leaving me feeling overcome with emotion. He was sitting in the hall directly across from the nurses' station with the other residents. It hadn't taken Dad long to adapt to the new routine. His face lit up as soon as he saw Chris. "Hey Lil' Monkey," Dad said. Chris immediately hugged his Papa as my heart melted.

Chris always loved seeing his Grandpa Lee. Likewise, Dad was always equally happy to see him. I had explained to Chris that Papa was sick and needed to be taken care of. He seemed to accept that explanation. Chris didn't pick up on anything different about his grandfather. Luckily, he hadn't witnessed a lot of agitation in Dad as I had gone to great lengths to shield him from this. As far as Chris was concerned, his beloved Papa was simply living somewhere new. Nothing else had changed.

Today Dad looked great. He seemed to be doing really well with his therapy. I had talked with one of his nurses on the way in. He was continuing to do the rehab every day, not only physical therapy, but also occupational and speech therapy. It definitely seemed to be agreeing with him. During the day, he was always in a good mood.

Nighttime, however, was a very different story. The nurse also informed me that Dad was sundowning. His typical routine was to slide out of bed and crawl on the floor until he reached the nurses' station at the end of the hall. It was a good distance for him to travel in this way. He would successfully bring his pillow with him each night. When he finally reached his destination, he would position himself against the wall and go to sleep. It was very similar to his actions back at Arbor Forest.

I was very surprised to find out that his agitation was once again becoming problematic. I had seen him several times at night when he was in the psychiatric hospital and he was always completely calm. I couldn't understand why this was happening. I didn't know if the nurse was exaggerating or if it was just the difference in the environments.

I decided while I was there to check on Dad's clothes. As I walked into his room, his roommate was again seated in his wheelchair. I began to look in Dad's closet and soon noticed that he had no clean pants. I bagged up the dirty slacks to come home with me. I didn't know how long it would take the facility to turn them around, but I knew it wasn't as fast as I could do them. I would have them back by tomorrow. I didn't ever want my dad doing without.

While I got the closet neatly in order, Dad's roommate decided to talk to me. "Your dad is keeping me up at night," he said.

"How is that?" I asked, turning around.

"He has outbursts and I can't sleep when it happens," he replied.

"Well, I'm sorry to hear that," I said. "He isn't used to this place yet. Hopefully, that will stop soon. Maybe you should get some sleep now while you have the room to yourself." I smiled at him. He continued to stare at me, but showed no emotion whatsoever, especially not a smile. I had tried on several occasions to be friendly with him as I would have wanted his relatives to do the same with Dad. So far, it had proved pointless. He had a very sullen disposition and I didn't seem to be able to break through that exterior. I smiled and waved at him as I walked out the door.

I found out this evening that Bob and Monica had decided to rent their home instead of selling it since the housing market was not doing well right now. Bob was busy trying to get the house ready which meant that he was working 24/7. Not only did he work fulltime and raise two boys, he was also busy packing the house up and painting the interior. Because the brunt of the move fell on Bob, he unfortunately wasn't able to visit with Dad but once a week, sometimes once every two weeks. He looked so sad all of the time, carrying such a heavy burden on his shoulders. I was worried about his health and what this move was inevitably doing to him. Unfortunately, I felt powerless to change it. All I could do was sit back and watch. It was breaking my heart.

Tuesday, September 20, 2011

As we patiently sat in the cramped office waiting for the case manager to arrive, I looked over at Mom. She had that exact same look of concern that I currently felt. One of the directors had arranged a progress meeting at Village Green first thing this morning. I knew that it was standard practice, but I had a bad feeling that there was an ulterior motive for this one.

The director soon handed me a copy of the medication list from Woodland Hospital. After briefly glancing at it, I noticed that the two medications for diabetes were missing. When I then brought it to the director's attention, she informed me that she knew nothing about it and I'd need to discuss it with Dad's nurse.

At this point, the true reason behind the meeting came out. The facility was not equipped or staffed to handle severe dementia patients that suffered from Sundowner's. They also didn't have any openings in their long term section. A lot of the patients from the facility that had its roof collapse earlier this year had been transferred to this location, my dad's roommate being one of them. He was currently in the rehab section, even though he wasn't receiving any therapy. They simply had nowhere else to put him. Regardless, they made it very clear that we would have to move Dad eventually.

After the meeting, I immediately went to see the nurse in charge of Dad's medicine. I had her check the log to see if by chance Dad was getting his diabetes meds even though they were missing from the list. I soon found out that they were indeed not being dispensed to my dad. "There is a problem," I said. "My dad has Type 2 diabetes. He has not been getting his diabetes meds since he's been here. That's ten days."

The nurse then looked through Dad's records. "His blood sugar was checked when he first arrived and it was fine," she replied. "The doctor had felt that it wasn't a problem." I wasn't sure if that was really what the doctor had said or if the nurse was just being lazy and trying to pacify me.

It wasn't working as I was livid at this point. "That isn't the doctor's call to make," I stated. "She doesn't know my dad's history. He has had diabetes for years. It doesn't just go away overnight. How come nobody notified his family about this?"

The nurse just looked at me with such indifference, her attitude absolutely astonishing me. "Well, those two diabetes meds need to be added back immediately," I emphasized. "It is not an option." I wasn't leaving this decision up to a doctor that had quite possibly only seen my dad a couple of times.

Unfortunately, the predicament wasn't that simple to remedy. The diabetes medication was not on the medicine cart. The nurse would need to contact the doctor about getting Dad's medications changed. Once the doctor approved the change, the pharmacy would need to prepare them and send them over. They also needed to start checking Dad's blood sugar on a regular basis. I knew based on the amount of red tape involved that it would probably be a couple of days before everything was finally straightened out.

When I got home, I promptly called Woodland Hospital to find out how the diabetes meds got left off of the list in the first place. The nurse assured me that Dad's blood sugar had indeed been checked and that he'd received his diabetes meds while he was there. She personally remembered doing it. Unfortunately, Dad's records had already been moved out of the geriatric wing. She no longer had access to them. For that, I would have to contact the Records Department.

The clerk in Records politely let me know that since I didn't have power of attorney for my dad, they couldn't release the records to me. They could however release them to Village Green if I got them to fill out a specific form. After going round and round, I finally decided that the point was moot. A mistake was clearly made by Woodland Hospital, but the bigger mistake was made by Village Green. They were the ones that neglected to compare the medicine list from Woodland Hospital with the medicine list that I had personally filled out. First and foremost, I needed to get Dad's current meds corrected.

Later that afternoon, I got a phone call from the pharmacy that handled the meds for Village Green. The doctor was contacted and okayed the change to Dad's meds. Unfortunately, a problem surfaced with the medication and the insurance company. The pharmacy needed me to contact the previous pharmacy that actually had active prescriptions for the two meds. I then called Collier Village Pharmacy and had them fax paperwork over to the new pharmacy verifying that

Dad was indeed on those medications.

It would take all afternoon to finally get this issue resolved. It was an absolute nightmare and all because a couple of individuals neglected to do their job properly. Was this in some way causing the extra agitation in Dad at night? All I could think about at that moment was whether any damage might have happened to him as a result of this?

June, 1974

I had spent some time away from home this summer staying with my cousin. While there, I received a phone call from my mom. Our stray cat had conveniently climbed into the sink in the hall bathroom and had her litter of four kittens. It was so exciting as we had never had a pet that had babies before. I was just sorry that I had missed the birth.

When I got home a week later, the first thing I did was check on the kittens. They were so tiny. As I gently picked each one up and held it in my hands, I decided on its name. I appropriately named them Grayish Gregory, Black Bart, Orange Oliver and Kitty Junior, all of them so precious.

Eventually, they grew old enough to go outside with their mama. We loved watching them friskily play. One day, Kitty Junior accidentally wandered off. We searched everywhere, but unfortunately never found her.

Mom agreed to let us keep one kitten, in addition to the mother cat. I knew that was a lot considering my mom was not an animal person. She actually did not care for the mother cat at all.

One morning months earlier, I had gotten up and looked out the sliding glass door in our Florida room. The mother cat was not there which was very strange. I had done this same thing every day since we first got her and she'd always been there. I then asked everyone in the family if they had seen her, but no one had.

For over a month, I religiously looked out the glass door every morning in hopes that she would magically appear, but she never did. Then, one day I looked out and got the surprise of my life. There before my eyes was Mama Cat. I couldn't believe it. "Mom, Dad, she's back!" I screamed with joy. I picked her up and lovingly held her in my arms, not wanting to put her down for fear she would disappear again.

Months later, I would find out that the mother cat hadn't simply run away. My mom had secretly put her in the station wagon and driven her all the way to Miami Lakes, which was over ten miles away. There, she had let the cat out and driven home by herself. The last thing she wanted was a litter of kittens and that was her way of dealing with the issue. She had intentionally never said anything to us about this incident. In her mind, she felt certain she had seen the last of that cat.

I had heard so many stories of pets miraculously finding their way back home, even when the distance was miles away. Mama Cat had somehow done exactly that. It was amazing. I began to think of my mother's surprise that morning. As she was in the kitchen casually cooking breakfast, she saw me make my way to the door and then heard me utter those words she undoubtedly never thought she'd hear. "She's back! Mama Cat is back." The thought made me chuckle. Sometimes life didn't play out the way we expected.

As I looked at the remaining three kittens, it was so hard to choose the one we would keep. One of them, however, had touched me in a very special way. We decided to keep Orange Oliver and give the others away.

1974 – 1976

Life with Orange Oliver was a true blessing. I became very attached to him and him with me, as well. We soon developed a very special bond.

He followed me everywhere. When I would take a bath, Orange Oliver was right there sitting on the ledge. Most cats would have steered clear of the water, but not him. He never let me get too far out of his sight. When I brushed my teeth, he lied right behind me on the floor and watched me. Each morning when I left for school, Mom would have to keep an eye on him so he wouldn't follow me. He even slept in my bed with me. He was basically my shadow. I had never had a pet like him *before. We were inseparable.*

Orange Oliver was your typical tom cat. One day, I came home from school just like any other day. He normally greeted me at the door. On this particular day, he wasn't there. I looked everywhere for him. The thought that he had followed me to school soon entered my mind.

When he still hadn't shown up the next day, I decided to make some flyers, stapling one to every pole near my home. I then went to John G. Du Puis Elementary and Palm Springs Junior High and did the same.

The next evening, I received a phone call from an English teacher at Palm Springs Junior High. When she had come out to her car after school, she had found Orange Oliver. He had affectionately brushed up against her leg and that was all it had taken. She then kindly took him home with her. She had also seen one of the flyers and thoughtfully called to let me know that he was doing just fine. The next day, we met and she returned Orange Oliver to me. I was so thankful that he had been found by such a sweet lady. Mostly, I was glad that he was back home with me.

There had been one other time that Orange Oliver had gone missing. On this particular occasion, I hadn't seen him for two days. I constantly went outside and called his name during that entire time.

Late on the second day, the man that lived next door to us suddenly appeared on our front stoop. When I opened the door for him, there in his arms before me was my precious Orange Oliver. It was such a happy moment for me.

Apparently, my cat had climbed inside of a huge, plastic container in the corner of our neighbor's backyard unbeknownst to him. As he securely placed the lid on it, he had no idea that Orange Oliver was already inside.

While he was working in his backyard today, he heard a cat meowing. He had followed the sound back to the plastic container where he found my beloved pet. Orange Oliver was famished, but he was once again home safe.

April, 1976

Orange Oliver had never been fixed. A cat on the next block over was currently in heat, Orange Oliver repeatedly getting into fights over this. On two different occasions, he had come home with multiple scratches on him. The first time had not been too bad with just a couple of small scratches on his face. This last time was much worse, the injuries looking like they might have been from the cat's owner and not the cat. I really worried for his safety, eventually reaching the point where I couldn't bear it anymore. I talked to Mom and Dad and we all agreed that the best thing to do for Orange Oliver was to get him neutered.

Within a week, we had the procedure done. Everything had been successful. The doctor had told us to keep him inside at night for seven days after which we could let him sleep outside.

As was instructed, we kept a close eye on him for the first week. After I had gone to bed that next night, Orange Oliver needed to go out. Mom had let him outside before she went to bed. Nothing seemed out of the ordinary.

The next morning, Dad left to go to work as he usually did. On the way to his car, he noticed Orange Oliver asleep near the driveway. He was in his normal spot lying the way he always did. Dad then bent down to pet him, after which he noticed that he was hard. He had apparently died during the night and rigor mortis had already set in.

Dad couldn't believe it, shuddering to think what it was going to do to me. I was still sound asleep at the time. All Dad could think about was how he was going to tell me. He then went inside and broke the grim news to my mom. They both agreed that it would absolutely kill me. At the time, they felt the best solution was to secretly bury Orange Oliver and not say anything to me. He had wandered off before, so there was a good chance I'd make that same assumption this time. Shielding me from this sad news seemed the right thing to do at the time.

My dad went into the garage and got a shovel. He then went to the side of the house and quietly dug a hole. He carefully wrapped Orange Oliver up in a bag and then placed him in the dugout area before covering him up with the loose dirt. From the outside, no one would have envisioned that a cat was buried below.

When I got up later that morning, I immediately noticed that Orange Oliver was nowhere around. "Mom, have you seen Orange Oliver?" I asked.

"No, honey," she replied, trying her hardest not to break down.

Throughout the day, I continued to look for my cat. I expected at any minute to hear his meow and for him to come running home, but he never did.

Later that day, the phone rang. I could tell by my mom's words that it was my dad. What I didn't know was what he had said. "Has she said anything about Orange Oliver yet?" he had asked. "Is she doing okay?" Dad was very worried. He was an animal lover just like me, so he understood how much this could hurt me.

For four days, I continued unsuccessfully to look for Orange Oliver, calling his name, walking around the neighborhood. I asked my parents repeatedly if they had seen him.

For four days, my dad had called home multiple times throughout the day to find out how I was doing. When he would come home at night, the first thing he would do was check on me.

Then on the fifth day, I again walked up to my mom. "Mom, I just don't understand what happened to him," I said. "He has never run away for this long. I don't have a good feeling about this. I think something bad may have happened to him." I intently looked at Mom, but she didn't say a word, the expression on her face clearly saying that something wasn't right. "Mom, did something happen to Orange Oliver? Do you know something that you're not telling me?" She just stared at me. I knew in that instant he was gone.

"Vanessa, we didn't know how to tell you," she said. "He died that first night we let him out. I'm so sorry." I closed my eyes and started to cry, deep, deep sobs from within. Mom gently took me in her arms and held me tightly as the cries became louder. I was inconsolable.

"Where is he?" I pleaded.

"Your father buried him on the side of the house, right outside your bedroom window," she replied.

I immediately ran outside, the broken up soil visibly showing where he was buried. I knelt on his makeshift grave and continued to cry.

Before long, the neighbor on that side of the house rushed over. She had heard my cries and was scared that something had happened. *After talking with my mom, she soon joined me in the backyard and tenderly hugged me. "Oh, mi dulce niña. No estés triste. Fue un buen gato y te amaba mucho." I didn't know what she said, but I knew it was loving.*

I lied in my bed for hours that day. When Dad came home that evening, he slowly walked into my room. "Pootie, I'm so sorry," he said. "I know how much you loved him. He absolutely adored you. In all my life, I had never seen a pet react to someone the way that he did to you." He then gently hugged me as I rested my head on his shoulders, the tears beginning to fall once again. I knew that my dad understood my pain.

"He's never coming back," I cried. "I never even got to say goodbye to him. He was so much more than just a cat. He was my friend." As I despondently looked at Dad, I thought I saw his eyes start to water. He was clearly broken up. He had loved Orange Oliver just like me.

Thursday, September 22, 2011

He was casually sitting in his bed, fully dressed, as we walked into the room. The blue and white striped shirt immediately caught my eye, hoping that it provided him a feeling of comfort in a world filled with so much uncertainty. The therapist had pulled me aside on the way in to let me know he had done well in his earlier session. I was so proud as I smiled at my handsome father.

"Hi Daddy," I said, kissing him hello.

"Hi Pootie," he replied. "Hi Mama."

"You look nice," I said. "Would you like to go out front for a little bit? It's really pretty outside." He shook his head yes and smiled. I knew he would absolutely love it.

I carefully wheeled Dad through the hallways towards the front door. We had taken him outside several times, but it was usually to the covered patio on the side. Today we were going to take him to the front of the facility.

As we soon made our way outside, I positioned Dad's wheelchair at one end right underneath a wind chime. Mom and I then sat in two rocking chairs immediately beside him. It was sunny, but not too hot, with a gentle breeze blowing. I looked over at my dad and he had the most peaceful look on his face, seeming so relaxed. We all leisurely sat together enjoying this special time. It was absolutely perfect. The wind chime was making such a beautiful sound. After today, I didn't think I would ever hear one and not think of my daddy.

His medicine had finally been corrected and he'd started taking his two diabetes medications today. He would also get his blood sugar tested four times a day. It had taken two full days to get this fiasco fixed. Today, he seemed fine, but I'd be watching him very closely to see if it really did have an impact on his current state.

On our way out of the facility later that afternoon, Mom and I stopped in the Director of Nursing's office. We introduced ourselves and asked for a minute of her time. She politely invited us in to have a seat.

"There was a mix up with my dad's medications that really concerned me," I said. As she shook her head, she obviously already knew about the mistake. "I had filled out a form listing all of the medications that my dad was taking. On the list were Januvia and Actoplus Met for his diabetes. The list of medicine that came from Woodland Hospital had left them off in error. I was told the purpose of me filling out the form was to ensure that my dad would be given the correct medications once he got here. Why did I go through that effort if it wasn't even going to be looked at? It really bothers me that the mistake on Woodland Hospital's list wasn't caught by someone here."

"We did notice it," she replied. "His blood sugar was checked and it wasn't high. We decided to just monitor it until we saw otherwise." She was giving me the same exact excuse that his nurse had given me.

"According to the nurse, his blood sugar wasn't being checked on a daily basis," I said. "How would you know if there was a problem?"

"There are certain signs if your blood sugar is too high," she responded. "Your dad wasn't exhibiting any of those signs."

"That is not how you handle diabetes," I stated. "You don't determine if there is a problem by looking for signs. You monitor it by checking the blood sugar." I couldn't believe I was actually having this argument. "It still doesn't matter. No one here had the right to take him off of medication that he had been on for years. My dad has an endocrinologist that specializes in diabetes. He felt that he needed to be on the medications. On top of that, you took him off of them and never even notified any of his family. You didn't call us and you didn't call Woodland Hospital."

"It really had not been a problem so far," she said. I just stared at this woman incredulously. Someone at this location had clearly been negligent. In all of the different facilities and hospitals that my dad had resided in, no one had ever boldly taken it upon themselves to take him off his diabetes medications. This woman was defending her staff when they were clearly in the wrong. She was obviously not about to admit that they had made a mistake. I was still livid. One thing was for sure. She would be watching my dad a little closer from now on.

I also mentioned the fact that he was so calm at Woodland Hospital, but was sundowning here. It didn't make sense to me. "We see that all the time," she replied. "It is the difference in the two types of places. This facility is a much more stimulating environment. It's like a hospital. There are people coming in and out constantly. There's a lot of noise. All of the hustle and bustle just seems to add to the dementia patient's agitation."

I wasn't sure how to take that information. Supposedly, this was the type of facility that my dad needed to be in. Yet, the very nature of it seemed to agitate him. What was the right answer? I had such mixed feelings about what type of place would be best for my dad.

I had started my search once again for another facility, seeming to never end. A brand new, state of the art memory care center for Alzheimer's patients, only fifteen minutes away from my home, was planning to open up in late October. I had optimistically scheduled a tour for this Tuesday. It sounded like it would be perfect.

I wanted more than anything to find the right place for my dad, one that he could stay in permanently. The constant moving back and forth was so exhausting, especially for Dad. I really hoped that this new facility would be the answer to our prayers.

Friday, September 23, 2011

I felt so discouraged upon hearing the latest news. It was completely unexpected as I had thought he was doing so well. While walking down the hallway towards Dad's room, I had run into his speech therapist. She informed me that the facility was discontinuing some of his therapy as he just didn't seem to be making any progress. He was also having some difficulty eating. "He hasn't had his upper teeth in for a couple of days now," she remarked. "It's affecting his ability to eat anything hard. I'm having to keep a close eye on him so he doesn't choke." As the disease was steadily progressing, Dad was requiring more assistance every day.

The insurance companies would only cover Dad at 100% for a certain number of days. Unfortunately, the days wasted at the first rehab facility had counted towards this number. In order for them to continue paying for Dad's therapy, it was necessary to thoroughly document his progress. If they weren't completely convinced that he was making strides, they wouldn't pay for the services anymore. Two of Dad's current therapists no longer felt that he was making any improvements. He was participating, but there just didn't seem to be any major development. As a result, they were discharging Dad from both occupational and speech therapy. This news was very disappointing. What chance did he have of getting better without the therapy?

When I saw my dad today, he was calmly sitting at the end of the hall near the nurses' station. He was looking down and hadn't seen me walk up to him. "Hi Daddy," I said, as I gently took his hand in mine. He suddenly looked up at me and smiled. "Daddy, your hair looks good." I had arranged with the staff to have the facility's barber cut Dad's hair and give him a much needed shave. The first one was complimentary and had turned out very well. He was clean shaven and his hair was trimmed nicely. In some ways, he looked like his old self.

We visited in the hall for awhile. Then, I carefully wheeled Dad back to his room so we could have some privacy. I positioned him next to the bed and I conveniently pulled a chair over. His roommate was nowhere to be seen.

Dad wasn't talking very much today. The few words he had said didn't make sense. He also didn't seem to have much energy. I checked with the nurse and made sure his diabetes meds and sugar level were okay. I also asked her about Dad's sundowning. She confirmed the story that several other girls had already told me. Dad had his days and nights mixed up which explained why he looked so tired right now.

While we were in his room, I began searching for his teeth. I had noticed from talking with him that his upper denture still wasn't in his mouth. I meticulously looked everywhere, but with no luck. I would let the staff know to be on the lookout for them. When he was at Arbor Forest, he had taken them out while eating one day and set them on the dining table. It was a much smaller facility and luckily, someone had found them. If the same thing had happened here, they might just be gone for good.

Dad's physical therapist soon stopped by to let me know that Dad had a session in about thirty minutes. Physical therapy was the only type of rehab that was still scheduled to continue. I promised to bring him down when it was time.

While sitting together, Dad and I soon heard a man's voice yelling, clearly coming from next door. I had never met this man or even seen him. He was usually very quiet. Today, he was completely irate.

"I want out of here!" he yelled. I could hear several things being moved or possibly thrown in his room. "Dammit, someone get in here and get me the hell out of here!" Dad and I cautiously looked at each other. Before long, a nurse hastily entered his room. She was trying to calm him down, but he wanted no part of it as his yelling continued. Another staff member soon joined them.

About this time, Dad's roommate nervously wheeled himself through the door. It was obvious from the look on his face that he had also heard the yelling next door. He hurriedly positioned himself on the other side of the room in front of the window.

The yelling seemed to get louder and the language more abusive. This was definitely not a job for the weak or faint of heart. I became very alarmed as the man sounded dangerous.

I decided it was time to remove Dad from the current environment. If they couldn't get this patient settled down, then we needed to leave. As I wheeled Dad down the hall, I caught a glimpse of the man doing the screaming. He was a much younger man than most of the others in this wing. He was currently sitting in his wheelchair, but wasn't able to get it to move on his own, causing him a lot of frustration. Three people were now in his room attempting to calm him down. I truly hoped that it would be under control by the time Dad's physical therapy was finished.

Later this evening, I invited my mom over for dinner. It felt very unusual sitting down to a meal without my dad here also. Mom was sitting in her usual spot at the table, but Dad's seat was vacant. I didn't think I would ever get used to it. They had both been regularly coming over for dinner ever since they had first moved here. It was always a very special time for us.

After dinner, we would always move to the living room where the boys would then select a movie for all of us to watch together. The volume was always turned up high so that my dad could hear it. It was just something we had gotten used to over the years.

As I now watched my mother eat, I was encased in sadness. It seemed as though every day something else was being taken away from us. This was just one more thing that was changing in our lives. Dinner with both of my parents was becoming a thing of the past.

Tuesday, September 27, 2011

Chris carefully placed the hard hat on his head and looked up at me smiling. "It feels like we're on a field trip, Mom," Chris commented. I laughed as I adjusted the bright yellow helmet on my head. We were about to tour Forever Hope Memory Care. The new facility was still under construction, so we had to wear the appropriate headgear. Chris had a big grin on his face as we walked from the trailer to the actual building to begin the visit.

The facility was privately owned and was actually inspired and built by three brothers who had a personal connection to Alzheimer's. One of the brothers was currently giving us the tour. He told me that they were even instrumental in starting the assisted living and memory care unit ideas. I had a feeling that what I was about to see was going to be revolutionary.

Historically, dementia care was usually in a separate wing of a building that was primarily used for assisted living purposes. I had never seen a facility that catered predominantly to dementia patients. Forever Hope Memory Care was the first place that I had ever seen that was designed solely to care for individuals afflicted with Alzheimer's and other dementias. In the Alzheimer's world, this was major.

Within a typical memory care unit, all of the patients were combined with little regard to residents at different stages needing different levels of care and activities. Forever Hope Memory Care was designed with four different wings or villages as they were called. The patients were strategically grouped based on the level of care that they needed. As their care needs changed, they wouldn't need to be moved to another facility. They simply moved to another village, with one even designated for hospice care. The need for someone to ever leave this center just didn't exist, even when the end was near.

The facility not only had exterior paths for walking, but also included a 24-hour interior walking path in one of the villages designed specifically for patients that wandered. Most homes that I had seen had an outside area for strolling, but I had never seen one that had an inside path. The halls were extra wide to accommodate this. I could imagine Dad using this extensively.

One of the common problems with dementia patients was that they sometimes dressed in many, many layers of clothes. I had personally witnessed this many times with Dad. To prevent that from happening, the main closet door was kept securely locked. The caregiver would routinely unlock the closet each morning and retrieve two outfits. Next to the closet was an open area with a small rod which was only about a foot wide. The two outfits would conveniently be placed here with the patient ultimately deciding which set of clothes they wanted to wear. This method prevented them from putting on several different layers, while still giving them the ability to feel like they were in control.

They also couldn't pull things out of their closet and accidentally put them in someone else's room or vice versa. That was a big problem in the other memory care unit that Dad had lived in. I was so impressed with the love and thoughtfulness that had gone into this facility's architecture.

The center had an RN and LPN on staff every day, available 24/7.

They also had a dedicated primary care doctor and geriatric psychiatrist that came to the facility once every two weeks to check on the patients. If necessary, their physician assistants could come out anytime they were needed. There wouldn't be any extra agitation due to the patient having to leave the premises. Instead, everything was brought to them which I considered invaluable. To have an all-inclusive facility would be the ultimate dream for a dementia patient.

A nurses' station was built at the end of the hall so that the hallway was completely visible to them. My dad had oftentimes wandered into someone's room and no one knew where he was. The idea of preventing that was very important to me.

Forever Hope Memory Care was designed to have a very serene atmosphere with murals on the walls and televisions that had relaxing videos playing throughout the day. Everything down to the smallest detail was designed with Alzheimer's in mind, obviously thought out by someone having lived through it themselves. No one else could have possibly understood the intricacies of the disease well enough to do it.

For every concern that I had, they invariably had something in place to handle it. The brother that I had met was so incredibly compassionate. My only concern was that the facility was still under construction, scheduled to open on October 24. It sounded like a dream come true, but without actually seeing it in operation, you just never knew.

The other consideration was that it was a little more expensive than what we were used to. It would probably cost around $5,000 a month. As Dad's care needs increased, so would that price. The rehabilitation facility that he was currently at had a long term care section. I tracked down some prices and for a semi-private room, it would be approximately $200 a day, the monthly amount considerably more. Even though they had more medical staff at the rehab facility, the setting was not conducive to Alzheimer's patients. The clinical environment actually seemed to make my dad more anxious.

I had gone on the tour today with some skepticism that maybe the memory care unit wasn't the best option for my dad. Several people had led me to believe that he needed to be in a skilled nursing facility. The visit today had opened my eyes, with this facility clearly having the best of both worlds. It was truly an amazing place. It gave me hope for the future, not just for my dad but for others suffering from this horrific disease. The world was definitely not ready for Alzheimer's, but this facility had taken a major step towards providing hope where there currently was none.

Friday, September 30, 2011

As I stood in the gravel parking lot looking at the work in progress, I had a good feeling inside. A lot of construction was still going on, but it was easy to imagine the end result. Only three days had gone by since my first visit, but I could see a substantial amount of headway. I had seen so many facilities this past month and most of them had left me feeling depressed. This place had felt different, filling me with hope for our future. I had spoken to Mom and Bob about it and we were all in agreement.

Today, I dropped a check off at Forever Hope Memory Care to reserve a spot for Dad. I felt so optimistic that it would be the perfect choice for him, potentially making such a difference in his life. The only concern I had was the timing. I would need to talk to Dad's case manager and make sure that they'd allow him to stay where he currently was until the facility actually opened.

When I walked into Dad's room, he was contentedly sitting upright in his bed. A woman was sitting next to him, trying to feed him a graham cracker and some juice. She politely introduced herself as one of the therapists at the facility. She had been working with Dad for awhile trying to help him eat. He was having a difficult time as was evidenced by the crumbs all over his blanket.

While carefully watching Dad, I noticed that he wasn't dressed. During the first two weeks that Dad was here, the rehab therapy seemed to have gone well, the therapists making sure Dad was up and dressed early every day. During that time, he was eating much better, too. Since the majority of his therapy had stopped, it seemed as though Dad was just left in his bed to sleep. The staff members didn't seem to make the same effort in getting Dad up now that he was out of most of his therapy.

As a result, he didn't seem to be making any progress. It was a no-win cycle for my dad.

The therapist asked me several questions about Dad's current state. She could apparently tell that the amount of attention Dad was getting lately was very upsetting to me. We talked for a long time. She was completely understanding about the situation and urged me to address the matter further.

Just yesterday, I was sitting next to Dad in his room. His roommate's daughter happened to also be visiting at the same time. When she arrived, she had found her father needing desperately to be changed. She had walked down to the nurses' station to let someone know. After several minutes had passed, she still saw no sign of anyone coming to assist. She was very upset. She then paged the nurse with the button on the bed. After about five more minutes, someone finally came in. "My father needs to be changed," she said. "This is ridiculous. How come nobody is checking on him? You can't just leave him back here and not look in on him." The girl had apologized and then taken her father into the restroom to assist him.

As I remembered the incident yesterday, I became more upset seeing my dad still not dressed in his bed. I could think of no excuse for the lack of care that these men were receiving. I then decided to page the nurse. Within a few minutes, she walked into the room. "Why isn't anybody getting my dad dressed anymore?" I asked.

"I'm sorry," she replied. "I didn't realize that he wasn't dressed yet."

"It seems as though ever since he was discharged from most of his therapy, nobody even bothers to get him dressed and out of bed anymore," I remarked. "It isn't good for him to just lie here every day. I feel like every time I've come here recently, that is how I've found him."

"Let me get someone to help me," she said. "I'll be right back." She then left to get another staff member to assist her.

"We're going to get you dressed, Daddy," I said. He smiled at me like he always did whenever I took care of him, a smile not only of love, but of trust and confidence. I then picked out an outfit from his closet and set it on his bed. The nurse soon returned with some help. Dad would be getting dressed today. It was tomorrow that I was worried about. I was slowly losing faith in this rehab facility, too.

Sunday, October 2, 2011

I had slowly crept downstairs to the basement, trying to be as quiet as I could as I brought Randy a bottle of water. Not more than ten minutes earlier, he had come upstairs and scared me to death. He had secretly walked up behind me and gently placed his hand on my shoulder, never saying a word. I had gasped in response. This was now his payback.

Randy and I were busy fixing up Mom's new home next door. Randy had done a lot of work in her basement. He was applying a special waterproofing paint to all of the walls to help prevent mildew. The windows needed blinds. The light fixtures had to be replaced. He also added some locks. I, meanwhile, meticulously cleaned every inch of the interior. We hoped to have the work done soon, as we continued moving Mom's belongings over.

An hour later, Randy, Chris and I drove to Village Green to see Dad. We arrived at 11:00 a.m. and found him in bed once again dressed in a hospital gown. It definitely seemed that he was not getting the attention lately that he normally got. Things were clearly more laid back on the weekend. I wondered if the staff was also acting accordingly. I was so thankful that we had made the decision to move Dad to the new facility. I had previously met some incredibly compassionate people in the memory care unit and I wanted Dad to experience that level of dedication again.

As soon as he saw us, a big smile spread across his face. He was in a very good mood and recognized all of us. "Hey guys!" he said.

Chris and I both kissed Dad on the cheek. Randy took his hand in his and gently caressed it. While we were talking, Dad suddenly began coughing. "Dad, do you need some water?" I asked. He nodded yes. I quickly got his cup from the nightstand next to his bed. I positioned the straw in his mouth and got him to take a few sips which seemed to do the trick.

"Come here and tell me what you've been doing lately," Dad said to Chris. As Chris happily sat on the bed to talk with Dad, I left the room and made my way down to the nurses' station to refill Dad's cup. Directly next to the desk was a cart that always contained snacks, a nurse pointing it out to me on my initial tour. I grabbed some graham crackers for Dad and Chris.

When I got back to the room, I opened up the package and handed Dad one of the crackers. As he was eating it, the coughing started up again. This time, it went on for awhile. I gave Dad some more water and it eventually seemed to get the coughing under control. I nervously looked over at Randy as he had that same look of concern on his face that I felt inside.

I knew one of the things that would affect Dad in this last stage of dementia was the inability to swallow properly. The damage to his brain would eventually cause him to lose the ability to coordinate his swallowing and breathing, the timing of that so crucial. Without it, food or fluids could aspirate or enter his lungs which could in turn cause aspiration pneumonia to develop. It was something that we took for granted in our everyday lives. It wasn't so with Alzheimer's. As with every other condition that we had faced, I cautiously looked at my dad and wondered. Was this just a fluke or was I witnessing yet another failure due to the disease?

We decided to get Dad up and dressed, quickly looking in his closet for a shirt and a pair of pants. I noticed that the bag of dirty clothes was full. One of the attendants had initially told me that the laundry required a 2-day turnaround. It seemed more like a 7-day turnaround. I ended up doing a lot of Dad's laundry myself so he wouldn't be without.

We then moved Dad to his wheelchair and took him down the hall near the nurses' station. It was currently lunchtime. The girl conveniently hooked the tray of food up to Dad's wheelchair. He had no trouble holding his fork by himself and actually ate several bites on his own. Then, he seemed to lose interest for awhile and sat still. I would then fix a bite and put it in his mouth which would get him going again. The assistance that he needed wasn't so much with the use of the utensils, but more with keeping him focused and on track with the eating. It was quite possible that he would lose interest long before he felt full. I worried that without someone watching him, he simply wouldn't get enough food in him. He had successfully managed to eat about a fourth of his lunch today.

Last night, I sadly thought about what the future would hold for my dad. I dreaded one moment far more than any other, the day that my daddy forgot who I was. I decided that I wasn't going to wait until he was on his death bed to tell him certain things. I wasn't guaranteed that I'd have that opportunity.

Today as I got ready to leave, I leaned down and gently kissed him on the forehead, looking so childlike and innocent. "You have been the best dad in the world to me," I said. My eyes soon filled with tears. "I love you, Daddy." He just looked at me with those blue eyes, but didn't say a thing. I couldn't tell if my words had registered with him or not.

I prayed so hard at that very second that God would give him a moment of clarity so that he could know how much he meant to me. I knew that irreparable damage had already occurred in his brain. All I wanted was one brief moment for my words to reach him. Let this precious man have some inner peace knowing that his daughter thought the world of him. Just one fleeting moment was all I asked for. Dad then looked at me and slowly smiled. It wasn't a huge grin, but just enough of one for me to know that my prayer had been answered.

We then all kissed Dad goodbye with Chris hugging him tightly. "Do you have to go?" Dad asked, looking directly at me. His words absolutely broke my heart. He was clearly alert and didn't want us to leave. I brushed his hair back off of his forehead for a few minutes. I knew that Bob and the boys were on their way over which made it a little easier.

"Daddy, Chris has school tomorrow and I need to take care of some things for him before then," I replied. He didn't say anything else. About ten minutes later, we again said our goodbyes and started walking down the hall towards the front door. I looked back at Dad and he was looking down.

On the ride home, I silently replayed those last moments with my dad over and over in my head, feeling so torn inside. Sometimes it was so hard to manage everything. I had needed to do some work with Chris before he went back to school tomorrow. It still didn't make it any easier to leave my dad. He had wanted us to stay with him. It was such a simple request. All he had wanted was to spend time with us. In the big scheme of things in life, what was most important? I didn't have the answer. What I did know was that today was going to be one of those moments that I would forever question. The image of my precious father as I slowly walked away from him would forever be engrained in my mind. I would always wonder whether I had made the right decision in leaving when I did.

Tuesday, October 4, 2011

He cheerfully hopped in the car, excitement written all over his face. It was noon and he was out of school for the day. Early release only happened twice a year, but when it did, it was special. The fact that he had no homework only intensified his happiness. After grabbing a snack from home, Chris and I quickly headed to Village Green to spend the afternoon with Dad.

We arrived at the facility at 1:40 p.m. and once again found my dad in bed. Chris immediately went to his side. "Papa, Papa," he said. Dad would flutter his eyes for a few seconds and then go back to sleep.

"Daddy, can you open your eyes for me?" I asked. Dad tried to open them, but was just too tired. I carefully pulled the covers back to check his body, heartbroken at the sight. His legs looked like sticks, completely emaciated. He had lost so much weight in the past few months. I then noticed that both of his feet were swollen. The right one was so swollen that you couldn't see any bones. I immediately paged the nurse.

Within a minute, she came into the room. "Look at how swollen his feet are, especially his right foot," I stated.

"Oh my, I hadn't noticed that earlier," she replied.

"Was his blood sugar checked today?" I asked. "Did he take his diabetes medications?"

"I'll double check," the nurse said as she swiftly left the room. She soon came back with Dad's chart. "Everything looked fine and he had all of his morning medications. I need to let someone know about this. I'll be right back."

The assistant director of nursing then came down followed by the original nurse. As she carefully checked Dad's feet, she shook her head, obviously very alarmed. "I'm going to call the doctor right away," she responded, as she walked out of the room.

About ten minutes later, she returned. "I got in touch with the doctor on call," she said. "He wants to put your Dad on a water pill for three days to help reduce the swelling. We'll start him on it today." She then checked both feet again before propping them up on a pillow. About that time, Dad opened his eyes. "How are you doing, Mr. Lee?" she asked.

He blinked several times, but didn't respond. "Hi Daddy," I said.

"Hi baby," he replied.

It was hard to tell how long it would have been before one of the nursing staff would have noticed the swelling if I hadn't alerted them. I knew that with his diabetes, it was important to always keep an eye on his feet. As I looked at both of them very thoroughly, I saw no open sores. I knew from previous reading that the swelling could be related to heart failure or possibly kidney failure. It was definitely a sign of something underlying.

It was also possible that his swollen feet were due to poor circulation. It seemed that Dad now spent most of his time in bed, at least when I was here. Now that most of his therapy had stopped, I didn't think Dad was getting enough exercise.

I gently rubbed both of his feet. "Dad, is this hurting you?" I asked. "Are your feet sore?" He shook his head no.

Chris and I remained by Dad's side all afternoon. Dad occasionally talked, but for the most part, he just rested. I knew he didn't sleep well at night. I hoped that was the reason he was so tired. I had offered to get him dressed, but he chose to stay in his bed. Until they got the swelling down, I really didn't want him up and about anyway. His feet definitely needed to remain elevated.

Later that afternoon, the nurse came by to check on Dad and let me know that his medicine was en route. "Please keep an eye on him," I said. "We're going to be leaving soon. I need to know that he's being looked after." She promised me that they would. I would be returning tomorrow to make sure.

Thursday, October 6, 2011

I couldn't remember the last time he had laughed so much. It was contagious. Every time he smiled, my heart melted. When Mom and I had arrived this morning, we found Dad relaxing in bed. This time though, he was fully awake and in a great mood. He continuously joked with me the entire time, sometimes saying off the wall comments. It didn't matter though as he was happy.

He soon looked at me and began calling me by my nickname, chuckling after each time. "Dad, why did you start calling me Pootie?" I asked. He had called me that for as long as I could remember.

"Well, why do you think I did?" he asked mischievously. He then smiled at me. I already knew the answer. It was basically that there was no rhyme or reason to the name. He simply called me by it one day when I was a toddler and the name had stuck. I was just curious what reason he would tell me now.

He continued to try to make me laugh and it was definitely working. "Pootie, Pootie, Pootie," he said in a sing song fashion. Then he laughed. He was acting so silly with me and I absolutely loved it.

Unfortunately, Dad was treating Mom very differently. It soon became obvious that he was mad at her for some unknown reason. I had no idea what was going on in his head, but he was clearly upset with her. There had been no problems the previous time that they had seen each other. I couldn't imagine why he was so disturbed with her now.

Mom had always received the brunt of the blame for Dad not living at home. The truth was that it was Bob and I that had made all of the hard decisions, along with input from his psychiatrist. Even though I had told Dad this on many occasions, he still sometimes took it out on Mom.

I noticed today that every time she said something to him, he had completely ignored her. It broke my heart. Mom had always been there for Dad and she didn't deserve this now. She eventually just sat back and became very quiet, clearly knowing when it was best not to rock the boat.

"Daddy, I want to check your feet," I said. He nodded and seemed completely open to the idea. I pulled the cover up and looked at his feet closely. The swelling had definitely gone down. I was extremely relieved.

This afternoon, we had to leave early as it was going to be a busy day for me. I needed to meet Chris at his school for a book fair. It was the last thing that he had mentioned to me before he left this morning. "Mom, are you coming to school today?" he asked. "Can you buy me a couple of books?" It meant so much to him and I just couldn't let him down.

After I picked Chris up from school, we would be heading over to Athens for a cross country meet. Shawn was racing at 5 p.m. Regardless of everything that was going on, I wanted their lives to continue as routinely as possible. Most of our days seemed unbelievably hectic, but I felt a sense of normalcy was important.

Mom's house next door was slowly starting to come together. Randy and I tried to do something to it every day. Even if the task was a small one, it made us feel like we were ultimately making progress, the work to be done seeming endless. On the weekends, Randy usually spent hours working on it. The dedication that he displayed towards my parents always amazed me.

We probably had another week's worth of work to do before some small pieces of furniture could be moved over. Mom was planning on thinning out her current house and then putting it on the market. Once she sold it, she would then move next door. I had a feeling that it was going to be quite awhile. Her current home was three stories and every inch of it was packed. Her new home was only two stories and a lot less square footage. She would definitely have to get rid of some things. We undoubtedly had a lot of work ahead of us to get Mom moved into her new house. Sometimes, I wondered how we were ever going to manage. I dreamed of the day it would all be behind us.

Friday, October 7, 2011

I closely watched her as we casually made the drive to see him, seeming completely happy. She was dressed nice and had her hair and make-up just right. I knew she did it for him. I thought about how necessary it was to continue on the journey every day, regardless of what had happened on the previous encounter. Mom's last visit was not a good one for her, but it didn't matter. She never once wavered about going back. Inside she may have wondered if Dad's demeanor would be the same, but on the outside, she still showed the same devotion as always.

I knew all too well what she was experiencing, sometimes having to dig so deep. You did it because it was the right thing to do. You simply

431

chalked the behavior up to the horrid disease and continued forward. The Alzheimer's road was a hard one to travel, eventually changing everyone that it came in contact with.

As we arrived at the facility at 11:00 a.m., Dad was still in bed fast asleep. We tried to arouse him, but he was too tired. His eyes fluttered, but he would fall back asleep each time. I pulled his covers down and carefully checked his body, Mom looking on in sorrow as I did. "Vanessa, he looks pathetic," Mom said. "He looks like someone in one of those pictures of a concentration camp."

It was appalling. I quickly found Dad's nurse in the hall. "Has my dad eaten breakfast today?" I asked.

"He ate about a fourth of his breakfast," she replied. "I actually was the one that fed him today."

My dad looked anorexic, nothing but skin and bones. I knew that he had lost a lot of weight during the past year. Prior to him getting sick, his weight had hovered around 195, give or take a few pounds.

"What was his last weight?" I asked the nurse.

She then opened Dad's chart. "He weighed 130.4 on October 4th," she said. "His initial weight when he was first admitted was 140."

I quickly did the math in my head. It was very disturbing. In just 25 days, he had lost almost ten pounds, almost a pound every other day. That also meant that in just over a year, Dad had lost over 64 pounds. He was rapidly withering away to nothing.

"Something needs to happen," I said. "He's wasting away."

"I'll contact the doctor on call," she replied. "He may want to try your dad on some appetite stimulants."

In seven months, my dad's diagnosis had alarmingly gone from early stage dementia to severe dementia in the last stage. His time frame had gone from 5 – 10 years down to 1 – 5 years. The disease was progressing more rapidly than anyone had ever imagined. Everything that was happening to my dad was text book. I inevitably knew what was coming from the vast information that I had read. It was just happening so much quicker than I had ever expected.

Mom and I returned to Dad's room. He was still very tired, but did manage to open his eyes. I kissed his cheek and tenderly held his hand. He soon drifted off again.

The rehab was not going well at all. Dad just didn't seem to have the drive to walk again. It seemed as though all he wanted to do was sleep, always appearing so tired. I had talked to Dad's case manager this afternoon and informed her that he would definitely be moving to Forever Hope Memory Care. She assured me they would do everything they could to make the transition a smooth one. We then discussed ordering a wheelchair for Dad. He had been using one that belonged to the facility, but I thought it was probably time to get him his own. I was slowly coming to the realization that walking again might not be a part of Dad's future.

I was so thankful that he still knew his family. I was also thankful that at times we could still bring a smile to his face. Nothing in the world warmed my heart more than to see my precious father happy.

Tonight, I stood at the kitchen sink doing dishes when I noticed that a car had pulled up in the driveway. I didn't recognize it. Looking down on it through the window, I could see two people inside. As the passenger door opened, I surprisingly watched Preston step out of the car. It was a wonderful sight.

I turned to Shawn who was standing immediately behind me. "Did you know he was coming home?" I asked. He just smiled at me. Preston was home for the weekend and had gone to great lengths to surprise me.

When he came upstairs into the kitchen, I hugged him tightly. His visit couldn't have come at a better time. No words could express the warmth that I felt at that very moment. I held onto my oldest son and hugged him in silence. It was these simple moments that I was coming to appreciate most in life.

Monday, October 10, 2011

I had peacefully lied on the couch with Chris last night as he read to me, covering ourselves with the bone colored afghan. It seemed as though every other page, I'd kiss his cheek. He never got distracted as he was clearly used to this type of behavior from me. Snuggling with him always put my life in perspective.

Before long, the phone suddenly rang. "It's Village Green," Randy said. As I quickly took the phone, I began to feel alarmed. The nurse informed me that my dad had two bedsores, one of them actually a Stage 2 bedsore. "What is being done about them?" I had asked.

"We're going to turn him so that he's lying on the other side and try to keep him that way," she responded. "We've dressed the areas and we'll be keeping an eye on them."

As soon as I had hung up the phone, I did some research on bedsores. That was when I discovered how serious they were. When a bedsore had advanced to Stage 2, it indicated an open wound. Depending on its size, the sore could have possibly already expanded into deeper layers of the skin. At this stage, some of the skin might even be damaged beyond repair. If the bedsore got any worse, it could cause an infection of the underlying bone or even worse, the blood.

As I continued to think about my dad's latest affliction, I became more upset every second. One of the primary causes of bedsores was leaving someone in their bed for an extended period of time without changing their position. That was exactly what was happening to my dad. If they didn't get the bedsores under control, he could be in serious danger.

Today, Randy, Chris and I went to visit Dad. We arrived at 11:30 a.m. and he was again lying in bed. I immediately pulled the covers up above his legs. The bedsores were definitely bandaged, but unfortunately, he was lying on his right side where they were located. The staff had not done what they said they would.

"Daddy, can you hear me?" I asked. This time, I saw no fluttering of his eyelids. I gently caressed his cheek as he was shaking. "Daddy?" He was completely unresponsive.

"Chester, can you open your eyes?" asked Randy, who had now alarmingly moved to Dad's other side. No matter what we tried, we couldn't arouse him. I immediately paged the nurse.

Within a couple of minutes, two nurses entered his room. One of them was the assistant director of nursing whom I had dealt with before.

"Something is wrong," I said. "He won't wake up." One of the nurses then checked his oxygen level which was low. Dad was having a hard time breathing. She quickly hooked him up to oxygen. Meanwhile, the other nurse checked his blood pressure. It too was low.

I stood back to give them room, tearing up as I watched everything unfold. "Did he take his blood pressure medicine this morning?" I asked.

"I'm not sure," she answered. "As soon as I can track down his nurse, I'll find out."

The nurses then carefully turned Dad to his other side so he wasn't resting directly on the bedsores. "Mr. Lee? Mr. Lee?" the nurse called. Dad still didn't respond.

After about ten minutes, his nurse entered the room. "Did you give Mr. Lee his medicine this morning?" the assistant director asked.

"No," she replied. "He's been asleep all morning."

"Was his blood pressure checked this morning?" I questioned.

"It was a little low," she responded, visibly starting to appear uncomfortable.

"I don't understand," I said. "You determined his blood pressure was low, but you didn't do anything about it? Did you tell anyone?"

She just shook her head no. I couldn't believe it. Apparently, the nurse had made the decision not to give him his blood pressure medications, but didn't notify anyone of his blood pressure. Why? She soon backed up against the wall and stood there silently.

Through it all, Dad continued to lie in the bed completely unresponsive. "You need to contact the doctor," I exclaimed. "Something is not right."

"I just did," the other nurse said. "He's not on the premises right now. I'm just waiting for him to get back to us."

"What are our options right now?" I asked.

"We need to run some tests on your father," she replied. "We can draw the blood here. Unfortunately, we have to send it out to a lab to get it processed. We're not equipped to do that here. You're talking at least a 24-hour turnaround. If we go ahead and do it now, we should have the results some time tomorrow." I really didn't feel comfortable about this news.

"The other option is to take him to the emergency room," she continued. "They would be able to run the tests a lot more quickly than we can. Once I talk to the doctor and get him up-to-date with your father's condition, he'll be able to advise us on what he thinks we should do."

We continued to stay by Dad's side as I gently stroked his cheek. He was currently getting the oxygen that he needed. I knew the lack of it could have serious ramifications. I hoped that was the cause of his unresponsiveness. I nervously looked at Randy. "I'm not sure what to do," I said.

"Why don't we take Chris home?" he replied. "He doesn't need to be here. Hopefully, by the time we get there, they will have heard back from the doctor. Then, we can make a decision." He then hugged me as I continued to watch my daddy.

"Mom, why won't Papa wake up?" Chris asked. He was rubbing Dad's arm, but Dad wasn't moving.

"I'm not sure, sweetheart," I replied. "He must be really tired." I gently kissed my dad on the forehead and whispered "I love you, Daddy" into his ear.

On the way out, we ran into my dad's nurse. "We need to take my son home," I stated.

"I'm so sorry," she said, as she hugged me. She then looked me directly in the eyes. "What is that perfume that you have on? I love it!"

My mind drew a complete blank. I had been wearing this perfume for many years. It was by far my favorite, but I couldn't for the life of me remember the name. "I can't think of the name right now," I replied.

On the drive home, I thought about the nurse's last comment, striking me as unbelievably phony. Here I was worried sick over my dad and all she could think to say was that she liked my perfume. And then it popped into my head. The perfume was Champs Elysees by Guerlain.

As soon as I got home, I urgently called the rehab facility back. It was now 3:40 p.m. I tracked the assistant director of nursing down. "Has the doctor called you back yet?" I asked.

"No, we're still waiting," she replied.

"I don't want to wait any longer," I said. "I want my dad taken to the emergency room immediately." In the short ride home, I had made the necessary decision. I felt this facility had neglected my father and I blamed them for his current condition. I sure wasn't going to depend on them to fix it. I had now lost all faith in Village Green.

I continued to call the facility every hour. My dad wasn't transported until 6 p.m. He was then taken to Brookview Hospital.

Hours later, I found out the disturbing results. They were not good. Dad had aspiration pneumonia. They found fluid in his right lung, fairly certain it was caused by aspiration which was probably caused by the dementia. He also had sepsis throughout his body, a complication related to the bedsores which was probably caused by the constant lying in bed.

Dad was not doing well at all. The decision to send him to the hospital when we did was the right thing to do. I felt confident that he was in good hands now. I shuddered to think what would have happened had we not seen him today.

I then closed my eyes and did the only thing left to do. I prayed. I prayed that it wasn't my dad's time. I prayed that God would save him and not take him from us. I couldn't bear to lose him. It was all in God's hands now. We desperately needed a miracle.

Tuesday, October 11, 2011

My heart caught in my throat as I cautiously walked into the room, not at all prepared for what I saw. My dad looked like a stranger. He was hooked up to oxygen, but was still having a hard time breathing. I could hear him as he struggled with every breath. He glanced over at me for a second and then soon looked away. I couldn't tell if he knew me or not.

The doctor soon came into the room. She was a petite Indian woman and very attractive. She politely introduced herself to me and firmly shook my hand. Her voice was very soft, but her demeanor was clearly one of authority.

"How is he doing?" I asked.

"I started your father on antibiotics," she replied. "The pneumonia has now spread into both of his lungs. There is also fluid in his heart." She paused as I took this latest news in.

"His kidneys have begun to shut down," she continued slowly. "He can no longer breathe on his own. He has to have the oxygen mask. He also has two bedsores. One is on his right foot and the other is on his right hip. The bedsores may be responsible for the sepsis which has spread throughout his body." I held onto the bed rail for support, the news devastating.

"His heart enzyme count is very high," the doctor explained. "It indicates that he will most likely have a heart attack. The blood tests also showed that your father has heart disease." That was the only thing so far that hadn't surprised me since the bypass surgery had only taken care of three of his arteries.

"Your father hasn't been able to talk yet," she said. "At times, he appears to be having chest pains. We've started giving him morphine to keep him comfortable."

My eyes soon filled with tears. Everything the doctor had just said left me feeling completely stunned, my dad not doing well at all. As I stood there watching him, my heart was breaking like never before.

"We are still doing everything that we can for your father," she stated. "I'm sorry to have to ask you this. I know you've just received a lot of information at one time. There is a good chance that your father could have a heart attack. If that happens, we need to know whether you want him designated as DNR. Would you want us to resuscitate him?"

I just stared blankly at her, unable to ask the many questions swirling in my head.

"Choosing whether your father is DNR or not only affects whether you want him resuscitated if he stops breathing or has a heart attack," she replied. "It has no bearing on the day-to-day treatment that we provide for him. It only has to do with emergency CPR. We would still continue to give him medication and treat all of his conditions."

"I'm not sure I understand," I said. "Why would we ever want to make him DNR?"

"It has to do with the quality of life," she responded. "If your father had a heart attack and he was not DNR, then we would attempt to resuscitate him. The longer that it took, the longer his brain would go without oxygen. There would come a point where the damage would be too extensive and the quality of his life afterwards would have been compromised. You have to decide whether you want your father to potentially live in that state. Is that what he would want?"

I was overwhelmed. "I need to talk to my mom and brother about this," I replied.

"That's fine," she said. "It's a big decision. Right now, we will resuscitate him if we need to. You just let me know what you decide." She was such a kind and compassionate woman. "I'll come back in a little bit and check on your father." She then walked out of the room.

I looked over at my daddy and started crying. It was not looking good. Nothing had prepared me for this moment. He looked completely different from the last time that I had seen him, seemingly dying right before my very eyes.

As the day progressed, he continued to look around the room restlessly. He had large medical mitts on both hands to keep him from pulling on any of the tubes. He wasn't talking and he certainly wasn't smiling. I had now been here for a couple of hours and I still didn't think he recognized me.

I then called Mom and Bob to let them know how Dad was doing. I hated to be the bearer of bad news, but they needed to know. I would bring Mom back with me to the hospital tomorrow.

A little while later, Bob walked into the room. He quickly walked up to Dad's side, but Dad didn't seem to recognize him either. I conveyed everything that the doctor had told me in detail to Bob. I then told him about the DNR decision that we ultimately needed to make. He was very quiet as he sat down in the chair by the window, undoubtedly as overwhelmed as I was.

About an hour later, Randy also entered the room. I had called him earlier and told him that Dad wasn't doing well. Randy immediately walked up to him. A few strands of Dad's hair had fallen down on his forehead. Randy gently brushed them back and started caressing his hair. Dad suddenly looked up at him with such love in his eyes. Randy was the only person today that Dad seemed to recognize. I stood back and watched this incredible moment unfold, the special bond between them so apparent. Once again, I teared up. To witness such love between my husband and my father was a gift from God. It moved me beyond words.

At this point in time, Dad was still not able to swallow. Until the doctor was certain that he could, she wouldn't allow him to drink anything. He was very dehydrated and his lips were dry. The nurse had previously shown me some medical sponge sticks that could be used with Dad to help quench his thirst. Randy took one of the sticks and soaked the sponge part in water. He then put it in Dad's mouth. Dad immediately sucked it, trying to get as much of the water from it as he could. Randy refilled the sponge with water and went through the same process several times, the sight reminding me of a mother bird feeding her young.

I stayed by Dad's side all day. He had remained alert the entire time. Although, I still wasn't sure he even knew who I was. So much was currently going wrong with Dad's body. I felt terrified that he wasn't going to make it.

Later that day, the doctor came back into Dad's room. She had scheduled an MRI for Dad earlier in the day. Based on the blood work that was initially completed on Dad, she suspected that he might have had a stroke. "The MRI results came back," she said. "It showed that your father did not have a stroke. This is good news." For the first time today, I felt a small ray of hope.

"I wanted to ask you something," I said to the doctor. Ever since I had found out my dad's condition, I couldn't stop thinking about us finding Dad unresponsive yesterday. What would have happened if we hadn't gotten Dad to the hospital when we had? Would we have received a phone call saying that he hadn't made it? I needed to know the answers. "If we hadn't found Dad yesterday when we did and he hadn't been brought to the hospital, do you think he would have died? How long do you think he would have survived with everything that was happening in his body?"

She looked at me with such a serious look on her face. "If you hadn't gotten him to the hospital when you did," she said, "he would have probably died in 1 – 2 days."

I then looked back towards my dad, tears streaming down my cheeks as I thought of how close we may have come to losing him. He still wasn't out of the woods yet, but at least here, he had a fighting chance. As small as it was, I felt determined to hold onto it with all my might. The thought of losing my precious daddy was unbearable.

Wednesday, October 12, 2011

I had been going through the motions ever since I had left my father, but my heart just wasn't in it. I made dinner last night for my family, but couldn't remember what we had. This morning, as Chris got ready for school, we had watched one of his favorite shows. I couldn't recall any lines from it though. I felt numb and empty inside.

Today the doctor gave us the grim news that all family members needed to make arrangements to come to the hospital as soon as possible. It might be their last chance as my dad's health was worsening. I called my uncles and let them know. They were going to try to fly up tomorrow.

The hospital had run more blood tests on my dad. His heart enzyme count was actually higher today than it was yesterday, the doctor feeling certain that he was going to have a heart attack.

I also found out that Dad tested positive for MRSA. He was checked when they initially admitted him into the emergency room. Since it was so contagious, anyone entering his room was advised to put on a paper gown and mask. In all the times Dad had been admitted into a hospital, he had never before tested positive. It was hard to tell where he contracted it, but my bet was on the last facility.

I walked up to Dad and gently kissed his forehead, his eyes open and somewhat alert. He would only look at me for a few seconds before he would swiftly look off in another direction, still very restless and continuing to move about. My heart was aching. I just couldn't stand to let go of him, but he looked so frail and tired. I didn't want him to suffer anymore.

I pulled up a stool next to Dad's bed so I could sit near him. I closed my eyes and begged God to allow Dad's brain to come back at least long enough for all of his family to tell him the things that would bring him comfort one last time.

A little while later, the doctor came back into the room. "Have you made a decision about whether you want your father to be DNR or not?" she asked.

I slowly shook my head yes. "We've talked about it and decided that we don't want my dad to suffer," I said. "It wouldn't be fair to him." I took a deep breath. "Change his status to DNR." With that, I lost my composure. As much as I knew it was the humane thing to do for my dad, I felt like I was giving up on him. It hurt so much to let go.

Later that day, Frances and her daughter came by the hospital. Frances had been a loyal friend to my parents for years. She immediately walked up to my dad. "Hi Mr. Lee," she said. Dad looked at her, but then quickly looked away. He didn't appear to recognize her.

I remembered how many times she had come to my parents' home to witness to them, even going to Arbor Forest several times and doing the same. She then walked over to me and tenderly took my hand in hers. Something had bothered me for days. "Do you think that my dad is saved?" I asked. I could once again feel the tears building up inside.

"Your father and I had talked a lot about dying," she replied. "He was very afraid of death." Then she smiled at me. "There is no doubt in my mind that the next time I see your Dad, it will be rejoicing in Heaven." I then hugged her tightly. As the tears fell down my face, I thanked God that he had placed her in my parents' path.

Later that afternoon, I called Village Green and informed them that my dad wouldn't be returning. They were holding the bed for him, but he absolutely wasn't coming back. I didn't know if he would pull through this or not, but I sure as hell wouldn't ever take him there again. They had almost killed him once. They wouldn't get a second chance.

An hour later, I left the hospital to pick Chris up from school. Then, the two of us drove to Village Green for the last time. We quickly made our way to Dad's room, finding it exactly as we had left it. I had brought several plastic bags with me to pack Dad's belongings. While in his closet, I ran across his favorite shirt, the blue one with white stripes that zipped up the front. I had so many wonderful memories of him in it. I held it up to my nose and slowly breathed in Dad's scent. I then closed my eyes and felt a tear fall down my cheek. I would be taking this shirt to my home as I wanted it with me always.

His roommate was sitting in his usual spot near the window. "How is your Dad doing?" he asked.

I stopped packing and looked directly at him. "He's not doing very well at all," I replied sadly. "He's actually in very serious condition."

"They don't take care of us here," he said. "They just leave us alone and neglect us." I nodded my head in agreement, remembering it wasn't that long ago that his daughter had said the exact same thing to me. "I hope your dad will be okay." I then smiled at him. He had turned out to be a very nice man after all.

As I continued to pack Dad's things, the assistant director of nursing came in. "How is your father doing?" she inquired.

"He is in critical condition," I replied. She just stared at me in shock. "Right now, there is fluid in both of his lungs and his heart. Sepsis has spread throughout his body. His kidneys have begun to shut down. He can't breathe on his own. They think that at any minute, he could have a heart attack." She didn't say a word.

"My father is dying," I said. "You all just let him lie here and never checked on him. You let it go on for too long. You should have done something about it sooner. Now it may be too late."

When it was obvious that she had no response, I turned around and continued to pack. I then heard her walk out of the room. How could they not have known how serious it was? How could she have looked so surprised at his condition?

When I finished packing, I said my goodbyes to Dad's roommate. Then, Chris and I each took a bag to carry to the car. As we walked out the front door, I felt a tremendous amount of anger at so many within its walls. I didn't know what the future would hold for my father, but I knew one thing for sure. He would never pass this threshold again.

Thursday, October 13, 2011

As I walked through the double doors, the first thing I saw was the sign on the wall near his name. In bold, black letters, it read "DNR", my heart skipping a beat as I stopped for a moment and stared. Somehow seeing it in black and white really hit home how close we could be to losing Dad.

When I stepped into his hospital room, Dad was awake and very alert as he looked over at me. He still didn't smile, but he didn't look away. I thought for a brief second that he might just know who I was.

"Hi Daddy," I said. "Are you doing okay?" He continued to stare at me. I then got one of the medical sponge sticks and soaked it in water, placing it on his lips as he eagerly opened his mouth. He was so parched. I then ran it over his tongue. I rewet the sponge and put it in his mouth to start the process again.

The doctor soon came in and smiled at me. "I have some good news," she said. "Your father's body has started responding to the antibiotics. It looks like the sepsis is under control, as well as the pneumonia."

"Really?" I asked. She happily shook her head yes as I stared at her in disbelief. I could feel my eyes filling with tears. This time though, they were tears of joy.

"In addition, his kidneys are looking better and he's breathing easier," she continued. "I'm going to keep him on the antibiotic and intravenous fluids. Also, I'll be adding a medication to help clear up the fluid in his lungs. Your father has improved a lot during the past 24 hours."

I looked back at my dad, realizing that a miracle had happened. God had answered our prayers. "That is the best news possible," I said. "Thank you so much, doctor."

As she was walking out of the room, I called after her. "I'm not ready to give up on my daddy," I stated. "I no longer want him to be DNR." She slowly nodded her head. As she walked through the door, I saw her take the sign down.

Dad appeared coherent several times today. He was also speaking for the first time in days. At one point, Mom asked him if he was in any pain and he answered her "No". Another time I had asked Dad if he knew who I was and he said "Sure". They were such simple responses, but had meant the world to us. They were just what we had waited for, signs of hope.

Later that afternoon, the nurse decided to get Dad sitting up in a chair. It seemed very ambitious, but she was determined. In order to do it, she had to get Dad to move his legs, which were currently bent and seemed to be locked in that position. As the nurse carefully tried to get him to stretch his right leg out, he suddenly said "Honey, Honey". It was so hard to watch as he was in terrible pain.

She continued to work with him and eventually was able to get Dad up. She then moved him into a chair where he calmly stayed for about an hour, leaving me completely amazed. My dad was sitting in a chair right next to my mom and me. We actually watched a judge show on television together. I never would have expected it when I got up this morning. What a difference a day had made!

While we were sitting together, he asked for water two different times. Unfortunately, the nurse had already said that he couldn't have any until they tested him to make sure he could swallow properly. I absolutely hated having to tell him no, his eyes appearing so sad. The speech therapist was scheduled to evaluate him again for sipping water. In addition, if the doctor could get the pneumonia completely cleared up and get him off of the oxygen mask, then the therapist might even try Dad on eating something soft.

He looked better today than he had ever since we had found him unresponsive that dreaded day. I felt an incredible warmth inside of me. God was so good. I knew it was going to be a long road ahead, but today was a positive step. I felt so blessed to have experienced it with my dad. My prayer was that he continued to improve with each passing day. For the first time in awhile, I felt hope from above.

Saturday, October 15, 2011

He immediately walked up to him and smiled, his little face full of exuberance. "Hi Papa," he said. Dad looked at Chris for a few seconds before looking away. He didn't appear to recognize him. I then looked at Chris and could tell by the look on his face that he was heartbroken, his little chin beginning to quiver. It was the first time that his Papa had not known who he was.

Shawn, Chris and I all continued to talk to Dad in hopes of his memory suddenly coming back. After about fifteen minutes, he still hadn't recognized any of us. As I moved the stool right next to Dad's bed, Chris hopped up on it. Dad was currently facing the other way looking out the window. As soon as he turned his head and laid eyes on Chris for the second time, something inside of him clicked. He smiled big and said "Lil' Monkey". It was music to my ears. Not only did he recognize Chris, but it was the first time that I had seen him smile in over a week. I looked over at Chris and he was beaming. It was such a sweet moment. God had given Dad back to us this afternoon for a brief instance in time.

The nurse soon came into the room to check on Dad. "Did the speech therapist test him yesterday for swallowing?" I asked.

"She did," the nurse responded. "She tried to get him to swallow some water. Unfortunately, he wasn't able to do it. The doctor is concerned about him being dehydrated and malnourished. For the time being, he'll continue on intravenous fluids."

We remained at the hospital for a couple of hours. Unfortunately, I didn't think Dad ever remembered Shawn or me during the visit. We witnessed no more telling moments of recognition as there had been with Chris. It was one of those rare and special moments of clarity that God sometimes gave Dad.

Before long, he fell asleep. The nurse mentioned that he was more restless at night which explained Dad currently feeling so tired. I attributed it to the Sundowner's, never letting up.

While I visited with Dad yesterday, I had written a letter documenting all of the incidents that had occurred at the last rehabilitation facility. Looking back, they were very lax with my dad's care. For the past several weeks, it seemed they just let him lie in bed all day. He had developed some bedsores which possibly caused sepsis which in turn caused the shutdown to some major organs. He had come very close to dying. If we hadn't stepped in and directed them to send my dad to the emergency room on Monday, he very likely could have died.

Today, I had sent the letter to a law firm that specialized in elderly neglect cases. The rehab facility was supposed to help my dad. They were supposed to take care of him. We had put our complete trust in them and they had let us down. I cringed at the thought of anyone else having to go through what my dad was going through. The next patient might not be found in time. Dad was clearly neglected at this facility and they should be held accountable for it. I would once again be my dad's voice.

Sunday, October 16, 2011

As we casually drove down the road, I looked over at Randy. "Thank you for coming with me today," I said. I knew of so many things at home that he had wanted to take care of this weekend. In the end though, he had put Dad first. He gently took my hand in his and brought it up to his lips and kissed it.

"Your dad has always been there for us," he replied. "Now it's our turn to be there for him. He needs us." I gratefully smiled at my husband.

"I love your dad, Vanessa," he continued, his voice starting to tremble. "He's always treated me like a son." With that, he suddenly teared up. Neither one of us knew what tomorrow would bring. What I did know was that I would never face it alone. Randy was my rock. He had been from the start. I couldn't imagine going through this without him by my side.

As Randy and I later walked into Dad's room, Dad immediately said "Hi" in a long, drawn out voice. It was such a happy tone without the slightest hesitation. Dad was sitting upright in his bed and had a huge grin on his face. He knew exactly who we were. It almost felt as though he was waiting for us.

"Hey Gump," Randy said as he walked up beside him. I then moved to his other side and tenderly kissed Dad's forehead. He was smiling. He was actually smiling.

I never knew from one day to the next what state I would find Dad in. Today's greeting was so unexpected. For a little while, he looked like his old self, just further proof to never ever give up.

Dad wasn't able to speak much today, other than a few one word responses, but he had clearly looked happy and peaceful. He had improved dramatically as far as his physical issues were concerned. His lungs, heart and kidneys were all looking better. The sepsis was also under control. I had hoped that once all of the infection was out of his body that his mind would return to the state it was in two weeks ago. Unfortunately, that hadn't happened yet.

The doctor had come in and talked to us about different feeding options for Dad as he still wasn't able to swallow on his own. Inserting a feeding tube in his stomach was out of the question. It would require anesthesia and he wouldn't survive it without further damage. The only other option was a feeding tube inserted into his nose which seemed to me very invasive. "Something needs to be done," I said. "He hasn't had anything besides fluids in a week. That can't be good for him. His body needs more than that."

I didn't like the idea of someone inserting a tube into Dad's nose, but I felt we had no choice. "Can you go ahead and start that process?" I asked.

"Absolutely," she replied. "I'll go ahead and get everything ready."

Later that night, Dad got a feeding tube inserted into his nose. They immediately started giving him Glucerna. I truly hoped that his body would absorb the nutrients and actually use them to his benefit. He was so malnourished and had gone without food for so long. I prayed that it wasn't too late.

Monday, October 17, 2011

He cried out in sheer agony several times as she tried to turn him. It was so hard to watch. His right leg was extremely sore. The nurses had to carefully turn Dad every two hours because of the bedsores. Mom and I were there today while they did it. We had witnessed them turning him before, but for some reason it seemed to be getting worse. At times, I had to look away.

Today was not as promising as some of the others were. I had a difficult time connecting with Dad. We would be looking at each other and then he would suddenly look away as if I wasn't there. He was also very restless. I tried talking to him throughout the day, but he just didn't seem to respond.

The feeding tube in Dad's nose was clearly bothering him. They had to keep the mitts on his hands so that he wouldn't pull it out. As restless as he was, I had no doubt that he would have had he not been wearing them.

The speech therapist was scheduled to test Dad with some food. She'd carefully watch where it went as he ate it to determine if he was aspirating. If he failed this test, then the only possible method he would have to get any nourishment would be through the tube. Based on how he looked today, that option just didn't feel right.

This afternoon, a woman from Humanity Hospice Care came by the room and introduced herself, wanting to discuss Dad's care. She had caught me off guard as I really wasn't ready to discuss hospice yet. I definitely needed some time to absorb it. We decided to meet tomorrow morning instead. Just the word hospice brought so many sad images to my mind. I had a hard time admitting that that might be where Dad currently was.

As I continued to watch my dad, the thought went through my head that this was not a quality life for him. Was God trying to prepare me for something? I hoped that the Glucerna would help his body to recover. I knew that it was just a temporary measure as it wouldn't be right to sustain his life indefinitely with a feeding tube. The crucial factor in getting Dad past this point would be whether his brain could remember how to swallow. Everything would be contingent on that. So far, he had failed every test he had taken. I truly hoped that tomorrow's would be different.

I felt so emotionally drained after today's visit. I knew that God was ultimately in control, feeling very strongly that He was leading this journey. I just wasn't sure where it was heading. Dad hadn't shown any improvement in days. Even so, I still held onto hope. My job wasn't to make those tough decisions. It was to be there for Dad and never give up. And I wouldn't. As long as he had fleeting moments of clarity, I would hold onto the belief that God wasn't ready for him to go just yet. When that time finally came, whenever it was, it would be God's call and not mine.

Later that evening, I began flipping through some of the literature about the hospice facility. On one of the pages was a quote. "How we handle our own crises shows our strength. How we handle those around us having crises shows our compassion." I hoped that one day Dad would be able to look at this difficult road that we had travelled on and be proud of how I had handled things. I hoped that he would understand the reasoning behind all of the tough decisions that were made. Most of all, I hoped that throughout all the ups and downs, the one thing that would stand out to him above all else would be how much I loved him.

Tuesday, October 18, 2011

As my eyes opened for the first time this morning, I felt re-energized, like I'd received a new outlook while sleeping. I knew one thing for sure. I wasn't ready to give up on my dad. I wanted him to live more than ever. I knew that when the time finally came to actually let him go, it was going to kill me. As I prayed this morning, I told God that I just couldn't do it. If He was ready to take my dad, He needed to hit me over the head with a brick. Otherwise, I wouldn't see it.

On the way to the hospital, the ring of my cell phone startled me. I recognized the phone number as that of Dad's case manager at Village Green. She had repeatedly called and left messages ever since Dad was first taken to the emergency room, the voice messages all the same. She was concerned about Dad's health and wanted to check how he was doing. She was actually a very sweet woman and I truly believed that she genuinely cared about Dad. I just wasn't emotionally up to talking to anyone from the rehab facility. Based on potential legal action, I knew that I'd need to refrain from saying too much. I honestly wasn't sure I could do that in my current state. I decided once again to let the call roll over to voice mail.

Dad had received Glucerna for two full days, the protein level in his body still very low. The doctor wasn't sure whether his body would use the nutrients or not. Unfortunately, he was so malnourished that the damage may have already been deemed irreversible. All they could do was give him the nutrients. Whether his body would use them and recover was out of their hands. Only time would tell.

He had also been very restless for the past two days, the feeding tube definitely bothering him. The only time he had really looked comfortable was when he was sleeping. I didn't know if Dad knew who we were today or not. At one point, it seemed like he recognized Mom's voice, but I wasn't sure he ever remembered me.

Dad was taken to radiology this morning to have a Barium Swallow test. He wouldn't open his mouth, so unfortunately they couldn't perform the test. In essence, he had failed it. This was not good news. The hospital felt as though they had done everything they could for Dad and his hospital care was slowly coming to an end. We needed to make a decision as to where he would go next.

At 10:30, Mom and I met with the woman from Humanity Hospice Care. I had dreaded the meeting ever since it had been initially set up. We originally wanted Dad to come home. Unfortunately, we were informed that hospice would not provide for someone coming out to their home every day. It would mean that the bulk of Dad's care would rest on Mom and me. We would need to manage his feeding tube and medications, in addition to dressing his bedsores and turning him every couple of hours. My hectic schedule wouldn't always allow me to be there. I didn't think that Mom could take care of Dad on her own.

"There is another option," the hospice representative explained. "Your father does qualify for inpatient hospice care. We have a facility not far from here. There are nurses and doctors there 24/7 that would be able to help with your father's medical needs and his care. He would have his own room and you all would be able to be with him anytime. Even his dog would be welcome."

"Would he be able to continue being fed through the feeding tube?" I asked.

"Absolutely," she replied. "If that is what you want to happen, we could continue that."

"What if he got better?" I then asked. "What if a miracle happened and he was able to remember how to swallow again? What would happen then?"

"Hospice isn't just for someone that only has a few days left," she responded. "Your father qualifies because his doctor feels he has less than six months to live. That's not to say that he couldn't survive longer. Our goal is to make him as comfortable as possible during his remaining time. If he was able to learn how to eat again and it changed his prognosis, then he eventually would need to be moved to another facility." She looked back and forth between the two of us as this news set in.

"I want to give you both some time to discuss this alone," the hospice rep said. "I'm going to make a phone call. I'll come back in a little bit." With that, she walked out of the room.

Mom and I carefully weighed the different options, both of us agreeing we just couldn't provide the level of care that the hospice facility could. I still held out hope that Dad could somehow remember how to eat again. In order for that to happen, we needed the expertise of a professional. By choosing the hospice facility, Dad would have that.

Before long, the rep returned to Dad's room. "We've decided to have him moved to the hospice facility," I said, my voice cracking.

She then compassionately took my hands in hers. "I promise you that we'll take good care of your father," she replied. "I know this is hard. You are doing the right thing." I then helped Mom sign all of the necessary paperwork.

"I noticed that your father is not DNR right now," she continued. "What do you want his status to be at the hospice facility?"

I absolutely hated facing this decision once again. This time, we had decided to put God in charge. "Make my dad's status DNR," I said. It was a decision that I had battled with so many times. In the end though, I had to do what was right for Dad.

Later that evening, Dad was discharged from the hospital and transferred by ambulance to the hospice facility which was conveniently only a couple of miles away. He was currently resting peacefully in his new room. The doctor had already seen him and was planning on testing Dad's ability to eat tomorrow. If at all possible, they were going to try to feed him. If Dad wasn't able to swallow, they would continue the Glucerna through the feeding tube in his nose. I knew he didn't like that. I prayed it wouldn't be necessary.

The test tomorrow was going to be pivotal, everything hinging on its success. If Dad wasn't able to swallow tomorrow, then he probably never would.

Wednesday, October 19, 2011

I was still filled with such hope through it all. We were driving to a hospice facility to see my father and I still felt hope. I knew that things were now at a different level and the situation was a critical one, but it just wasn't within me to ever give up on him.

As Mom and I walked into his room, he was lying in bed sound asleep.

The room was on the first floor and was huge, containing several chairs, a television on the wall and a private bathroom. A large window on the far wall provided a beautiful view.

Dad appeared very peaceful and didn't seem to be in any pain. They currently had him on morphine three times a day to keep him comfortable. He was still receiving Glucerna through the feeding tube in his nose, the protein level in his body remaining very low. It was questionable whether the Glucerna would actually make a difference.

Dad was unsuccessful in his attempt at eating earlier today. He had ultimately lost the ability to swallow properly. It didn't appear that it would be coming back. In the days to come, we would have to make the painful decision whether or not to remove the tube. The doctor would be leaving that up to us. I knew that Dad was not doing well, but I was still not at that point.

Dad was currently lying in the bed on his back, his legs not nearly as bent as they had been in the hospital. It meant that the nurses wouldn't have to turn him every couple of hours. The ordeal was a very painful one for my dad. I was happy with anything that reduced his suffering.

Before long, one of the staff members entered the room. She needed to change Dad and also redress his bedsores. Mom and I were politely asked to wait outside. As we sat on one of the couches in the lobby, the undeniable serenity that surrounded us left me amazed. I had gotten so used to the noisy environment at the hospital and previous rehab facility. This place was completely different, so quiet and tranquil.

Upon returning to the room, Mom put the television on. She excitedly found an old movie and thought Dad might like it. He was in and out of sleep the entire day. When he was awake, he didn't seem to notice the TV, remaining fixated on the view from the window in his room. The sun was currently shining in and Dad was soaking up every bit of it with his eyes.

I periodically would sit next to him and gently caress his hand in mine. He never said a word or smiled, just looked around. I doubted very seriously that he knew his daughter was sitting next to him. How was my daddy supposed to know that I hadn't abandoned him if he couldn't even recognize me? I felt like a stranger as the tears ran down my face.

Mom and I remained by Dad's side all day. He was so different the last few days. Physically, he was doing so much better. Mentally, he just wasn't there. He didn't seem to know his family anymore. We were just taking things one day at a time, my heart beyond broken. I still couldn't comprehend letting go of him. As long as he had a breath in his body, my hope would remain alive.

Thursday, October 20, 2011

She slowly walked into the room, steam rising above her cup of hot chocolate. As she sat down, looking so calm, she then pulled out her book. Every few seconds, she'd lovingly glance up at him. After a few moments had passed, she'd then return to her reading. I wondered if she truly understood the severity of what was happening. Dad had remained much the same as he had yesterday. Mom and I had sat with him for a couple of hours now. I still detected no recognition on his part, simply lying in bed peacefully. I softly kissed him on his cheek before leaving his side.

A meeting had been scheduled this morning with the doctor and his staff. As Mom and I walked into the conference room, we were amiably greeted by several people. Not only was the doctor present, but one of the nurses, the case manager, the office manager and a couple of volunteers were there as well. The chaplain was also seated at the table. It was his presence that saddened me the most. I knew but one reason for him to be there.

The doctor soon began the meeting, covering the medications he was giving to Dad, his daily care and the feeding attempts. He had a very kind demeanor and tried to be very honest with us. As he began talking about Dad's feeding tube, it became obvious that he was not in agreement with it.

"I cannot tell you what to do," he said. "If it was me, I would remove the feeding tube from your father's nose and allow him to die with dignity. Believe me. He gets absolutely no enjoyment or taste from the tube in his nose. It is sustaining him by giving him something he cannot get on his own." I had honestly never looked at it that way.

He then paused a moment before cautiously approaching the next subject. "There is something that we often do with patients that can no longer eat on their own," the doctor continued. "We feed them with a spoon. It's usually soft foods like ice cream or pudding. Your father can't swallow, but he can still taste. Even though there is a danger that he could aspirate, we feel it's worth the risk to give him something that comforts him. Our goal is to make his remaining time as comfortable as possible. Allowing your father to taste food is something that may give him a lot of pleasure."

"Are you saying that he doesn't have much time left?" I asked. No sooner had I gotten the words out than the tears started falling. The office manager walked over and kindheartedly handed me a tissue.

"I can't tell you how long he has," he replied. "No one knows that. All I can tell you is what I would do in the same situation. The truth is I once was in that same predicament with one of my parents. I made that hard choice. I can tell you from my personal experience that the look on my father's face as he recognized and savored the ice cream on his tongue was one I'll never forget or regret."

"It is a terrible situation to be faced with," he continued. "You have to ask yourself what your Dad would want. Would he want to be kept alive by a tube in his nose? I personally don't believe that is the right thing to do, but it isn't my father lying in there."

I was at such a loss. Was the feeding tube more for me than it was for my dad? I kept telling myself that it was to give him a chance in case he remembered how to swallow at a later point. Now, I wasn't so sure. If something could give my dad some pleasure, shouldn't I allow that? How could I deprive my dad of this? "I need some time to think about this," I said.

"You don't need to make a decision right now," he replied. "Give it some thought and talk to everyone that needs to be involved. If you decide that you want us to feed your father with a spoon, we'll remove the feeding tube. You need to understand though that once it is removed, we will not put it in again. It would be too uncomfortable for your father and just wouldn't be humane to put him through that."

As we gradually walked back towards Dad's room, I felt depleted. It was a very sad meeting, the doctor very clear on his standing. Did he know more than he was saying? I didn't want to give up on my dad, but I didn't want him to suffer either. I was so torn.

When we walked in the door, I noticed that Dad was awake and looking out the window, staring into the sunlight. I walked around the bed to the other side in the direction that he was looking. My dad suddenly looked up at me and without the slightest hesitation said "Hey sweetheart" just as he had done a million other times in my life. My heart skipped a beat. I felt as though I couldn't breathe.

"Hey Daddy," I responded. "I love you." I smiled at him as tears filled my eyes. His words had been so effortless. As I stared into the eyes of my precious daddy, I had no doubt that he knew exactly who I was.

A short time later, the moment had passed, but it didn't matter. For a little while, my dad had come back to me and it was just him and I sharing that special moment. No one would ever be able to take that away from me. When the time finally came for my dad to leave us, he would go knowing that I had been by his side.

An hour later, Mom and I were standing next to Dad's bed. I looked over at her and she blew my dad a kiss with her lips. I then looked back at my dad and what I saw was yet another miracle. He put his lips together and tried to blow a kiss back to my mom. I knew in that moment that Dad understood without a doubt that he was staring at his wife. He would have never done that with anyone else but her. He then smiled lovingly at my mother.

This morning, I had begged God to show me a sign. For the past four days, we didn't know if Dad knew us or not. For a few minutes today, all of that had changed. God had given him back to us just long enough to share the special love between us one more time. It was a miracle and a blessing that I would cherish forever.

Friday, October 21, 2011

An eerie feeling enveloped me as I walked down the long hall of the funeral home. Peering into the rooms on each side, I imagined the events that took place in them. They were currently all empty, but I knew that tomorrow, they might very well be occupied. A lot of sadness occurred within these walls.

Mom and I had decided to meet with the funeral director this morning at 10:00 a.m. We had put it off for awhile and decided to go ahead and take care of it today, truly hoping that we wouldn't actually be using them anytime soon. I just wanted to have all of the decisions behind us.

We provided all of the necessary information to the director. When the time came, we wanted Dad to be buried in Georgia National Cemetery in Canton. Dad had told me several times that he absolutely did not want to be cremated. I had promised him every time the subject had come up that we would honor his wishes.

The director confirmed what we had already been told previously. We needed Dad's discharge papers from his time in the Air Force. In order to be buried in a national cemetery, we had to prove that Dad had been honorably discharged and that he had served during wartime. We explained that we were still trying to locate the papers.

Then, we made our way into the massive showroom. We eventually chose a slate blue casket with a light blue insert. On the inside of the casket was a picture of Heaven with the words "In God's Care". Dad wouldn't have wanted anything fancy. I think he would be happy with all of our choices today.

We then went back to my parents' home. Mom had taken Dad's discharge papers months earlier and secretly hidden them. Unfortunately, she couldn't remember where. I had come over on two previous occasions and searched for them to no avail.

I had even contacted the VA office, but a tragic fire had long since destroyed my dad's records. They were having to reconstruct the records from other offices. I had filled out a form a month ago specifying the city that Dad joined the service in, the city he was discharged from and the appropriate dates, but I had never heard back from them. I had asked Mom several times, but she couldn't remember receiving anything in the mail. It was turning into a nightmare.

I soon started searching the house. The first item I looked for was a response from the VA's office. I found several piles of old mail in the family room. After about fifteen minutes, I actually found the letter I was looking for. Apparently, something on my initial application was amiss. I then made a phone call to their office, but the clerk informed me that it needed to be done in writing. Before I went down that discouraging road again, I tried for a third time to find Dad's discharge papers.

I began by looking in my dad's desk. I meticulously went through every drawer, but found nothing. Then, I moved onto the wooden file cabinet. Unfortunately, they weren't there either. After an hour, I moved my search into the bonus room which was currently a mess, papers everywhere. I honestly didn't know where to start.

Mom had repeatedly told me that she remembered putting the papers in a file which was what I had looked for this whole time. For some reason, I decided to start looking through anything and everything, regardless of what it was inside.

An hour into the pursuit, I curiously came upon an old envelope with a very weathered look to it. When I flipped it over, I absolutely froze. On the front of the envelope was the Great Seal of the United States, the top portion of the seal reading Department of Defense. Stamped across the front were the words "Official Records". I didn't even have to look inside, knowing that I was holding my dad's discharge papers. I was never so happy to see anything in my life, mouthing a silent thank you while looking up towards the sky.

As I carefully went through the envelope, I began to cry. On the top of the first paper in big letters were the words "Honorable Discharge". It went on to read "This is to certify that William C. Lee, Jr. Airman First Class Regular Air Force was Honorably Discharged from the United States Air Force on the 10th day of December 1954". Now, we had the actual proof for this man that we knew was honorable his whole life to be buried in a national cemetery with military honors. We would now be able to do the right thing by my daddy.

I immediately texted Bob to let him know the good news. He had also tried to find the papers previously. I felt such a tremendous weight off of my shoulders.

Mom and I then decided to take care of her gas account for the new house. We had made a lot of progress today and decided to forge ahead. Unfortunately, the line at the gas company was very long. After about an hour, we successfully opened up an account for Mom and arranged to have the gas turned on in her new home.

I then quickly took Mom back home and picked Chris up from school before we headed over to Athens. Preston had called me last night and wanted very much to see his Papa Lee. I was planning on taking him early Saturday morning.

I called the hospice facility later that night to find out how Dad was doing. One of the nurses told me he was currently sleeping. He had apparently had a good day. They were still giving him pain medicine around the clock which allowed Dad to rest peacefully. I was so thankful for this comfort. I still hadn't decided on the feeding tube. Part of me knew that the doctor was right. The other part just couldn't bear to let go. It was a decision that I dreaded, but knew needed to be made soon.

I hated that I missed seeing my dad today. So many things needed to be accomplished and some of them could only be done during the week. The entire day was spent doing things that were in some way necessary for my parents. I had wanted to get everything taken care of at once. I told myself that if my dad was in his right mind, he would have been so appreciative of everything that had happened today. He would have understood why we hadn't seen him.

I would also hope that the errands today would have provided Dad comfort in knowing that I was looking after Mom. My dad worried about my mother so. One of the last serious conversations that I had with him was about watching over Mom. He hated that he wasn't able to do that anymore. "Take care of your mother for me," he had said.

With tears in my eyes, I had nodded my head in assent. "I will, Daddy," I had replied, "always." He had seemed satisfied with my answer, but his sad eyes had said otherwise. He was brokenhearted that he wasn't the one to be taking care of her.

Saturday, October 22, 2011

He had a determined look on his face as he sat at the bar eating his breakfast. I had no doubt that he would excel. After taking Shawn to his ACT test, I arrived back home around 8. Preston still wasn't up. I looked forward to him seeing Dad so much. The mutual respect that had always existed between them was endearing. It always warmed my heart to watch them interact. I knew today's visit would be very different from the last time Preston had seen his Grandpa. It meant so much to me that he wanted to be there for him. I prayed that at some point Dad would recognize him. I also couldn't wait to see Dad myself, having really missed him yesterday. I planned on giving Preston a few more minutes of sleep before I woke him up to head over to the hospice facility.

Not much later, the phone unexpectedly rang, Mom's voice clearly implying that something was wrong. "Vanessa, I just got a call from Humanity Hospice Care," she said. "Your father passed away this morning at 8:10." Everything suddenly went dark. My world stopped. I dropped down to my knees and began crying. "Noooooo, Daddy, noooooo". It couldn't be. It just couldn't be. My precious daddy was gone and I never got a chance to say goodbye to him.

I continued to cry for what seemed like an eternity. I don't remember seeing anything around me. I was in my own world, the pain inside killing me. I never knew anything could hurt so much. It didn't matter how many times I had played this moment out in my head. Now that it had actually happened, I realized that nothing could have ever prepared me for it.

I found out that the nurse had checked on Dad at 7:45 a.m. He was awake and doing fine. When she went back into the room at 8:10, she noticed that he had passed away, going very peacefully.

I soon looked up at Randy, tears running down his face. I stood up and we closely held onto each other. "He's gone," I cried. "I can't believe he's gone. We were just getting ready to go see him." We both continued to cry as we firmly held each other up. "The worst part was that he died alone. Did he know that he was dying? Did he wonder where we were? Was he scared?"

"There's a reason why everything happened the way it did, Vanessa," he said. "Maybe you're looking at it the wrong way. Maybe he wanted to spare his family any more pain and that's why he decided to go peacefully by himself."

I thought about Randy's words. Is that what had happened? My dad was the most unselfish person I had ever known. Was his last act here on earth again one of selfless love?

"We don't know how it happened," Randy continued. "Maybe Jesus and Curtis and your dad's mother and father were all waiting for him with open arms." I continued to weep in my husband's embrace.

Chris soon walked into the room. "Mommy, why are you crying?" he asked.

I then sat down as Chris got up on my lap. "Your Papa Lee passed away this morning," I replied. I watched Chris' face as his mouth started to quiver, his innocent, blue eyes soon filling with tears. I hugged him tightly as they began to flow down his cheeks.

Before long, Preston got up, the look on our faces revealing what had happened. I then stood up to hug him. "I wanted so much for you to see him one last time," I said. "I guess it just wasn't meant to be."

"I'm so sorry, Mom," Preston said. I put my arms around my oldest son and hugged him closely as I continued to cry.

A little while later, I drove my mom to the hospice facility where we met Bob and Aaron. We went inside to say our last goodbyes. Dad was lying in the bed and looked like he had so many times before as he slept peacefully. This time was different though. I gently caressed his face and his arms, just wanting to touch him. When it came time to say goodbye, I couldn't do it.

I then walked towards the offices. I found the man that had initially come down to Dad's room when we had first arrived. He was sitting at his desk and looked up at me so compassionately. "How did he die?" I asked.

"His heart just stopped and he quit breathing," he replied. "Nothing out of the ordinary happened. I don't think he was in any pain. The look on his face was one of peace. He was just tired." He then paused for a couple of seconds. "It was time."

I thanked him and then walked slowly towards the lobby. As I passed Dad's room, I thought about stepping inside once again. The others were still saying their goodbyes, but I just couldn't do it. I continued on to the lobby where I sat on one of the couches and buried my face in my hands. I then cried. How could I say goodbye to this man who lived inside of me? A part of my heart had his name on it. It was his and that wasn't ever going to change. How was I supposed to let go of him?

Later that afternoon, I drove to the funeral home. The director soon came out. "I'm so sorry about your father," he said, apparently already having received a call from the hospice facility.

"I found my dad's discharge papers yesterday," I said, handing him the envelope. He then called the cemetery to finalize the arrangements. The service would be held on Tuesday. Mom would need to bring Dad's clothes up later. Everything was in order.

I then went home and tried to contact everyone about the funeral. I also needed to provide some stories about Dad to the pastor giving the eulogy. I was on autopilot all day trying not to think about my dad being gone. So much still needed to be done and I knew that I wouldn't be able to get through everything if I didn't continue in this manner.

Later that day, I lied on my bed thinking about the journey that I'd travelled with my dad. I thought back to the meeting with the hospice doctor on Thursday. I think he invariably knew that Dad was dying, but just couldn't tell us. Then I thought about my dad's words to me that same day, "Hey sweetheart". Those would inevitably be his last words to me forever. God knew then that it would be his last time seeing me. Everything that had happened yesterday had clearly happened for a reason. God was in control directing everything. I just didn't know why at the time.

As I closed my eyes and cried, I thought about one of my favorite songs "There Will Be A Day" by Jeremy Camp. It had never spoken to me as it did now. I thought about the beautiful lyrics, now so fitting, of a day when all pain would disappear, a day when all tears would be wiped away, a day when all suffering would be no more.

My heart was hurting so much. I realized at that very moment that amidst all of my pain, one feeling was no longer there. It was a scared feeling that I had experienced every day for over a year, an ever present uneasiness inside of me over what could be happening to my father at any given minute. I never rested easy. I knew that Alzheimer's was relentless and I lived every single day never knowing what it would take next from my father.

I realized in that instant that that terrified feeling was gone. My dad's battle was over and the disease couldn't hurt my precious father ever again. He was finally at peace. Today, his suffering had ended.

Sunday, October 23, 2011

As I looked through a lifetime of photos, they moved me to tears, feeling so unbelievably blessed to have had him as my father. He was such a good man. Everyone who ever knew him loved him. I had no idea how I was to go on. I simply couldn't imagine my life without him. I spent the day going through old pictures of Dad, filling several frames which I planned on displaying in the funeral home during the visitation.

I felt a tremendous amount of guilt inside over not seeing my dad on Friday. No matter what I did, I couldn't seem to shake it. We had made the decision to handle some critical matters that day, having no idea just how close the timing was. Mom and I had gone to see Dad every day since he was taken to the emergency room, never missing one. Had Dad wondered where we were? Was he coherent enough that day to have noticed? It absolutely broke my heart to think that he might have been sad over it. I had no doubt in my mind that God was in charge that day. He had his hands on us and led us in everything that we did. Still, I felt guilty.

Today, I received a letter from a dear friend that was there for me every single day of the journey. We had been friends ever since the 2nd grade, but I had not seen her since I left Miami as a teenager. We had reconnected a few years back and I was now convinced that there was a definite reason why. She had given me such strength when I needed it the most, filling my heart with love. Only God could have known to bring us together after all these years. Only God could have known that she would have the wisdom, experience and compassion that I would need during this time in my life.

Vanessa,

My heart is breaking for you. So many memories of my mom's horrible disease and all that we went through with her and the guilt I still feel to this day. I am reading about your last encounter with your dad. What a dear, sweet memory for you and your mom to have of him. He loved you both. God is so kind and full of mercy and grace to give that piece of your dad before he passed. I didn't have that with my mom. I believe God had all of this planned. Your dad being of his right mind to send you and your mom love and then you finding the discharge papers the day before he died. That is God!

I am sure that you find great comfort in knowing that although your dad is gone from this earth, he is at peace and he will be buried in the proper way....indeed a man of honor. You may not have known how close the timing was in all of this, but rest assured that God did. He is in control. He is walking with you and when need be, He is carrying you. Please try not to feel guilty.

I believe that Curtis and your dad are rejoicing together right now. Please always know that I love you dearly and if I could be there for you at the funeral, I would be. I will be thinking of you and praying for you. You did everything you were supposed to do for your dad. God had it all worked out. It isn't your fault. I am sure your dad knows without a doubt that you and your family love him immensely. Everything you did, you did unselfishly and because of your love for your dad. You are a good daughter, Vanessa. Your dad knew that and God gave you a special gift when your dad said those precious last words to you..."Hey Sweetheart." You are so blessed. I'm here always.

Love and prayers,
Laurie

Tuesday, October 25, 2011

No one else was currently in the room as I slowly walked up to him, looking so different from the man I had always known to be my father. The past year had been devastating for him. It felt so surreal as I stood watching this precious man lying before me.

My dad's visitation was scheduled to start at 9:00 a.m. I had arrived at the funeral home early so that I could set out all of the framed pictures of Dad. It had also given me some much needed time to be alone with him.

I had so many things that I wanted to say to him, but I couldn't stop myself from crying. Never before had my father been so close and yet so far away at the same time. All I wanted to do was bend down and hug him.

"I don't know how I'm supposed to go on without you, Daddy," I said. "I have spent the last year taking care of you and now that you're gone, I just don't know what to do." I paused for a moment to catch my breath, holding on to the side of the casket for support. "You were the best dad in the world to me. I am so blessed to have had you in my life. What happened to you wasn't fair. It just wasn't right. You deserved so much better, Daddy." I again wiped the tears from my eyes. "I hope that I did right by you, Daddy. I hope you now understand everything that happened and why. I am going to miss you so much." I gently caressed his cheek. I then felt the softness of his hair. "You will live in my heart forever. Wherever I am, you'll be. I love you so much. Rest, Daddy. I will see you in Heaven."

I then placed my hand directly on top of my dad's hands, praying that he could feel my love for him. As I continued to stare at my dad and cry, I felt a hand gently touch my back. I turned around to find my sister-in-law, Vicki, and my nephews, Chad and Trevor. I hugged her tightly as the tears continued to fall. This was going to be a very difficult day to get through.

People continued to enter the room. As I slowly looked around, I saw so many present that loved my dad so dearly. From his wife, children and grandchildren to his brothers, cousins and friends, Dad was surrounded by so much love. Even friends of Randy and mine had come to pay their respects. It had meant so much to us.

I watched as everyone joyously looked at the many pictures of Dad around the room, bringing smiles and sometimes even laughter to their faces. I wondered if Dad could hear the many stories being told about him. I wondered if it warmed his heart as it did mine.

At one point, I stood back and looked at my dad lying in the casket, a brightly colored flag draped over the bottom portion. The miniature Alf doll that had been in his truck for as long as I could remember and the collar from his beloved pet, Porky, were resting inside next to his body. It just seemed fitting that they be with Dad. I then watched Chris walk up and stand next to his beloved Papa. He began touching Dad's hands. I couldn't imagine what he was going through. It must have been so hard for someone so young to fully grasp what was happening.

As it neared time for the actual service, the funeral home director informed us it would be our final opportunity to say goodbye to Dad before the casket was closed forever. I watched as, one by one, his many loved ones respectfully stopped at his side. When everyone else was done, I slowly made my way to Dad, trying to visually take in every inch of him. It would be the last time I ever saw his earthly body. I then bent down and tenderly kissed my precious father's cheek for the very last time as a tear dropped down on his shoulder.

The service was held at 10:30 in the chapel at the funeral home. Everyone soon made their way inside. The eulogy was a warm and special dedication to my dad. The pastor told of so many wonderful stories in dad's life, some even had us laughing. His brother Shelby had spoken next, his heartfelt words bringing tears to my eyes.

The interment would be held at Georgia National Cemetery at 2:00 p.m. Everybody met at Golden Corral to have lunch before embarking on the trip to Canton.

As we later drove into the cemetery, we were directed to an area to line up. The hearse carrying my dad's body was the first car in the procession, all of the other cars respectfully lining up behind it. A group of men riding on motorcycles would lead. As they rode, they carried flags that waved freely in the air. It was such a moving moment.

Soon afterwards, we arrived at a covered pavilion. As we walked towards it, I noticed the many men and women standing on both sides. I counted well over fifty of them, all standing at attention saluting us, a United States flag by each of their sides. I had heard about a group of veterans that graciously volunteered their time to recognize members of the military during their funerals called the Patriot Guard Riders. As I passed by these amazing people, I wondered if they were a part of that group. Members of the Honor Guard were also present. The idea that these strangers were paying such tribute to someone they had never even met left me feeling incredibly moved. It didn't matter to them. Dad had proudly served his country and that had been enough.

As we all took our seats, I looked to the front of the facility. There rested Dad's casket, the flag I had seen earlier now draped over and completely covering it. The blue field of the flag was placed at the head of the casket, over the left shoulder of my dad. It was a custom that had begun back in the late 18th and early 19th centuries.

The pastor that had given the earlier eulogy again led a short service. At its conclusion, a gun salute involving the firing of three volleys each by seven service members ensued. I listened to the command "Ready, Aim, Fire" being repeated loudly before each volley. As each firing occurred, I cringed, feeling the vibrations inside. It was truly explosive. When it was over, a young man holding a bugle began to play "Taps". I bowed my head and cried, thinking about how much my dad would have cherished this memorial. How I would have loved to have sat next to him experiencing this amazing service. Instead, the service had been for him. It was all for him.

At the end of the ceremony, several service members folded the flag that had been lying on top of my dad's casket. When it was completely tucked in, the stars were positioned so they pointed upwards towards the sky. It was meant to remind us of our national motto "In God We Trust". One of the service members then knelt in front of my mother and said "On behalf of the President of the United States, the United States Air Force and a grateful nation, please accept this flag as a symbol of our appreciation for your loved one's honorable and faithful service." He then handed my mother the flag and stood to salute her. A few minutes later, another gentleman handed my mother a bag containing the shell casings that were fired during the gun salute.

After the service, we drove to the burial site. We weren't allowed to go to the actual area at that moment. Instead, we watched from afar as the crane began to dig the hole. We then saw a vehicle bring Dad's casket over. This would be his final resting place.

As I looked around, the sun was out in full force. Dad would have absolutely loved the feeling of serenity. We were up on a hill with lush greenery all around us. I knew based on the environment that Dad would be well taken care of here. It was such a beautiful place. Dad would be happy with this choice.

On the long drive home, I replayed the visitation, the service and the interment in my mind, all of them so moving. I realized as I leaned my head against the window and looked outside that the hardest part was now beginning. Now I had to figure out how my life was to go on without my daddy in it. Family would travel back home. Lives would try to continue as normal. Tomorrow when everyone went back to work and school, reality would set in. That was when I would realize how much I was truly going to miss him. Part of me would be empty, a part of me now gone. I didn't know how I was ever going to fill the void that he left. I already missed my daddy so much.

Epilogue

Monday, October 31, 2011

As I was going through some of my dad's things from his stay at Arbor Forest, I came across his name plate that had hung on the wall outside his room. It had remained boxed up until now. The name tag read William Lee. All of the places that he was a part of this past year had all referred to him by his legal first name, William. My dad never went by his first name. Anyone who knew him well knew him as Chester.

The first time I had heard someone refer to him as William, I had corrected them. It had started happening so often that after awhile, I stopped mentioning it. Looking back, I wondered if maybe there was a reason that he had been known as William throughout this past year. So much of my dad's behavior was not my dad at all, but that of a stranger. Maybe that was why he had been known by another name. The name Chester would always be the one I associated with my loving, caring daddy.

My days were now spent taking care of my mother. Between social security, insurance, my dad's tombstone, his will and the new house, so much still needed tending to. A lot of it was dependent on the death certificate. The funeral home was still waiting for the doctor at the hospice facility to sign off on it.

Mom was slowly doing better. I think she felt a certain relief that her husband was no longer suffering. It was so hard to watch your loved one going through something that you felt powerless to stop. I knew that if my dad could say one thing to me right now, it would be "Take care of your mother". And I would until the day they could be together again. Doing that helped me because not only was it the right thing to do, but it would have made my dad incredibly happy. And nothing in the world meant more to me than that.

Not a day had gone by that I hadn't thought back over everything that happened during our journey together, questioning every decision that was ever made. If things had occurred differently, would my dad still be with us? Should he have had every surgery? In the end, how important were they? Was there a way I could have taken care of Dad at home? Could I have found a fulltime nurse to live with us? How would we have paid for it? What would the impact to my children have been? The questions were endless. They were inevitably the same ones that I had asked myself over and over the entire year. I doubted that they would ever be answered now. I also wondered if the guilt would ever subside, finding that it was a terrible thing to live with.

Today was Halloween. This evening had been very difficult. For the past several years, we had taken Chris and Andrew over to my parents' home, Dad proudly walking his grandsons around the subdivision. He loved to show them off to all of his neighbors. Tonight would be the first Halloween without him.

We decided to take the boys around our own neighborhood instead. Some traditions were best left unchanged. The truth was I hadn't gone over to my parents' home too often since Dad passed away. The few times I had gone, it was very painful. I saw him everywhere. I knew that as I pulled up into their driveway, I'd see Dad sitting in the wrought iron bench waiting for me. Or maybe I'd find him mowing the lawn as he did so often. As I walked down the basement stairs, I'd hear Tom T. Hall playing as my dad puttered around. I'd also see him sitting in his recliner watching one of his favorite shows or lying in his bed taking a nap or at the kitchen table deciding what to make us for lunch. He'd be in every single room because he lived there. Still. It would forever be Dad's home.

Friday, December 2, 2011

Today would have been my dad's 80th birthday. Sometimes it just didn't seem real that he was gone. I kept waiting for the day when I would wake up and the pain would have subsided. I had come to accept that it would be a long time before that happened.

I still saw my dad everywhere. When I looked out my kitchen window and saw his red truck parked next door, it hurt knowing that he would never drive it again like he used to do so many times. I could never casually call him on the phone. He'd never come over to my house to visit. I'd never find him sitting in his recliner when I went over to see him.

Nothing was the same without him and I knew it never would be. Our lives had somehow continued forward around the void that he left. The only thing that made any of the pain worth it was believing that Dad was finally experiencing a peacefulness that he hadn't felt in years. I couldn't bear for him to suffer anymore.

I tried to concentrate on the wonderful and loving memories of my dad. The truth was that I had a lifetime of them. I couldn't have asked for a better Dad. We were always so close. I was his little girl and he was my daddy. He had always taken care of me and that hadn't changed with age. It was such a comfort knowing that no matter what happened to me, he would always be there to see me through it.

Even though throughout the last year the roles had been reversed, I never really looked at my dad any differently. Somehow, just having him next to me, whether it was at the memory care unit, a rehab facility or one of the many hospitals that he frequented, had given me the strength to carry on. I had taken for granted that my dad would always be there for me to hug his neck or gently kiss his cheek. I missed being able to stare into his blue eyes and tell him how much I loved him. In an instant, it was all taken away. What I wouldn't give to have just one more moment with my dad.

Not long ago, I found myself driving near Arbor Forest. Before I knew it, I had pulled into the parking lot. I soon found a spot on the end and turned the engine off. I didn't know why I was there, but I couldn't leave. As I sat in the car, I was suddenly flooded with so many memories of times I had shared with my dad. An inexplicable feeling soon swept over me, like he was so close. It almost felt as though all I had to do was walk inside the building and make my way to the memory care unit. As I'd slowly walk down the hall, I'd see so many special people that I knew.

Alexandra and Susan would smile at me as I passed the common area, the parakeet happily chirping in the corner. I'd reach my dad's room and find him calmly sitting in his blue recliner. He'd look up and lovingly smile at me as he had so many times before. I'd then bend down and tenderly kiss his cheek.

As I lowered my head, the tears streamed down my face as I realized that my dad wasn't inside. No matter how much I wanted it, he was no longer inside. All that was left of him within these walls was a lone picture on the bulletin board and so many precious memories.

I received a very special message from my uncle today. As I read it over and over, I felt the tears well up inside. It was the bright spot in my day.

Merry Christmas Vanessa, my wonderful niece. You have had some very difficult years, and you make me very proud to be your uncle. Take some comfort in believing that adversity, while never easy or asked for, makes us stronger, more appreciative and more understanding for enduring the hardships. I have no doubts that your life will be blessed and honored and an inspiration to others.

I love you.
Shelby

Thursday, February 3, 2012

As I sat on the steps watching Riley run around in the backyard, I suddenly heard the phone ring inside. The call was from a lawyer that I had contacted shortly after Dad had passed away. The first law firm had never gotten back with me, so I had soon contacted a second. They had actually responded within one day.

Over the past several months, I had had several lengthy conversations about Dad's entire medical history spanning the past couple of years. I had to go back through some painful times and answer a lot of questions. I had dreaded having to relive those times, but I had to do it for my dad. He needed me to once again be his voice.

I had gone to Brookview Hospital and obtained the complete set of Dad's medical records during his stay. I had also requested records from the hospice facility. Those, in addition to Dad's death certificate, had been sent to the law firm.

They would be reviewing everything. If necessary, they'd even forward the records to a medical expert for review. Based on the information, they would decide if there was sufficient evidence to prove neglect. One of the lawyers had already told me that there was insufficient proof for a bedsore case. They would have needed to be more than a Stage 2 at the time of his admission to the hospital. However, it did appear that there might be a medication, dehydration and malnutrition issue.

The procedure had been a lengthy one. Reviewing Dad's records involved a lot more than just reading them. They had to be analyzed in detail. In order to win a case in court, there had to exist blatant proof of negligence. Dad may very well have been neglected, but proving that in a court of law was different, the burden a lot greater.

Today, I had received the long awaited news. I honestly wasn't sure what I had hoped for. Did I want the negligence to be so great that it could easily be proved in court? Or did I want to find out that there just wasn't enough proof and that maybe Dad wasn't as neglected as I had thought? I was completely torn.

The lawyer proceeded to tell me that her decision was in no way indicative of Dad being neglected. He indeed may have been. In her expert opinion though, it would have been very difficult, if not impossible, to have proven. There just wasn't enough evidence. Based on the hospital admission records, it appeared that Dad was simply an elderly gentleman with a lot of health problems.

I still couldn't decide whether it was good news or not. I deeply wanted to blame someone for what had happened to my dad. I had known that Alzheimer's would one day take his life. What I didn't know was whether the rehab facility had caused it to happen sooner than it should have. I definitely didn't want them to be able to do it to anyone else. The other side of me wondered how much of his death was just inevitable because of the disease. In the end, we decided to finally put the concern over Dad's negligence to rest. We had already endured so much. We decided it was time.

Saturday, November 10, 2012

As I stared at the note, a feeling of anguish over the tragic news enveloped me. I was in disbelief to find that some dear friends of my parents' recently passed away. After the husband was diagnosed with dementia, they had decided to move into a smaller home together where she would care for him. I knew the stress involved with being a primary caregiver was serious and sometimes fatal. It was a difficult position to be in and one that had always concerned me with my parents.

A little over a week ago, my mother's dear friend passed away, actually dying before her husband whom she was caring for. A week later, her husband also passed, as often happened when one spouse died. In a week's time, the children had sadly lost both of their parents. I thought back about our decision to put my dad in a home. Had we continued to allow my mother to be my dad's primary caregiver, would she have perished before my father as well? Would we have lost both of our parents, too?

Today, I saw some pictures online from the Forever Hope Memory Care facility where I had planned on moving my dad. I loved viewing the different photos, the residents seeming so happy there. As I carefully looked through them, I came upon one that left me speechless. I knew this man. I smiled as I found myself looking at a picture of Joseph whom I remembered well from Arbor Forest.

Joseph and Dad had shared the same dining table the entire time my dad had lived there. Joseph was still alive. Tears sprung to my eyes. I was so happy to see him. I had become friends with this man and sat next to him myself for so many meals over the months. He was such a kind man. At the same time, I was also very sad, sad that my dad wasn't still here as well.

As I continued to look at Joseph's picture, I was soon flooded with so many memories of a time when my dad was here, a time when we could talk and carry on conversations, a time when we could eat together, a time when we could sit and lose ourselves in the beauty surrounding us, a time that seemed a lifetime ago.

It had now been over a year since my daddy was taken from us. Not a day went by that I didn't miss him terribly. In those months, I had learned how to cope with his death. I had learned how to go through life and not dwell on the painful parts. I had learned to accept it. I had yet to learn how to live life to the fullest without him.

These days, when I thought about my dad, I imagined his smiling face with so much love in his eyes, his voice as he affectionately called me by my special nickname. I remembered a time when there was such laughter, when our lives were so rich with love, when the future seemed endless. I remembered a time when illness didn't prevail. Most of all, I remembered a much simpler time when he was my daddy and I was his little girl.

Afterword

As I look back on my father's life, things appear so clear to me now. There were so many warning signs. I even had someone pointing the finger at Alzheimer's for years. I ignored them all, refusing to believe that anything was wrong with my dad. Instead, I chose to minimize the signs and blame them on aging, thinking it was just a normal part of senility. I will never know what difference early detection would have made in my father's life.

The truth is I believe my dad had been suffering from dementia for many, many years before we ever found out. He went to great lengths to hide it from all of us. He knew something was wrong, but had no idea what it was. The last thing he ever wanted was to burden his family, especially his children. So, he kept it quiet.

Not long ago, I ran across some notes that my mother had made. They were dated March 22, 2010, many months before we ever knew there to be a problem. She had noticed changes within my father. He could no longer remember how to operate the microwave. When he needed water heated for coffee, he would have to ask my mom to do it. He also couldn't remember any of his work experience from 1956 to 1977. The only barber shop he remembered working at was the last one that he owned in Pensacola. My mother had the insight to know that something was terribly wrong. Had I listened to her the many times she came to me with her claims of Alzheimer's, we may have been able to have slowed it down.

By the time the first symptoms appear, Alzheimer's has already been actively destroying the brain for years. When these warning signs emerge, the nerve cells that process, store and retrieve information have already begun to degenerate and die. It is critical that we know the early signs and not ignore them or attribute them to something else. Had I been more aware of them, I may have recognized what was happening and been able to do something about it. Being proactive could have made a difference.

After living through my dad's ordeal, I am convinced that this world is not ready for Alzheimer's. This horrible illness will eventually touch most people's lives in some way or another. Still, there is a lack of awareness. Every 68 seconds, someone in America develops Alzheimer's, the numbers staggering. We like to think that there is justice in this world. We like to believe that horrid diseases such as Alzheimer's are reserved for only the worst of people, that if you live your life in the right way, you won't be subjected to it. The truth is that it hits some of the most wonderful people in the world. It doesn't matter what good deeds you've previously done or how you've lived your life. It doesn't matter how much money you have. It doesn't even matter what race you are. No one is immune. It can happen to anybody.

We are living longer now than any previous time in history. As a result, so many more people are being afflicted with this relentless and horrendous ailment. There is currently no cure, but there may be things we can do to slow its progression and make the journey a little easier for everyone involved.

- There needs to be more awareness about this disease, especially in the medical field. Every decision made for a dementia patient needs to take it into account. I found that some of the most proficient doctors in their specialized fields knew very little about Alzheimer's. As a result, some of the decisions made for my dad were not in his best interest. It is crucial that every caregiver be involved with all decisions. Question everything. Don't rely on others as I did because they may actually know less about Alzheimer's than you do.

- Every person that cares for someone with dementia, whether it be a skilled nursing facility, rehabilitation facility, hospital or memory care unit, needs to be specially trained on how to best care for them. They need to be able to redirect a patient when needed. Treating a person the wrong way can sometimes add to the agitation and possibly make the disease progress even more.

There are basic techniques in dealing with dementia that can make a world of difference.

They also need to be more vigilant in recognizing common symptoms in someone with dementia. Something as simple as a UTI can cause extreme agitation, but it is oftentimes overlooked. Having the skill sets to recognize it and catch it early can reduce the suffering tremendously. Simple tests like taking someone's temperature or a urine sample can go a long way in detecting serious problems with little effort. Undetected UTIs in a dementia patient can lead to serious complications.

- Be more involved with your loved ones. Make an effort to know their medical history. Don't assume that just because they are under the care of a doctor, the right decisions are being made and they are receiving all the care that they need. If something doesn't seem quite right, question it. There were definitely red flags with my father. He was taking three different medications for high blood pressure, yet he wasn't under the care of a cardiologist. By the time he started experiencing chest pains, his arteries were already substantially blocked. Could the blockage have been detected earlier? Could that have prevented the vascular dementia?

- Take care of yourself. It may seem selfish at the time, but in the long run, it is crucial. If you are caring for someone, you need to be in the best physical, mental and emotional state that you possibly can. You'll be less effective in caring for your loved one if you're not. It is very easy to give your all to someone else, but it is important that you keep some for yourself.

I read something the other day that really struck a chord with this point. Whenever you fly on an airplane, a flight attendant will instruct everyone on the use of their oxygen mask. We are told to always put our mask on first before attempting to help someone else put on theirs. For someone that puts others first, especially their children, this seems backwards. The reason is very simple. If you run out of oxygen, you can't help anyone else with their oxygen mask. Likewise, if you don't take care of yourself, you can't take care of your loved one with dementia. The stress from burnout will eventually cause your own set of health issues.

- Don't be afraid to ask for help. Alzheimer's is bigger than most people can imagine. It is a 24/7 job. There is sometimes a feeling that if you're not managing everything on your own, you're not measuring up. That is simply not the case. Taking care of someone suffering from Alzheimer's can be devastating. Doing it at home, especially by yourself, isn't always an option. Sometimes the best course of action is one where help is sought out. It isn't a reflection of failure on your part. It may just be a sign that the disease has become too monstrous to handle alone.

- Make sure that your loved one has a living will outlining exactly what life prolonging medical treatments will be allowed should the need arise. When the time finally does come, it may be too late to discuss it with them. Facing tough decisions such as a feeding tube, breathing tube or even resuscitation will be made much easier knowing what their wishes were. It will allow for decisions to be made without feeling as if you are giving up on your loved one, but instead allowing them to pass from this life with their dignity still intact and their wishes honored.

  I battled excessively over the feeding tube in my dad's nose, unwilling to let him go even though it was probably obvious to everyone else that his condition was terminal. Had I had the foresight to discuss it with him sooner, it would have made the decision to keep it in or remove it much easier. It would have also taken away the guilt. I will never know whether I made the right decision or not.

- We need to advocate for our loved one when they cannot. Chances are we know them better than anyone else. Alzheimer's will eventually take away a person's ability to communicate effectively with words. It is up to us to stand up for them when they need us to. We need to be their voice. It makes a difference.

- Most of all, enjoy every precious moment as if it was their last. I cannot stress this one enough. I would give anything in the world to just have one of those moments back.

I watched Alzheimer's take my father from me, little by little. It changed him every day until one day, he was simply a shell of the man I knew as my daddy. It made him a stranger. On the outside, he looked the same, but on the inside, he was completely different. This vile disease had slowly taken and taken until nothing was left of him.

My ultimate dream is that there will come a day when there will be no more Alzheimer's or dementia of any kind; when people will be able to live their lives with every precious memory intact until the very end. I realize that it may not happen within my lifetime. Until that wondrous day, my hope is that this book helps to bring awareness to this terrible illness. The more we as a society learn about this disease, the better we'll be able to handle Alzheimer's. Everyone afflicted with it should have a fighting chance. I pray that my father's suffering and his untimely death were not in vain and that something good will come from it. I hope that his story will in some way help others affected by this tragic ailment, whether it is in providing helpful information, support or simply words of encouragement. May our many tears be the fortitude that helps others deal with the adversity from this devastating disease.

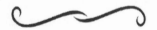

Thank you for reading my book. It truly means a lot to me. The experience within these pages has forever changed me. I hope that it has made a difference in your life as well. Please take a moment to leave a review. I would appreciate any comments you may have. Your opinion may be the deciding factor for whether others choose to read this book.

Thanks so much!
Vanessa Luther

Acknowledgements

First and foremost, I would like to thank my Heavenly Father without whom, I am nothing. You led me through this devastating time when I was directionless. You have blessed me beyond words and will always live within my heart.

To the many angels that surrounded my dad on this journey, words cannot express my gratefulness for everything you did. My dad was a stranger to you, but still you cared for him with a deep sense of love. Not because you had to, but because of who you are. You truly made a difference in his final year.

To Shawn and Preston, thank you for believing in me. It was so difficult to take that first step, but your encouragement and support gave me the strength I needed. I am forever grateful for you seeing the writer in me.

Thank you, Suzanne Jenkins, for your guidance through this daunting world of publishing and for your friendship. Yours is a tremendous talent which I truly respect.

To the many people who read the book and gave me insightful and invaluable feedback, I thank you from the bottom of my heart. Preston, Shawn, Randy, Bob, Mom, Vicki and Laurie, I am grateful that you took the time to do this.

Thank you, David Shenk, for allowing me to share your compelling words. They helped me at a time when I desperately needed understanding. I hope they help others just as much.

To my sister-in-law, Vicki, thank you for your guidance during this journey. No matter what my questions, you were always there for me with necessary and timely information. I cannot thank you enough for your kind words and invaluable critique of the book.

A heartfelt thank you goes to my dear friend, Laurie. You stood beside me every single day. A lot of those days were not pleasant, but your friendship never once wavered. Your love helped to bring me through this terrible ordeal. I will forever be grateful that our paths crossed again after so many years.

I want to thank my Uncle Shelby and Uncle Ronnie for being the best brothers to my dad that anyone could ever ask for. Your endless devotion to my father meant the world to him and me as well. Never once did you allow his refusal to travel to stop you from seeing him. You both made the trip to visit him faithfully, regardless of the impact to your own lives. I also want to thank my cousins, Jeanneen and Johnny, for making the trips as well. The smile on Dad's face and laughter in his voice from your times together will be forever etched in my memory.

To my beloved older brother, Curtis, even though you weren't physically with me, I felt your presence every day. You've never left me. Knowing you were always watching over us gave me incredible strength. Knowing you are with Dad now gives me incredible comfort.

To my younger brother, Bob, thank you for always being there for me, regardless of what I needed. Ours was a tough road to travel, but we did it together. The special bond between us has only grown as a result of this journey. I am so thankful that you are still two doors down.

To my precious sons, Preston, Shawn and Christopher, you are the light of my life. You have and continue to grow into incredible people. You selflessly gave of yourself and spent so much time with your grandpa during his last year. I'm so very proud of the young men you have become and I know Dad is as well. You approach everything you do in life with a loving heart. You are a true blessing.

To my loving mother, you are my pillar of strength, enduring so much to protect your children. Your everlasting love for Dad shone through as it still shines forth today. You have taught me by example what a mother and wife should be. I have been blessed to have had the perfect role model in my life.

To my wonderful husband, Randy, you are my rock. For over 34 years, you have stayed by my side giving me love beyond words. The last year of Dad's life was very trying. You stepped up and helped with whatever needed doing, treating my daddy as your own. Words cannot express what that means to me. I love you dearly.

Lastly, to my precious father, I owe so much of who I am to you. When I look in the mirror and look past the exterior to my inner heart, I see you. You have instilled in me the importance of living life with a kind and open heart. No matter what I was going through in my life, you were always there for me. I couldn't have asked for a better dad. Your last few years were extremely hard on you. What happened wasn't fair. I only hope that you can now understand the decisions that were made and know they were all made out of love for you. Not a day goes by that I don't miss you terribly or feel that ache inside that never seems to go away. For now, I can only dream of the day when we will meet again in Heaven. What a glorious day that will be. Until then, you will forever live on within my heart. I love you, Daddy.

References

Atkins, Charles MD (2008). *The Alzheimer's Answer Book*. Naperville, Illinois: Sourcebooks, Inc.

What is Alzheimer's Disease? Writer/Dir. David Shenk. Film. Web. http://www.AboutAlz.org/

http://www.alz.org

http://www.alz.co.uk

http://www.alzheimersreadingroom.com

http://www.medicalnewstoday.com/releases/121816.php

http://sundownerfacts.com/sundowners-syndrome

VANESSA LUTHER is the author of *A Life Stolen*, the true account of the devastating, but inspiring journey that she and her father travelled through Alzheimer's.

She grew up in Hialeah, Florida and later moved to Pensacola, where she met and married her husband. After graduating from the University of West Florida with a Bachelor's degree in Computer Science, they moved to Atlanta, Georgia where she worked as a Consulting Software Engineer for 17 years. Vanessa put her career on hold to raise her three sons and eventually became her father's primary caregiver.

She currently lives in Lawrenceville, Georgia with her husband, three sons and their dog. She also cares for her mother, who lives directly behind her.

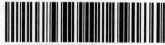

19310895R00301

Made in the USA
San Bernardino, CA
20 February 2015